To Marilyn Hawkins and Marsha Parker whose commitment to interdisciplinary shared governance resulted in the publication of the first edition of this text. Their personal effort laid the foundations for the implementation of interdisciplinary shared governance at Community Hospitals of Central California upon which the applications in this text are based.

Contents

Preface   xiii

Acknowledgments   xix

About the Author   xxi

About the Contributors   xxiii

CHAPTER 1: HEALTH CARE IN A QUANTUM AGE 1

Tim Porter-O'Grady

A New Understanding   2

The Emerging Value of Knowledge   2

A New Context for a New Age   4

A New Reality for Organizations   8

Changing Context for Healthcare Service   9

The Evolving Nature of Work   10

    Technology   12

    Economic and Financial Shifts   13

Social Reengineering   15

Changing Healthcare Structures and Models   16

    Managing Demand   16

    User-Driven Models   17

    Overcoming Medical Separatism   17

    Consumer-Driven Care   18

    The Quality Movement   19

    Value-Driven Care Delivery   21

Principles for a New Age   22

    Partnership   23

    Needed: A New Kind of Leader   25

Creating a Learning Organization   26
Equity   27
Accountability   30
Ownership   33
The Interdependence of Everything   35
Creating a Real System   36
Suggested Reading   36

CHAPTER 2: INTERDISCIPLINARY SHARED GOVERNANCE:
A MODEL FOR INTEGRATED PROFESSIONAL PRACTICE 39
   Tim Porter-O'Grady, Marsha Parker, and Marilyn Hawkins
Building on Foundations   39
Why Shared Governance?   41
Building to Support the Point of Care   44
The Premises of Shared Governance   45
Teams: The Foundation of All Work   47
      The Different Kinds of Teams in a Shared
          Governance Context   49
      The Population-Based Continuum   51
Councils: The Basic Unit of Organized Decision Making   53
Shared Governance and Decision Making   55
Decisions and the Locus of Control   56
Councils and Representation   57
Service Pathway Leadership   58
The System Councils   58
Distinguishing System Accountability and Service Accountability   59
The Patient Care Council   61
The Operations Council   65
The Governance Council   67
      Information Support   70
New Constructs . . . New Mindset   71
Suggested Reading   73

CHAPTER 3: BUILDING THE FOUNDATIONS: TRANSFORMING
THE ORGANIZATION 75
   Tim Porter-O'Grady, Marsha Parker, and Marilyn Hawkins
The Integrating Process   75
The Inadequacy of Structure   77
A Focused Work Group   78
The Shared Governance Steering Group (Design Team)   80
      Shared Governance Steering Group Membership   82

The Initial Developmental Process for the
    Shared Governance Steering Group   84
Conceptual Design for Shared Governance Implementation   85
Nursing Shared Governance   87
Interdisciplinary Shared Governance   90
Shared Governance Steering Group Basics   90
Understanding the Limits   92
    Budgetary Availability   92
    Deadlines   93
    Workload   93
Individual Differences   93
Other Resources   94
Development and Training   94
Authority and Decision Making   95
Information Access   95
Determination of Boundaries   95
The Planning Process   96
    Expectations   96
    Functional Components   97
    Roles and Positions   97
The Work of the Steering Group   98
The Change Process   101
Suggested Reading   102

**CHAPTER 4: CONSTRUCTING INTEGRATED CARE DELIVERY:
    BUILDING A SERVICE CONTINUUM 105**
Tim Porter-O'Grady and Marsha Parker
The Patient Pathway   106
New Realities   107
Building the Continuum of Care   109
Relational Service Design   109
Linkage Defines the System   111
    Horizontal Linkage   112
    Provider Linkage   113
Organizing Around Populations   114
Defining Linkages   114
Building the Vision   115
Structural Linkages   116
New Values   117
Delineating the Pathways   119
Systems Linkages   120

The Need for Information   120
Pathways and Information   123
Communication Linkages   124
The Process of Building Linkages and Teams   127
Interactions in the System   128
Organizing Around the Patient   129
Making the System Functional   131
References   135
Suggested Reading   135

CHAPTER 5: DECISIONS FROM THE CENTER:
BUILDING A SUSTAINABLE INTERDISCIPLINARY
MICROSYSTEM AT THE POINT OF SERVICE 137
Kami English, Curtis Takamoto, and Tim Porter-O'Grady
Patient Care: The Foundations of Health Service   138
The Fundamentals of the Patient Care Council   140
    The Purpose of the Patient Care Council   143
    The Patient Care Council Membership   144
    Defining the Work of the Patient Care Council   147
Service Pathway Council and Team Accountability   148
    The Accountability of the Service Pathway Council   152
    The Work of the Service Pathway Council and the
        Pathway Teams   155
    The Accountability of the Patient Care Council   156
The Transition from Nursing Shared Governance to
    Whole-Systems Shared Governance   160
    Expanding the Nursing Practice Council   161
    Interfacing with the Medical Staff   162
Patient Care Integration   164
Suggested Reading   167

CHAPTER 6: THE OPERATIONS (MANAGEMENT) COUNCIL:
LEADING ENGAGEMENT, MAKING SHARED GOVERNANCE
WORK 169
Jeff LeFors and Tim Porter-O'Grady
Ensuring Effective Decision Making   170
    Empowerment   171
Changing Concepts of Management   171
Technology-Driven Systems and Work   173
    The Knowledge Worker   173
Distinction of Accountability   175

Management Accountability 175
The Two Levels of Management 176
The Foundation of the Operations Council 178
    Support for the Management Role 180
    Purpose of the Operations Council 181
    The Role of the Operations Council 183
    The Operations Council Membership 184
    Making the Operations Council Work 187
    The Operations Council Process 188
Clarity of Issues 189
Clarifying Operations Council Accountability 190
The Operating Budget Process 193
The Capital Budget Process 194
    Capital Project Presentations 195
    The Primacy of Financial Accountability 196
    Setting Targets 196
Operations Council Commitment 196
Consensus-Based Decision Making 198
Shared Vision 199
Systems Accountability and Support Accountability .. 201
Linkage to the Other Councils 202
Cautions about Control 203
Support from the CEO 204
Other Administrator Changes 204
Other Manager Transitions 205
Conclusion 205
Suggested Reading 206

**CHAPTER 7: TRANSFORMING GOVERNANCE:
LINKING STRATEGY WITH PRACTICE** **207**
Tim Porter-O'Grady and Kathryn McDonagh
Linking the System 207
New Notions of Leadership 208
Governing Boards in Transition 209
Linking Governance and Function 210
Translating Board Accountability 213
Translating Direction 214
    Governance Council Membership 217
The Role of the CEO 217
Role of the Consulting Partners 218
Governance Council Accountability 221

Breadth of Accountability   222
The Question of Systems   223
The Governance Council and the Cascade   224
Challenges to Effectiveness   228
Shifting the Focus of Work   229
Interface with the Medical Staff   230
Enhancing Effectiveness in Shared Governance   231
Checks and Balances   232
The Importance of Governance Culture   232
Conclusion   233
References   234
Suggested Reading   235

CHAPTER 8: INTEGRATING PHYSICIANS AND BUILDING
PROVIDER PARTNERSHIPS: A COMMUNITY HOSPITAL
SYSTEM APPROACH. 237
Phil Hinton, Marsha Parker, and Tim Porter-O'Grady
The Formal Medical Staff   237
A Physician's View of Barriers to Shared Governance   239
    Informal Structures as Barriers   239
    Changes in Incentives   240
    Physician Disconnection from a Systems Perspective   242
Visioning Whole-Systems Shared Governance   245
    The Vision   246
    Structuring to Support the Vision   248
    Seeing the Future   250
    The Implementing Experience   250
    Inviting the Medical Staff   252
Integrating Physicians into the Whole System   252
    Physician Roles in the Corporate Shared Governance Councils 254
    The Medical Staff, Governance, and Operations   255
    Medical Staff Integration into the Pathways   256
    The Medical Staff and Decision Making   256
    Physicians at the Point of Service   257
    Physicians and the Critical Path   258
Becoming Inclusive   259
Communication: Trying to Reconnect   259
    Critical Communication   260
Resolving Conflict   262
Governance for the New Vision   262
    Strategy Priorities   264

Shared Governance and Value-Driven Care   266
A Few Questions for the Physician's Shared Governance Journey   268
What Seems to Be Working So Far   269
The Future for Physician Partners in Shared Governance   269
Conclusion   270
References   270
Suggested Reading   270

**CHAPTER 9: INFORMATION INFRASTRUCTURE FOR
INTERDISCIPLINARY DECISION MAKING** **273**
Marsha Parker, Lynn Neimeth, and Tim Porter-O'Grady
The New Information Infrastructure   273
The Implications of Shared Governance Principles and
   Structures for Information Management   273
      Information as a Resource   275
      Shifting Control   276
      Structure   277
      Culture   278
      Training   278
      Information   279
      Systemness   280
Information Flow among Shared Governance Entities   280
      Self-Directed Workgroups and Information Management   282
Information Project Team   283
The Trouble with Vendor Partners   284
Real-Time Information Access   286
      The Superusers   287
Information Management Philosophy   287
Good Information Management Strategies   289
Tactical Implementation: Some Sample Projects   290
      Virtual Office: New Ways to Work   291
      Clinical Information System   292
Roles and Accountability   293
The Changing Role of the Chief Information Officer   294
      Board Support for the New Information Infrastructure   296
Integrated Health Network Core System Design   297
Information Development as Evolution   305
Conclusion   306
References   306
Suggested Reading   307

**CHAPTER 10: CREATING SUSTAINABLE COMMUNITY IN
HEALTH CARE** **309**

Tim Porter-O'Grady and Marsha Parker

Health and the Community   309
The First Community: The Membership Community   310
The Basics   311
Linkage Is Key   313
The Information Infrastructure   313
    Creating Useful Information Systems   314
    Supporting the Point of Service   315
    Clinical Support   316
    Reduced Provider Competition   317
    Information for Evaluation   317
    Linking the Internal and External Communities 317
    Community Health Information Networks   318
    Linking to the Political Structure   320
Making the Community Connection   321
Community Partnership Activities   325
    Getting Started   325
    Partnership for Children   326
    A Community Dream   326
    Shared Governance and Community Health   327
    Broader Notions of Health   327
    Organizing Around the Community   329
    Community-Driven Service   331
Conclusion   332
References   333
Suggested Reading   334

Index   335

Preface

It goes without saying that we are in the midst of major social transformation. The pace of change is accelerating in ways unanticipated. No matter how small the activities related to this challenge of transformation, the demand for effectiveness, value, efficiency, and strong meaningful outcomes accelerates daily. Much is already affecting the healthcare system in ways that have transformed it forever. Since 2000, the move from a disease basis for medical practice toward genomics and DNA-based therapeutics has ushered in an entirely new age for medical practice. Still, the ushering in of this new age also promises an entirely different framework for the delivery of health care and for the application of therapeutics within the context of the 21st century.

Within the context of this transformed age there is an increasing need for new leadership and organizational structures within which to offer a constantly moving and changing rubric for health service delivery. Along with the changes in therapeutics is a necessary shift in the infrastructure of health care to adjust to a digital age and the realities that this move creates. The pace of change in all aspects of life has a tremendous impact on the application of that change within the context of health care. The digital age has brought with it mobility and portability of healthcare services and reduced intensity of intervention as well as creating a faster-paced therapeutic process. The need for building interdisciplinary relationships and integrating the therapeutic process as well as the practices of the various disciplines is accelerating at the same pace as the change in technology and clinical applications.

New models of healthcare processes for delivering care call for a new infrastructure and different relationships as the healthcare system becomes more difficult to hold together. The need for linkage and interdisciplinary integration serves as the only counter to the growing potential for fragmentation and discord along the healthcare continuum. In 1985, the first text on nursing shared governance documented a new model for governing professional practice within the organization and provided an opportunity for practice-driven decision making to be a major construct of the organizational infrastructure. Since that time, shared governance has matured and become the operating infrastructure for many nursing organizations throughout the world. Indeed, the Magnet Recognition Program of the American Nurses Credentialing Center, which recognizes organizations of clinical excellence, requires nursing shared governance approaches as a fundamental construct of the infrastructure necessary to support excellence. Although the concepts of shared governance have been applied to nursing for the past 20 years, the principles of shared governance are universal. The principles relate to the governance of any professional discipline in the exercise of its work and in the relationships and interactions necessary to sustain it. It is this need to recognize an overlapping and integrating infrastructure for clinical practitioners that this book is directed.

Interdisciplinary relationships and interactions are becoming increasingly necessary to ensure synthesis and integration of clinical care across the patient experience as he or she interacts with the healthcare system. As digitalization and specialization grow in complexity and uniqueness, it becomes increasingly important to incorporate mechanisms of relationship and interaction between the disciplines and along the continuum of care to ensure that the patient's needs are not continually fragmented. Interdisciplinary relationships, clinical interaction, integrated care, and management of the continuum of care all serve to underpin the need for a new integrated model for relationship, interaction, communication, and facilitating the patient's health experience. Indeed, a constant necessity to prevent the fragmentation of the delivery of care creates the need for an effective infrastructure that provides a frame for the interaction and communication necessary to facilitate professional practice in an expanding digital reality.

Simply pulling people together in a new relationship that reflects the need for interaction and communication does not mean that they either want to or know what to do with it once it has occurred. Clearly, within the context of this new healthcare delivery framework, all kinds of new opportunities must emerge and be coordinated in a way that addresses this changing milieu and helps to create a framework not only for learning but for application and relationship building in the usual incremental way. Components of this transformation have already been addressed (such as the work on contemporary notions of microsystems), but very few organizations have taken the time to undertake the work of addressing health care as an interactive dynamic and complex system of relationships. Sustainability is inexorably bound together with the need for comprehensiveness and for interdisciplinary relationship within the context of complexity thinking. No one part of any system can be altered without ultimately affecting all parts of the systems. Implementing nursing shared governance cannot simply be an end in itself.

Ultimately, if care is to be advanced and the therapeutic process is to be successful, unidisciplinary approaches cannot be the sole means of structuring the delivery of care while ignoring the relationships necessary to sustain it. Simply taking on the mechanisms of patient care will not effectively create a more viable patient care service without building an infrastructure that demands and creates a framework for sustaining the necessary relationships. If the structures, relationships, interactions, and interdependencies between all parts of the political and social system are not included and advanced in the change, the change simply cannot be sustained.

It is often fascinating to see many of the same mistakes made over and over again with regard to human dynamic change. Consistently, there has been, over the years, even in the process of implementing shared governance, a flagrant disregard of the wide variety of fits that have to be achieved to ensure that an organization remains effective in the midst of dramatic and comprehensive change. Simply adjusting one's service components or resources does not create the conditions necessary to ensure sustainable change. Any approach to the adjustments an organization needs to be relevant and applicable depends on how comprehensive the view from the center of the system is and how well it is configured and organized in a way that represents the response to change and to make sure that response has been considered and carefully addressed. It is this lack of integration, integrity, and coordinating the complexities of clinical practice that have kept many consultants employed today, even some who should not be.

This book focuses on the interdisciplinary integration and the infrastructure necessary to support it. This text focuses on the creation of a model or framework for transforming healthcare services in a way that addresses the need for an interdisciplinary infrastructure. Experience has taught us that nursing shared governance is a strong and viable foundation upon which to create the framework for excellence and to address the needs of a nursing practice–driven environment.

Still, it is necessary to recognize that systematic planning and engagement of all key stakeholders from every discipline are necessary to ensure the vitality and viability of a truly effective clinical system. Through systematic planning and a model for comprehensive redesign, the interdisciplinary frame for effective practice can emerge. Through using a set of principles as a foundation for transformation, organizational leadership in health care must now ground their efforts in a detailed understanding of synthesis of clinical relationships and the application of the processes associated with creating continuity and congruence not only in patient care but between and among the disciplinary stakeholders necessary to advance it. The leadership of the organization, both in administration and clinical practice, must evidence a willingness to embrace the emerging quantum realities and the quantum applications in a sociotechnical framework necessary to ensure the formation of new relational forms and structures that advance the clinical practice and therapeutic dynamics in a continuously transforming healthcare system.

For effective transformation to occur a new model of service integration and interdisciplinary relationship must ultimately drive the system. The fundamental and sustaining principles of partnership, equity, accountability, and ownership define the foundations for creating this new infrastructure. These core elements form the centerpiece for all the relationships and activities of integration necessary to sustain comprehensive clinical practice. Every component of the design of the point of service (the microsystem) now must focus on a construct for the effective organization and integration of healthcare work and the disciplines that provide it. A conception of the continuum of care driven by a strong set of interdisciplinary relationships and infrastructures helps create a framework for building an integrated continuum of care.

Human dynamics and relationships now must include the linking of technological and digital realities necessary to support them. Structure must also serve to provide an enduring linkage between micro- and macrosystems across health care. Also, as the information infrastructure increasingly becomes the architecture of the future of health service construction and relationship, a prevailing structure that frames the human dynamics associated with the action of health service will be essential. Recognizing that a evidence-driven, sustainable, comprehensive, and truly health-based construct must be created in the healthcare system drives the notion that if it is to be created, it cannot be done without incorporating and investing all the disciplines in this concerted effort.

The reader is advised, as always, that some approaches described in building an interdisciplinary infrastructure in this book are simply that—models, descriptions, ideas. Although shared governance certainly represents a commitment to sound principle, good theoretical foundations, and time-tested applications, the related principles reflect the unique application of emerging thought about the integrity and integration of services around which infrastructure can be built. It is not recommended that any particular one of these ideas or notions be replicated as a single or preeminent notion applicable to all situations and circumstances. This book provides ideas, experience, and notions that can be tested and replicated in any number of settings. The editor and authors hope that this book will serve as a template for principles that guide transformation and integration of the disciplines in a construct that advances patient care and ultimately has an impact on creating new models for health.

This book continues to focus on a range of pertinent ideas and notions related to preparing organizations in the disciplines that do the work of health care.

For a transformed healthcare script, however, the reader must recognize that the information contained herein is not an exhaustive treatment of the topic of integration and interdisciplinary decision making but is simply a beginning point from which to deepen one's understanding of applications in the creation of truly integrative interdisciplinary models of relationship and infrastructure that support it.

All transformation continues as a journey. This book outlines the content and framework necessary for a journey toward interdisciplinary collaboration and integrated decision making in a relevant organizational structure. It is recommended that other works also be accessed and be incorporated into a complex array of ideas and notions that guide the thinking and actions of the change agents as we all collectively construct a more creative, substantive, and sustainable delivery model for interdisciplinary integration and practice-driven decision making as an effective vehicle for transforming patient care.

As always, nothing is fraught with more danger and difficulty than attempting to create a change in the order of things. The "noise" in the system that results is at times unbearable and even untenable. Every person's role is effective in every place in the organization when transformation drives the effort to create new models for meeting the needs of a changing system. True transformation addresses as much the requisites of changing activities in the boardroom as it does in the patient's room. The political interactional and structural challenges that are necessary as a part of addressing transformational change must be incorporated into the planning and design of a new infrastructure.

The effort on the part of the leaders from every place in the system is at minimum Herculean. This kind of a transformation is a major structural change and requires a level of commitment from leadership and from clinical staff. It calls for faithfulness to the process of transformation that demands continual commitment and personal perseverance. Even though the results may be inspiring and the change clearly meaningful, the need to persevere and to sustain cannot be understated. The skill and talent of participants in maintaining a high level of effort and energy in the creation of a truly functional integrated and interactional healthcare system will require access to talents and gifts in places where there was no expectation or sign that they might be present. The wonder of shared governance and integrated shared decision making in the past 20 years has been the discovery of the secret and hidden places in organizations where can be found leadership, creativity, innovation, and new thinking. The investment of the stakeholders in every place in the system bears much fruit and brings much value to the organization, sustaining a new dynamic in delivering health care in a value-driven and evidence-based construct.

Of course, time is the best test of whether any strategy, creative venture, and transforming activity brings meaningful results. In the past 20 years of building toward an interdisciplinary model, the efforts have resulted in many viable integrated shared decision-making structures that could not have been previously successful. There are times in history where the characteristics of the age and the demands of the time converge to create the conditions for successfully implementing models and processes that could not have been implemented at an earlier time. The foundations already laid now serve as a firm basis upon which to build and transform the next stage of integrative health care. The need now clearly exists for a seamless dynamic and truly health-based script emerging as the prominent condition and circumstance for a truly effective system. It is in the spirit of building toward this effective system of health service that the notions, ideas, and insights found in this book are directed.

Acknowledgments

No work of this kind can ever be put together without the assistance of numerous participants. We wish to thank all those involved in the earlier publication introducing shared governance titled *Whole-Systems Shared Governance: Architecture for Integration*; Marilyn Hawkins and Marsha Parker, my co-editors; contributors Kami English, Phil Hinton, Jeff LeFors, Lynn Neimeth, Bruce Perry, and Curtis Takamoto. Their work at Community Hospital in Fresno more than 10 years ago provided the template upon which the future of interdisciplinary shared governance could build. This revised text extends their original work. We are appreciative of the foundations they laid in the first text on bringing shared governance to the whole healthcare team. Thanks also go to Kathryn McDonagh whose work on the chapter on governance has made a significant contribution to the quality of this book. Special thanks go to Mark Ponder whose editorial guidance, modeling, and mentoring, as always, contribute to the quality of this final product. As I always do with each text that I am associated with, I want to thank my colleagues and partners in clinical practice and leadership who have supported and sustained me during the years of struggle and creativity in the design, implementation, and documentation of new models for guiding professional practice and professional decision making in a transforming healthcare system. Their continual commitment and struggle to make possible every day the realization of a truly effective community-based healthcare system remains a source of inspiration and encouragement to me. I am forever thankful to share the journey toward truly interdisciplinary practice with them.

About the Author

Tim Porter-O'Grady, DM, EdD, FAAN, has been involved in health care for 38 years and has provided both administrative and consulting services to a wide variety of healthcare agencies internationally. In addition, Tim is currently Associate Professor and Leadership Scholar at Arizona State University, College of Nursing and Healthcare Innovation. He has written more than 160 professional journal articles and has published 17 books. He resides in Atlanta, Georgia, in the Blue Ridge Mountains and enjoys reading, writing, and hiking.

About the Contributors

The chapter authors, Kami English, Marilyn Hawkins, Phil Hinton, Jeff LeFors, Lynn Neimeth, Marsha Parker, and Curtis Takamoto, were all members of the Shared Governance Leadership Team at Community Hospitals of Central California at the time of the publication of the first edition of this book. Kathryn McDonagh is a governance consultant in private practice in Atlanta, Georgia. Tim Porter-O'Grady is a health systems consultant in private practice in Atlanta, Georgia, and was lead consultant in the shared governance project at Community Hospitals of Central California.

CHAPTER 1

Health Care in a Quantum Age

Tim Porter-O'Grady

The future is like heaven;
everyone exults in it but no one wants to go there now.

—JAMES BALDWIN

The social context for health care is changing in dramatic and radical ways. It is essential for leaders to be able to recognize the change in context that is driving it. The transformation from the industrial age to the sociotechnical edge now calls leadership to perceive the experience, organization, and delivery of health care in a fundamentally different way. It is essential for leaders to see these changes in a much broader context. The very foundations and framework of society in a global community are being shaken by a shift in reality—a quantum shift.

The world is undergoing significant change. We have moved into an age in which some parameters look nothing like those of the age that we have lived through. The industrial age is ending, with all that that implies. The journey into this new age requires a great deal of adjustment—an "unbundling" of old behaviors, old structures, and old ways of thinking. This transformation into the sociotechnical age, or quantum age, will challenge your understanding of the journey, the work of health care, and what will be required of each of us.

There are broad indicators of the significance of this change from the industrial age to the sociotechnical age:

- An information explosion in the movement to digitization of all data is transforming the way people communicate, interact, and share information.
- The globalization of the economy is creating new fundamentally altered relationships between communities, nation-states, and international regions and is redefining the boundaries for everyone.

Newtonian thinking and the reductionism that it represents are being replaced by recognition of a unified global community and the idea that all issues are, at some level, structurally integrated and represent the fundamental quantum infrastructure (complex and adaptive systems) that changes the way in which people perceive relationships, interactions, and communication. Quantum reality reflects the constant "dance" at the intersection between the external environment and internal life of the organization, reflected in the response people make to this relationship and how they shape their behavior to advance the life of the organization. Leaders respond to this reality by creating responsive and adaptive strategies and engaging all elements and stakeholders in the system in a collective dynamic to positively impact each other, the system, and the individual.

Universal ways of performing information management and the technology of data transfer and portal access are becoming more fully understood and more incorporated as a part of our lived experience. It is increasingly recognized that information and digitization are dynamic and that all processes and relationships related to communication are built and sustained for the foreseeable future and upon how decisions are made in ways that will affect lives across traditional boundaries.

A NEW UNDERSTANDING

In the context of this significant change, new developments of relationships and intersecting structures are forming a construct for the new age. This new quantum context is challenging the foundations of many of our social, political, business, and service organizations. At every point and level of human behavior and relationships and at every intersection of human community, the principles that once defined who we were and what we were have now given way to a broader view of humanity, experience, and the science which underpins our knowledge: what we believe and the way in which we behave.

> **Knowledge is the newest form of capital and now plays as great a role as finances in the sustainability of systems.**

THE EMERGING VALUE OF KNOWLEDGE

Knowledge workers' competence is becoming the fundamental construct of all organized systems. This knowledge becomes the foundation for economic progress and for productive work. It also is the major medium of exchange in the global community. Those with specific and unique talent and knowledge are necessary resources to innovative enterprises and to changing systems. They can probably determine what the future of the enterprise will be and will even drive much of the generation of new knowledge and power relationships in organizations and systems. It is now understood that those who have knowledge, manage knowledge, create knowledge, or use knowledge are critical to the sustenance of society and the globe. Indeed, the very value of a knowledge-driven world is moderated by the understanding that those who manage knowledge manage all the fundamental quantum constructs, such as chaos, complex adaptive systems, the whitewater of constant change, and the need for synthesis (predictive and adaptive) in both human systems and behaviors.

The recognition of the unfolding reality related to knowledge creation and knowledge management is sufficient alone to create a new shift in the power and relational equation in social, political, and work systems. The application of knowledge affects whole industries (indeed, every aspect of our life), increasing their social, financial, and political stock and at the same time diminishing and perhaps even eliminating the value of previous knowledge as new foundations are laid for it. The relevance and applicability of knowledge are not its only central values. As knowledge loses relevance and diminishes in value, it loses its impact and calls us to shift our frame of reference and what we know to be more relevant and appropriate to the time.

Whether intended or not, the emerging information and knowledge society has already altered the circumstances of how people live and work around the globe. The circumstances that we now experience require us to conceive our social constructs as a people, as communities, or as whole societies in entirely different ways. Problems, however, are associated with this emerging need to live our experiences in different ways:

- A knowledge society requires a shift in the locus of control and in the distribution of power. Knowledge challenges those who currently hold power and requires them to locate it differently from the places and in the ways it has traditionally been distributed in organizations. The knowledge worker is now the source of power.
- Knowledge workers historically unfamiliar with the use of power have a difficult time understanding how to obtain and use it appropriately. Not only are knowledge workers unfamiliar with the way in which knowledge needs to be used and expressed, but they must learn how to use knowledge in a way that advances and increases the value of power.
- A generation moving more strongly toward knowledge-based organizations requires a growing focus on outcomes and results. Evidence-based work drives the fundamental constructs of the value of work. Workers' attachment to process, function, and activity now simply impedes their ability to adjust as outcomes, evidence, and impact demand.
- The structures shift dramatically in knowledge-based organizations. Systems must make it easy for knowledge workers to apply what they know, translate knowledge systems, use the technology of knowledge, and manage the infrastructure of knowledge, loosening up the application of tight controls in the system. This need for broader distribution of structure, power, and relationships challenges many hierarchical infrastruc-

tures and challenges their ability to facilitate the innovation and creativity necessary to sustain and maintain the effectiveness of the system. Having many hierarchical levels of decision making in an organization impedes the speed and fluidity with which knowledge and decision making can flow.

Many of these circumstances are now converging to create a serious cascade of events both globally and locally. What is occurring in health care is simply a subset of what is occurring across all systems. These changes create the same set of challenges in every segment of human life. What is important for healthcare professionals to realize is that much of what is unfolding in health care falls within a broader system and gives meaning and context to many of the dynamic changes that are occurring. These changes must continue to occur to make healthcare delivery more effective and relevant.

> **Knowledge is more than power; it is a medium of exchange as important as any other commodity in the workplace.**

A NEW CONTEXT FOR A NEW AGE

Interdisciplinary shared governance is used to create an organizational structure in a context for managing the shifting and highly interactive changes affecting the provision of healthcare services. Many of the demands of the healthcare system, as in other parts of society, require different organizational constructs, an emerging set of relationships, interactions not based on a hierarchy but on partnership, and, ultimately, different ways of making decisions and implementing them if effectiveness is to be sustained.

Newer knowledge regarding complex adaptive systems and their implications for organizations is having a significant impact on the design and structuring of human systems. These systems must accommodate several converging forces that interact to create the conditions necessary for systems to change, adapt, and thrive. Active agents in the systems continually interact in frequently random ways rather than in planned and controlled approaches. Out of the convergence of these actions and interactions, patterns emerge which both inform the behaviors of the agents and represent the impact of that convergence. Through following a few simple but central rules, wondrous levels of complexity and social architecture emerge in highly intragroup and interconnecting ways, resulting, if positive, in continuous improvements.

Every system exists within its own specific environment as well as represents its place in the larger environment. As that environment shifts and changes, systems also need to shift and change in order to maintain an effective fit between the external environment and the internal operating system. Effective complex adaptive systems learn from this interaction between the system and its environment, adapting and changing in a way that improves the situation for both the system and its people. In this interaction, effort does not need to be perfect; in fact, it can be suboptimal, just good enough, sufficient to stimulate and maintain movement to either increased efficiency or greater effectiveness.

Diversity and variety add to the system's strength and effectiveness. It is out of paradox and ambiguity abounding in the complexity where contradictions and changing forces converge to create new and different possibilities, enabling the system to adapt to changes in its external environment and within. This connectivity is indicative of a continuous and dynamic network of actions, elements, and forces working in conjunction with each other, such that a change and adaptation in any one part of the network has a dramatic and significant impact in other parts.

In complex adaptive systems, simple rules prevail. Simply because systems are complex does not mean they are complicated. Emerging patterns in the system have a level of complexity and a rich variety but reflect their relationship in a kaleidoscope that demonstrates both the simple rules that drive it and the visual complexity that represents it. These rules are generally broadbased or universal (e.g., all water finds its own level), yet can yield all kinds of complex applications. Also, complex adaptive systems are self-organizing. Hierarchies are uncommon in these systems. Interactions and intersections in these systems are constantly reconfiguring and rearranging as they adapt to changing conditions and circumstances; working diligently to create relevant form and action that meets immediate need and lays the foundation for change and adaptation. This process often appears uncontrolled, chaotic, and uncertain. Yet, embedded within it is a pattern of organization and order that continually moves through a system ensuring its continual adaptation and sustenance.

Shared governance and shared decision making both represent human dynamics and behaviors as they respond within the context of complex adaptive systems. Shared governance serves as a simple vehicle for engaging systems and their members and creating the necessary forums and intersections to assure the decisions and actions remain dynamic and as close to the point of service and productivity as possible. Separating function and contribution, councils and decision-making forums focus on relationship and responsiveness and build in the infrastructure the dynamics necessary for full and essential engagement of every component of the system. It also invests its stakeholders in those efforts and obligations necessary to assure the systems vitality and viability.

Whatever the change process, it will continue to be complex and high intensity (see Table 1-1). The structural underpinning for interdisciplinary decision making is a model that reflects this necessary response to the ever-changing paradigm, moving systems to the interdisciplinary infrastructure necessary to successfully operate outward from the point of service and giving form and structure in a way that supports the function and outcome of integrated health-

Table 1-1 The Changing Healthcare Marketplace

Old	New
Single payments	Contracts
Physician manages care	Third party manages care
Do more, make more	Do more, make less
High hospital occupancy	Shifting hospital occupancy
Referrals, money maker	Referrals, money loser
Primary care, low status	Primary care, high status
Treat disease	Improve health status
Institution centered	**Community centered**
Free-standing facility	Integrated facility/systems
Physicians and hospital separate	Physician-hospital organization
Patients one by one	Patients in groups
Solo practice	Group practice
Tertiary care, money maker	Tertiary care, money loser
Physician centered	Patient and family centered
Curing	Healing
Patients come to providers	Providers go to patients
High profit margins	Value-driven returns
Physicians	Physicians and physician extenders
Traditional medicine	Alternative medicine
Providers as revenue generators	Providers as value centers
Reactive medical care	Health needs assessment; innovation
Emphasis on treatment	Emphasis on prevention

Table 1-1   The Changing Healthcare Marketplace (continued)

Institution centered	Community centered
Vertical organizations	Complex adaptive systems
Inpatient care	Continuum-based health care
Ignoring waste	Designing out waste
Assumption of provider competency	Competency/improvement report cards
Community practice	Critical pathway standards
Assumed outcomes	Outcome measurement
Patient as recipient	Patient as participant
National reform	National, state, and local reform

care delivery. Although it is unique to the healthcare system, shared governance is based on a sound foundation in complex adaptive systems and systems thinking and reflects the emerging principles of the quantum age into which we are quickly moving. Shared governance is well documented in the literature and has been implemented, especially in nursing organizations, across a broad multitude of healthcare organizations throughout the United States. Shared governance takes the characteristics and principles that reflect the format for operating in a complex and adaptive system and gives them a structural component that builds the structures and infrastructures that promulgate full engagement of stakeholders in the support of new relationships, intersections, functions, and activities operating in a truly interdisciplinary and interactive healthcare system.

The healthcare system is constructed predominately of knowledge workers (professionals) who historically apply their skills and talents in the very strongly vertical, compartmentalized hospital structure. As health care changes and becomes more decentralized, a much broader format is needed to view the breadth of services emerging along an increasingly diverse continuum of care. Leadership in health care can no longer look at the services provided within a narrow, vertical, institutional format. In an effort to create sustainable outcomes it is now necessary to bring together many diverse players. A wide range of providers facilitates the clinical outcomes necessary in an evidence-based framework, linking activities, functions, relationships, and intersections as the effects of sustainable and achievable clinical outcomes. Achieving all of this requires an entirely different way of thinking in an organization, one that is designed in a meaningful way and that will actually produce the interdisciplinary evidence-based frame for truly effective health care.

> **Leadership is no longer managership. The whole role of leader is directed to facilitating the growth of leadership in all roles in the system.**

A NEW REALITY FOR ORGANIZATIONS

Reallocation of power in health care parallels the reallocation under way in most other parts of American and global society as evidenced in the business and service constructs of work. Hosts of changes currently affect the design of healthcare organizations (see Figure 1-1). In many ways, as these organizations change from their hierarchical infrastructure and management-driven framework toward more knowledge-based and point-of-service-driven designs, their operations, services, and governance functions must also be reconfigured so that strategy, tactics, direction, policy, and process as well as point-of-service decision making can intersect in a much more meaningful and sustainable way.

Also, the ever-increasing focus on effective decisions made by those who impact them at the point of service requires an entirely different construct for the function and operation of healthcare organizations. In complex adaptive systems, service integration along the continuum of care forces organizations to revise their infrastructures and to think in new ways about how health care

Figure 1-1   Developments in Health Care That Are Influencing Quality and Effectiveness

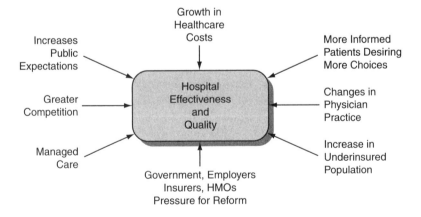

should be delivered; how professional relationships should unfold; how inter-disciplinary infrastructures are created to sustain these relationships; and how environments, structures, and processes affect the delivery of meaningful, value-driven services.

Building a point-of-service system means reallocating power in the organization to those who do the work of health care.

The changes in the organizational relationships and in people's understanding of what is effective affect the design of healthcare systems and services. New rules and circumstances are beginning to have a dramatic and measured effect on how healthcare services are being offered, managed, and evaluated. For example, many hospitals have moved from paper-based processes to entirely digital infor-mation systems. Along with these more horizontal ways of communicating, these organizations have modified their vertical lines of authority and have begun to unlink vertical control and create new links of horizontal relationships, intersec-tions, and interactions across a system driven by the point of service.

The kinds of services provided in the new marketplace are new and creative, with interesting new service mechanisms creating an entirely different construct for how that work will be completed. Furthermore, self-directed and integrated structures will continue to emerge as the context of a much more seamless and horizontal continuum of integrated healthcare services provides a better ser-vice framework for a population-driven healthcare system. The creation of inte-grated and interdisciplinary structures means that the organizations themselves cannot be managed in the same way as they were in past generations.

CHANGING CONTEXT FOR HEALTHCARE SERVICE

It is important, therefore, for leaders to be clear about the environmental factors that suggest workplace readiness to explore self-directed, seamless, and integrated structures in a delivery system that integrates every point of deci-sion making along a continuum of services and must measure its results and value all along the way. The primary role of the leader is to determine the ways in which the old frameworks and behaviors (industrial age hierarchy, parental management style, for example) must give way to more contemporary notions about operations and the application of systems models. And we must break the old rules (see Exhibit 1-1).

This chapter outlines primary principles that exemplify the new Sociotech-nical age and must constitute the foundation for any sustainable change in struc-

Exhibit 1-1   The Old Way

For every dollar spent on direct patient care, we spend three to four dollars

- waiting for it to happen
- arranging to do it
- writing it down

ture (partnership, accountability, equity, and ownership). Without these principles or their application, structure will be built on shaky ground and will collapse quickly with the next major shift in direction and function. Furthermore, leaders need to be challenged to redesign and reconfigure organizations in ways that reflect a much more point-of-service-driven, empowered, and information-based system.

> **The role of leadership is primarily directed toward breaking down old frameworks and practices, making organizations and people ready for newer configurations.**

THE EVOLVING NATURE OF WORK

As part of the healthcare transformation to a new age, the traditional delivery infrastructure must be reinvented to support a new understanding of work, health, information, quality, outcomes, relationships, and intersections within an organized delivery system (see Exhibit 1-2). These changes will result in fewer managers and will alter managers' roles and functions, as well as the expectations and functions of those who provide services. They will challenge current practices and will generally turn organizations and perceptions of work upside down and force us to think about meaning and purpose in relationship to function and activity. There are a number of shifts that are already under way:

- Hospitals are being deconstructed to do two things: diminish the focus on bed-based activities and create efficiencies in the organization.
- Healthcare services, traditionally scattered throughout different settings, are now being reconfigured into an integrated service pathway, some of which is hospital based and some of which is not.
- Linear administrative hierarchies are diminishing in value as more effective point-of-service designs are created. They are being transformed into equity-based models characterized by collaborative decision making, management support, and consultative roles as more decentralized point-of-

Exhibit 1-2   Problems with the Traditional Structure

- Fragmentation of care
- Turf issues and duplication
- Nonproductive downtime
- No coordination of care
- Task orientation versus outcomes orientation
- No accountability for big picture
- Cost management instead of producing value

service decision making arises and knowledge-based ownership of work processes emerges at the point of service.

- Competition is now moving to the systems level. Systems are competing with each other to provide a wide range of services to as broad a population as can be served. Each system, in a sense, is also competing with itself in trying to increase its ability to provide cost-effective high-quality services and maintain the satisfaction of its patients and providers.
- A short-term, fix-it mindset is not appropriate for addressing constant change. Fad surfing and fashion shifts in health care, so often seen in the past, must be replaced by a willingness to consider whether fads or fashions make any difference or facilitate sustainable cost-effective service relationships.

Besides the immediate signs of a shift in practices and processes in health care, there are other key influences that define a comprehensive scope of change accompanying the preceding challenges. These external and internal environmental factors create the conditions that require sustainable shifts:

- The local impact of global forces of change
- Building infrastructure for complex adaptive systems
- Contemporary systems theory (quantum versus Newtonian thinking)
- The emergence of performance-driven payment schemes
- The movement toward a focus on creating health
- The growing competence and decision-making role of subscribers (patients)
- The demand for change and the organizational readiness to respond

Furthermore, three major forces are converging to create conditions that have made avoidance of significant change no longer a viable option: technology, social reengineering, and economic reconfiguration.

Most restructuring must occur between people's ears.

Technology

The computer chip and the Internet have both become the major vehicle upon which we are traveling into the new age. Indeed, their applications affect almost every aspect of life, from the minute our digital alarm clocks wake us up in the morning, through the management of our information and life during the day, to the arming of our home security systems when we go to bed at night. Information and communications technology will link all service components and all stakeholders at the point of service, making it both possible and necessary to locate most decisions where the providers and consumers meet.

Technology is not simply changing how we work; it is changing how we live.

Technology has created mobility in health care. One of the effects of technology is to reduce the demand on once-necessary functions and activities. Examples include procedures such as cholecystectomy, laser surgery, chemotherapy, and monoclonal antibody therapy and gene therapies. All of these reduce the intensity of interventions, the lengths of stay in hospitals, and the need for dependence on beds. Each also significantly reduces the activities of one or another healthcare provider. Many applications of technology make care more portable and less invasive, thus radically altering the service structure. The impact of the techno-infrastructure is exemplified in almost every area of healthcare delivery.

Instant Access

Key components of the technological revolution are to a great extent driving the transformation of society and the emergence of a new age. In communication, technology alone is connecting humanity in ways that could never have been anticipated in the past. Boundaries and borders no longer have significance or meaning now that technology integrates people across artificial barriers of any kind. People of every culture and circumstance can now connect and communicate with each other across national boundaries. Further, they can generate unlimited volumes of information and almost instantly send them over phone lines and wireless channels to any part of the globe.

Technology has created an opportunity to connect the world in ways only dreamt of in past generations. As a result, we have become a global community—and are confronted with all the attendant options and problems.

Technology in the world of commerce has already altered forever the way in which business is conducted. Companies have created so many useful technological products that we simply cannot survive without them. Although we might take them for granted (older generations are still suspicious of technology), we can watch them transform every part of human experience in many subtle and not-so-subtle ways.

Technology means instantaneous access to anything that any person might want or need. Very little information is out of the reach of individuals who know how to use communication technology. Not only can most information be accessed, it can be integrated in ways that permit a breadth and depth of view only previously imagined. Information provides a framework for flexibility and gives everyone the opportunity to link with others in the time it takes to say a word or strike a key. In the past hundred years, we have gone from train travel to fiber-optic travel to wireless networks, and we can now connect with others around the world without ever leaving home (think of MySpace, FaceBook, YouTube, and others).

Economic and Financial Shifts

Clearly, nothing has a greater impact on the U.S. healthcare system and culture than the changes in economics and finance that are currently occurring. Although the economics of health care is complex, simple conditions are converging to create the need for a major shift in the orientation and structuring of the healthcare system. What is currently happening in the United States is the direct result of a lack of control in spending over the last 30 years. We are simply expending too much for the health care that we are getting in return. In fact, healthcare expenditures are outstripping other social expenditures by a factor of 3 to 4. Without experiencing a net improvement in the health of the nation, we continue to watch healthcare costs spiral above every other economic indicator.

> The prevailing reality affecting all parts of the economy is that resources are finite. Therefore, good stewardship means careful allocation and use of resources.

Growing Costs

Health care in the United States has grown from a $100 billion industry in 1965 into over a $2 trillion industry today. Despite increases in technology and the availability of services, we still have not conclusively addressed the basic health issues of the nation. It is suggested that the improved health many Americans enjoy is a result mostly of improvements in public health (e.g., excellent sewage systems, immunization campaigns, and other community services) not of the services provided by our "illness care" system.

A good portion of our economy is tied up in providing or paying for healthcare services. Healthcare leadership has a powerful influence on what happens to the system and the political and economic decisions that are made about it. If there is no generalized commitment to transformation and reconfiguration, chances are that costs will continue to grow at or about the same rate they have in the past, creating an overwhelming demand for economic and financial retooling of the system. A new way of looking at service provision—accounting for health care, paying for it, and costing out the expense and financial outlays for service—becomes a critical focus for the healthcare system. Although Americans have historically been opposed to creating an integrated, federally designed plan to address the issues of economics and finance in health care, those issues still need to be addressed, even if it means addressing them at local, regional, and state levels throughout the nation.

Fortunately, much of the healthcare leadership is already involved in the retooling and restructuring of the delivery system in a way that is increasing the cost-effectiveness and efficiency of service provision and changing the character of the relationship between cost and value. Controlling costs and capping expenditures require that every system and institution that provides healthcare services tighten its belt and begin addressing the following questions regarding the appropriate delivery of health care: What do we provide? How much will it cost? What will our work be? What are the cost-benefit trade-offs of the initiatives that we undertake in creating meaningful health care? What are we getting for what we pay? Are we getting real value for the work of health care? Much of the work of transforming health care can be seen as an attempt to respond to these questions.

Healthcare-related activities eat up a large share of the gross domestic product in a way that negatively affects the economic balance of the country. We cannot ignore the consequences of overspending on health care and and its impact on our ability to thrive as a nation.

Changing the structure means changing the way healthcare services are provided. This affects both behaviors and expectations.

SOCIAL REENGINEERING

The shift from national to regional and global power relationships is forcing social and work institutions to look critically at their own structures, relationships, functions, and purposes and to reconstruct them within a broader context. Politics is now about international relationships, and economics is now about international interfaces on a global business, manufacturing, and service stage. Increasingly, decisions about competition, products, services, profits, trade, boundaries, and politics are being radically influenced by an operating set of variables that are international in character. No nation from this time forward can make decisions for itself without taking into account the context of its relationship to other parts of the global community and hope to have a sustainable future. The intersections between regions and nations on the international stage are now as critical as the activities that occur within any one nation.

The transformation we are experiencing is affecting every place on the globe. No one is exempt from the impact of this change, and our world is altered forever.

Learning is altered by technology. We now have an educational system that is no longer adequate for the needs of those it is intended to instruct.

At the social level, service structures that promote the future of society are also shifting and adjusting. Immigration, education, employment, entitlement programs, crime, and social health are all arenas where radical adjustments have emerged with significant implications in scope, social process, and community construction.

For example, the increased role of computer technology in the education of children has created a conflict in the framework and structure of education in American society. Through the use of interactive technology and computer systems, children can learn in 5 to 15 minutes what used to take 5 hours of didactic, one-to-group teaching activities to instill. However, to fully implement the technology already present would require a shift in the kinds and numbers of teachers, the design and format of the classroom, and the design and structuring of education in America.

The complex, critical issues of role, outcome, employment, and relevance all influence the viability of the response to the educational crisis created by the possibilities of technology and the emerging need for its socially relevant use. This, joined with the other issues identified earlier, creates a major social challenge influencing the reconstruction of the social paradigm both in the United States and other nations around the globe.

CHANGING HEALTHCARE STRUCTURES AND MODELS

The medical model of health care is fraught with serious problems and issues. Medical intervention is clearly "situational" and dependent on the identification of illness for the generation of services and payment. The historic problem with the medical model is that it offers too little too late and that the treatment activities are reactive rather than proactive. Because technology makes it possible to intervene earlier and to reduce the intensity of interventions, it begins to alter the character of practice and create the conditions that provide a different framework for valuing healthcare delivery.

> **The American model of health care is dying on the vine. A new more fluid and integrated approach to providing healthcare services is essential if an effective and efficient system is to be created.**

Managing Demand

In the future of the healthcare delivery system, there will be a growing dependence on primary and preventive services. Accessing the consumer earlier in the cycle of life, before high-intensity and costly illnesses appear, will be an important part of the design of the system (see Exhibit 1-3). This means, however, retooling every element of the system in a fundamental way to permit early service provision. This retooling serves as the underpinning for reconfiguring the structure, administration, and integration of healthcare organizations (including the formation of shared governance structures).

Exhibit 1-3   Managing Demand

- Who will get sick?
- When do people seek health service?
- What are the "user" characteristics?
- What do we need to do to address early demand?

User-Driven Models

The goal of capping costs can lead to the creation of a user-driven healthcare system. In a user-driven system, individuals take on the obligation to pay more for services that address their health and illness care needs. Managing the price of health care means that healthcare providers must adjust services to respond to an increase in the cost of doing business. In other words, they will have to learn to develop services and offer them in a way that is ever attendant to the cost of those services yet flexible enough to ensure patient satisfaction and good medical outcomes.

Overcoming Medical Separatism

Historically, in the United States the practice of medicine has remained relatively free of broad-based and integrated accountability. Shrouded in the mystery of incomprehensible quackery, and then Newtonian-based science, the practice of medicine has developed without having to provide much evidence of its efficacy for achieving desired outcomes. The individual rights of physicians have been protected by broadly permissive state practice acts and a legally protectionist physician-patient relationship. Indeed, a whole range of laws and regulations has emerged that insulate physicians and shield them from the consequences of poor practice. Although this is now changing, the only way to break through this shield has been to use the legal system (i.e., to sue physicians and other healthcare providers based on evidence of incompetence or gross neglect).

We are watching the end of the practice of medical care as we know it in the United States. The independent, nonaligned unilateral practice of medicine is dead.

Physician practice has remained relatively independent thus far, but now that impact and outcomes have become the driving factor and value has become the measure of viability, physicians can no longer remain outside of the circle of accountability. Increasingly, physicians are becoming partners in a number of different arrangements, either through shared risk, ownership, or other kinds of contractual or service relationships between service providers and across the continuum of care. The growth in such arrangements changes physicians and their relationship to the healthcare system. Although there is much noise involved in this shift, it is essential for fully establishing an accountable, cost-effective, and service-based system. Integrating physicians as partners in the organizational system places special demands on the design of the system. Shared governance becomes a requisite structural design that integrates physicians, creates decision-making partnerships, and provides a framework for continuously facilitating and managing these partnerships.

Consumer-Driven Care

As part of the effort to get control over both care and cost and to create a care delivery system that integrates cost, service, and outcome, newer managed care approaches to organizing care delivery and health services are quickly emerging as the favored models for delivery in the United States. Shifting payment risk to the consumer has grown significantly in response to the belief that it improves services, increases consumer accountability, and reduces the costs of delivering those services. Although there is still much work to do to produce sufficient evidence of quality and cost control, it appears that cost shifting to the consumer lowers insurance company costs, influences consumers to use less health service, and increases the individual's obligation to pay for what he or she uses.

> Managing lives is different from treating sickness—you must know the person before you can be successful in keeping him or her healthy.

It is equally important that consumers be incorporated into the decision-making framework. Consumers must have access to the same range of services in consumer-driven care that they might in any other approach. However, the consumer access for services must reduce the total amount of cost to the system and still provide a continuous linkage of services in such a way that consumers can access the system early on, before they need major interventions, but at their own expense. To ensure attractiveness and draw appropriate consumers into the market, insurance providers are therefore forced to offer high-deductible competitive services that meet their demand for cost efficiency, consumer cost control, and some evidence of positive outcomes.

We can never again make decisions for consumers; instead we must make decisions with them—they "own" their health and must be accountable for it.

The Quality Movement

Nothing in the United States has had a greater impact on work, business, and health care in the past decade than the introduction of the quality movement. Deming and his associates have made Americans aware of the fact that, in the global community, competition is not just a matter of price but also of quality. And because healthcare professionals do not live their lives in isolation and are dependent upon the satisfaction of those they serve, quality is an essential component of health services.

Americans have jumped on the quality/patient safety movement bandwagon and have achieved some remarkable results. However, we are still early in the process. What we do and what we produce and how we manage costs are all now thrown together into a focus on process that is dramatic in its detail and an inspiration with regard to its impact on outcomes. Those who have taken on the task of achieving real customer orientation, process engineering, quality delineation, quality improvement, and team-based systems have shown dramatic results in terms of quality and marketability (see Table 1-2). Indeed, these results have set the level for organizational expectations.

Quality is about achieving sustainable outcomes. Outcomes are what we use to measure the value of processes. Our actions have no meaning separated from the ends to which they are directed.

The quality imperative also leads to the conditions that create a demand for a shared governance structure. Quality cannot be sustained or even obtained except at the point of service, where an organization lives out its service life. Therefore, quality must be an ongoing construct of any work. That being so, the organizational structure must be one that empowers those accountable for quality to make effective meaningful decisions interdependently and free of the supervising, controlling, and approval levels of past organizational structures.

Although much effort has been put into ensuring quality and safety, especially during the past decade, there is still precious little evidence that the focus

Table 1-2   Transition to a Customer Focus

Traditional Focus	Customer Focus
Professional teams	Multidisciplinary customer-focused teams
Clinical standards	Customer satisfaction, priorities, and value outcomes
Manage customers around department's routine	Manage resources for customer
Task oriented	Improvement/outcome oriented
Call appropriate personnel oneself	Do not pass off work one can do
Complicated organizational structure	Simplified organizational structure
Multiple customer contacts	Limited customer contacts
Documentation by profession	Multidisciplinary patient record
Point finger	Fix structure/process/impact
Work faster	Work smarter/better
Narrow job scope	Broad role scope

is bearing dramatic results across the system. As the quality initiatives have grown across the system, and quality offices have grown in size and scope, the accountability for quality has shifted to the office of quality in the organization away from provider ownership of it. The separation of quality from provider ownership, with the majority of quality initiatives driven outside of the point of service, has assured that healthcare organizations cannot yield the results obtained by those who own and do the work of providing health service. If those at the point of service providing care do not own the quality of their work, it cannot be obtained by others who do not do the work, regardless of their commitment. You simply cannot produce a quality you do not own.

Furthermore, the quality imperative includes all of the stakeholders, and getting board members, physicians, administrators, nurses, and other providers in the same room to delineate issues of quality and service, indeed to "sing from the same sheet of music" with regard to service and quality, requires a new type of organizational structure. Shared governance creates a framework for ensuring that the right players are in the right place and make the right decisions about what they do and the impact of what they do—in short, are able to control the quality of their work.

Innovation means making new—essentially renewing the system around a new set of principles for creating 21st century health care.

Value-Driven Care Delivery

Finally, the evidence-based, value-driven movement has created the conditions for reorienting the point of service in a much more functional, cost-effective, and service-efficient manner. The demand for outcomes (value) ultimately focuses on the performance of those upon whom outcomes depend. Building team-based relationships, integrating the disciplines, creating equity at the point of service, designing around the patient population, and creating continuums of relationship, linkage, and integration across the system are all fundamental ways of reconfiguring a healthcare organization to be more tightly fitted and to be able to answer the value question.

It is becoming increasingly clear that old structures no longer serve the needs of patients or providers, nor are they appropriate for providing care in a value-based organization. As a result, in health care there has been much exploration of alternative designs for patient-focused activities. Designs are emerging that better support the provision of satisfying service and the achievement of meaningful and cost-efficient outcomes.

This means, however, that old departmental, functional, "silo-based" approaches to the work must be let go. Old rituals and routines will be challenged and people's work relationships and attachment to activities and functions of the past will be severely tested. The result will be structural and political "noise" (see Exhibit 1-4). New roles will be developed, interactions and functions will be closely examined, and processes and relationships will be assessed to determine their contribution to the achievement of patient outcomes and specific cost outcomes. Certain roles will not survive the analysis or the change, and the integration of roles will call for new kinds of players and practitioners.

Required is a new focus—a focus on discovering where service is best provided and how integration can create a linkage that has imbedded in it the necessary value-driven processes. Compression of the organization creates a leaner system with fewer managers, better-prepared practitioners, and a clearer delineation of functions and expectations around the organization's core of clinical activities. This creates a demand for a new administrative service and organizational structure, one that can act as a vehicle for linking the stakeholders together and can provide a decision-making framework that produces desired outcomes without sacrificing equity, investment, empowerment, and ownership at the point of service. Shared governance is one such structure.

Exhibit 1-4   Structural and Political Considerations

- Team attitudes
- Turf battles
- Career goals
- Manager versus leadership roles
- Corporate culture
- Change quotient
- "Risk" quotient
- Current and future performance
- Current and future external environment

> **Structure in complex adaptive systems now must be fluid and flexible to respond quickly to new relationships and services in the continuum of care.**

> **Shared governance is about shared decision making and building equity within a complex adaptive system.**

PRINCIPLES FOR A NEW AGE

It should be apparent that the constructs and foundations of the 21st century into which we are further moving are fundamentally different from those of the age out of which we are passing. One of the obstacles to progress when we move into a new age is what we think we know and understand. The constructs we have in place—the current organizational designs and structures and even the tools of our mental model—are inadequate for conceiving how we might behave or develop in the emerging new age. As we watch technology alter our conditions and circumstances, we see it create the need for a new script. Many of the constructs that carried us to this point are not adequate to carry us to the next point.

> **Quantum thinking replaces vertical and linear thinking about work and relationships. It dramatically alters the way we see reality and build partnerships.**

As a result of these realities, a new set of principles is being forged, and these principles will constitute the basis for new forms and structures, such as shared governance. The movement away from the Newtonian underpinning that characterized the industrial age and the linear understandings that represent it is creating the foundation for new ways of thinking and conceiving and doing in contemporary complex adaptive systems.

The emergence in the last 40 to 60 years of quantum mechanics and the recent understanding of its impact on structures, organizations, and human systems creates a different foundation for the emerging age. A focus on whole systems and the ability to integrate across them (versus a focus on parts) requires a method of application that is fundamentally different from that used to date. Thinking about "wholes" is characteristic of the new age; thinking about "parts" is characteristic of the industrial age. Our entire framework for thinking about organizations is changing dramatically, and questions about how organizations (complex adaptive systems) will function in the future and what they will actually become with the emergence of a global culture are being raised.

The new age is represented by a set of principles that exemplify it rather than simply define it. Because the new age is unfolding, in essence "being born," as we live through it, it is very difficult to establish parameters that define it clearly. And in fact, it is not necessarily appropriate to do so. In the midst of a move into a new age of understanding and application, the ability to *discern* is better than the ability to *define*. In addition, leaders can put form to what is seen only when discernment is a part of their skill set. However, in reading the emerging signposts, you can see that certain principles can give us a clearer indication of what the underpinnings of the new age might be and what form some of the responses to it might take. These are the same principles that support the concepts of shared governance—the principles of partnership, equity, accountability, and ownership, the central characteristics of life in contemporary complex adaptive systems.

Principles guide our thinking about the foundations for our action and serve as a baseline, a template, for measuring the consistency of our actions with our beliefs.

Partnership

It certainly does not take much effort to realize that partnership will become an increasingly prevalent organizational model. Older nationalistic and dividing-line models of social and political organization are quickly disappearing as the world reorganizes itself into far broader and more regional relationships. However, even in the midst of the growth of regional entities, compartmentalized national and ethnic groups are attempting to hold back the future in protecting their own narrow interests at the expense of their relationships with other groups. The Middle East serves as a most recent example of this dynamic.

> **Partnership is essential to relationship building and is the foundation for constructing the future of organizations.**

As globalization moves forward, it provides a motivation for nations to form economic, social, and political coalitions that strengthen their global economic viability. Isolationism and exclusivism are simply untenable in a world characterized by an entirely different set of constructs, but the effort to create broad-based partnerships is filled with risks and some danger. Overcoming old barriers; dealing with old relationships; and working through discordant experiences, the judgments of history, the circumstances of war, and a host of other regional and national issues require painstaking effort and mind-bending patience. The rewards of doing all these tasks are significant, of course. Broader economies show greater strength, greater potential, and longer-term viability.

Partnerships are clearly arising at every level of society. The principle of partnership applies to small local communities and to large nation-states. Small companies and major enterprises are forming alliances, networks, and other new types of conglomerates. Many are now becoming partners in an effort to consolidate around a certain group of products or services through which they can excel. Larger entities are designing themselves to become lean and effective and thereby increase their competitiveness on the global stage. Smaller entities, on the other hand, are amalgamating to extend their power base and be able to challenge larger entities.

> **The principle of partnership is driving changes at every level of the social order. Political, social, economic partnerships are necessary for thriving on the global stage and building sustainable relationships.**

Partnership will clearly require the dismantling of old approaches and models of hierarchical isolationism and vertical integration. Obviously, more horizontal linkages between companies, services, structures, and systems will be required to sustain the networks necessary to compete on a broader stage. Increasingly, the work structures that develop in complex multifocal organizations must be more centered around the point of service so that the issues of service and product can be more clearly defined by those who produce the outcomes.

The growth in the role of partnership is evident in the increased use of work teams, integrative work arrangements, interdisciplinary models of organization, and multifocal service structures. As organizations form partnerships, they must increase their effectiveness in order to thrive. Lean design, more efficient functions, stronger networks and relationships, and clearer delineation of quality and outcomes become the foundation for achieving successful outcomes.

It must also be remembered that partnerships occur when the parties to the partnership have something unique or significantly different to bring to it. Partnerships occur when the need to aggregate unique contributions advances values in ways that could not be done unilaterally. This value of difference is a critical element of building effective partnerships. It recognizes in the differences the unique and specific contribution each member of the partnership brings to the table and how that unique contribution, when aggregated with the contribution of others, advances the value of the whole.

Needed: A New Kind of Leader

Leadership is an adult-to-adult interaction, not a parental role. New skills will be necessary to extinguish old "boss" behaviors.

The work of building partnerships and making them sustainable offers a new challenge for leaders. The new processes of integration and organization and the shift in work structures support new models of leadership responsibility. The content of the leadership role is altered forever, and the tolerance and talents of persons making the journey toward the revised role will be sorely tested. Partnership demands dialogue about the relationship between players and the way in which work is structured and completed. Because of the problems likely to occur in the journey from one construct of organization to another, leaders must show a willingness to lay the issues on the table before the stakeholders, gather them around those issues, and facilitate their attempts to find solutions to those issues.

Old constructs and structures in an organization do not support the transfer of the locus of control to the point of service unless the structures themselves shift (see Exhibit 1-5). One of the greatest challenges in transforming professional organizations is to restructure the point of service or productivity and at the same time alter the decision-making framework, administrative structure, and governance structure in ways that increase the organization's ability to support the organizational changes. The demand for shared governance grows because the old structures are inconsistent with an organizational format in which leadership is mainly located at the point of service.

Exhibit 1-5   New Rules

- Patients first, departments second
- Simplify, simplify, simplify
- Create relationships where they do not already exist
- Integrate disciplines and roles where appropriate
- No budgetary increases
- No decrease in quality

The locus of control in empowered organizations is at the point of service where most of the decisions are made.

Creating a Learning Organization

In moving toward partnership, an organization must become a learning center in which creativity, problem solving, solution seeking, integration, functional proficiency, quality improvement, relationship building, process enhancement, and outcome determination are the fundamental elements. A learning organization is continuously and dynamically shifting and adjusting what its members know and evaluating what they apply. The structures of such an organization must be as fluid as the ebb and flow of relationships necessitated by changes in the work and the organization's economic situation. New models require shared risk, shared leadership, and shared governance.

The application of the concept of partnership can create a different context for operating and functioning in the organization and can alter its relational milieu and its service structure. Command and control systems will no longer facilitate functioning, especially if the majority of decisions is moved to the point of service. Empowerment becomes not simply a concept but a modus operandi in a point-of-service organization. Furthermore, partnership demands that all of the members of the system, defined by their relationship, be linked in a way that facilitates their common commitment to achieve desired outcomes. There can be no role ascendance, no vertical integration that allows a single person or unit to captain every effort along the continuum of relationships. In health care especially, multiple provider relationships contribute greatly to the character and quality of the care. No one player can know about or control all of the elements of the relationships necessary to consistently achieve desired outcomes along the service continuum. Sustained achievement of desired outcomes requires interdependency—a web of complex relationships between players that facilitates their identification with each other. Again, history and previous expectations and relationships ensure that the transition to real partnerships will be challenging. Such a shift requires the leadership to act increasingly as facilitators of the efforts of others as well as exhibit exceptional skill and patience in creating the required structures and support systems.

> **Command and control systems are the vestiges of a system long since past. Unilateral decision making is not the most effective or sustainable approach to good decision making.**

Partnership in these new organizations calls for a level of openness and honesty not formerly evident in most workplaces. The quality and safety movement has already forced organizations to look critically at their work. The next step—the revising of structures and service systems—demands that the relationship between work and the outcome of work become increasingly more important. Ameliorating the relationships imbedded in work requires a commitment to build the intersections needed to overcome the powerful barriers to true partnership.

> **Health systems must now build a host of noncompetitive relationships. The health of an organization depends on the strengths of its horizontal relationships with partners along the continuum of care.**

Equity

Equity is more than a measure of equality. Equity assumes equality. The foundation of equity is value. Indeed, equity is an indicator of the presence of value. It demonstrates that there is an effective and meaningful relationship between parties—a relationship from which value is obtained by all parties. Equity further involves recognition of the contribution of each role necessary to an outcome. Equity assumes that all outcomes are dependent on the integration of the roles directed toward achieving them. Rarely are outcomes sustained through the activities of any one individual. In systems thinking, equity is a measure of the integration of all players' contributions to outcomes.

> **Equity is not a measure of equality but instead is an indicator of value. Every role has value to the extent that it contributes to the purposes and work of the organization.**

To be effective, every effort in a healthcare organization must be devoted to restructuring, renewing, and redesigning the structures and services of the organization to better define health and produce health through the efficient delivery of healthcare services. Currently, health care is being driven more by fiscal issues than by any other factor. However, quality and sustainable outcomes are emerging as clear elements of the value equation. It is important to recognize that each contributes to long-term viability and to understand what needs to be in place to achieve a healthy future.

> **Equity demands a commitment on the part of all partners in the organization and a recognition of the contribution each makes to the success of the system. No outcome is sustained through the activities of any one person.**

Equity assumes that there is commitment to effectiveness on the part of all players. Furthermore, equity validates the belief that different roles contribute in different ways to outcomes but that no role is clearly more important than another. In the past, roles were defined by their location in the hierarchy and by their job content. In an integrated whole systems approach, roles are merely distinguished by the activities of the individuals who are acting within the roles.

> **The knowledge worker at the point of service is as important to the success of an organization as anyone else and must be invested in decisions that affect the work he or she does and the outcome of that work.**

Clearly, different roles are necessary to sustain an organization. There are those who must administer and those who must provide services. Further, there is a need to delineate the different contributions of those who provide services and those who manage. It should be assumed by anyone reviewing an organization that roles that have no clear accountability and no specified relationship to the desired outcomes should simply not exist. This principle provides a realistic basis upon which to look at roles along a continuum of services in a nonhierarchical and integrated system with a point-of-service design. Because control, leadership, function, activity, determination of quality, and value are mainly located at the point of service, the relationship between the players there becomes more important.

In a point-of-service organization, the success of the organization depends on the judgment and activities of those who live at the point of service. Collins, Hamel, and others have pointed out that over this next decade leaders must increasingly realize that an organization's human capital—the persons who do the work of the organization—actually determines its level of performance. As Drucker succinctly puts it, it is not only financial capital that ensures the ability of an organization to thrive over the next millennium, it is the understanding that human capital is the vital variable that ensures continuing ability to thrive over the long term. This growing notion of check and balance between fiscal and human capital creates a new equation in the workplace that requires a distribution of emphasis and value in creating effective constructs and structures for work. It is upon this premise, as well as that of partnership, that shared governance begins to take more legitimate and specific form.

> **Decentralizing the structure of an organization does nothing if the decisions are not decentralized to the point of service. Unilateral control at any place in the system is just as destructive as it is at the top of the system.**

Inevitably, providers and their partners will function in a more decentralized interdependent continuum of services across a broad-based service structure. That will demand empowerment, independence, interdependence, and an ability to understand the application of value at the point of service and between and among the players. The viability of the organization, its cost-effectiveness, and the efficacy of service provided will depend on the competence of the worker. This concerns not only technical proficiency but also the integrity of the provider relationship.

Also important is the interdependence between the providers and other professionals as well as the effectiveness of their decisions without the kind of supervision so evident in the past. A decentralized broad-based delivery system unfolding in a number of different sites, highly mobile and consumer driven, simply cannot afford or sustain enough managers to supervise and approve the activities of these workers. Practitioners therefore must become interdependent and independent in their activities and relationships. The question that arises is, how does one build a structure that (1) makes that possible and (2) creates sufficient checks and balances to ensure that defined outcomes are obtained and sustained?

Equity, therefore, is more than simply a concept or a belief. It is the best mechanism for integrating relationships at the point of service in a service-based organization. It forces the organization to stay focused on its services and customers. It is represented in the organizational structures, processes, and mechanisms. Equity is evidenced, among other ways, by a strong organizational commitment to supporting people's involvement and investment in the point of service.

Equity is clearly enhanced through inclusive processes at every place decisions are made. It also demands accountability and ownership. And, as already mentioned, organizational and administrative constructs must exhibit commitment to equity as a fundamental principle.

> **Integrating relationships means committing to the linking of all persons around the roles and intersections necessary to build the system.**

Accountability

The most significant transition occurring in organizational systems is from responsibility to accountability. In the industrial model, command and control strategies define the decision-making construct for the organization. Subordinating relationships were essential to the character of the system.

> **Accountability is generated from within a role, not delegated from one role to another.**

Indeed, satisfaction of the "boss" was the paramount consideration in the work relationship, no matter how it was characterized. If the boss was satisfied with the employee's work, the employee was well rewarded (and ostensibly also satisfied). If the boss continued to be satisfied, the employee could thrive and advance up the organizational ladder.

> **Accountability is about outcomes. Rather than being accountable to someone else, an individual is accountable for performing to a level of expectation clear to all the stakeholders who shared in defining it.**

The main problem with the worker-manager relationship, besides the fact that it does not much benefit the organization, is that it rarely creates ownership, investment, and commitment on the part of the worker—except in regard to the worker's own purposes. It tended to polarize workers and managers and was one major cause of the labor movement in the United States.

Organizational parentalism became the essential model for human relationships in an organizational system, but the increasing availability of outcomes data, which gave everyone access to information about work and its products, put a strain on this model. Eventually the constructs of the "work environment," advanced information technology, and systems understanding converged to create the demand for a different context for the relationship between people and systems.

> **In the case of accountability, all stakeholders share a role in evaluating the performance of others upon which their roles depend. Accountability creates the need for a real 360° evaluation.**

Further affecting work relationships is the fact that organizations are steadily becoming more dependent upon the knowledge of workers at the point of service. As already mentioned, the knowledge possessed by workers is now one of the major mediums of exchange in the workplace. In the old industrial model, organizations unilaterally owned the means of production. As organizations become more technologically and knowledge dependent, the means of production and the mediums of exchange are passing into the hands of those who do the work. A different kind of work relationship must exist when the tools of work and the mediums of exchange are no longer owned solely by the organization. The conditions for real partnership are created and produce a demand for increasing levels of accountability.

> **Broken accountability in any one place in a system is brokenness in all parts of the system. Integrity requires the linkage between all the places where essential decisions are made.**

Furthermore, in the professions (especially the health professions), ownership of the professional mandate for specified work is assumed as a subset of effectiveness. The licensed professions in health care ostensibly act in the best interests of society in ways that members of society would normally act for themselves but, when sick and under duress, entrust those decisions in partnership to the professionals whose unique and specific knowledge is essential to their recovery. With a unique body of knowledge and its application on behalf of patients, health professionals reflect their delineated accountability in every level of their professional activity. Because of the unique ownership of their knowledge and the organization's dependency on its accountable exercise, the partnership between the professions and the organization is essential to the viability of both.

Accountability, rather than being delegated (as is responsibility), is specifically imbedded in roles. Indeed, accountability cannot be delegated away. People are always accountable for something, not accountable to someone. Accountability relates to outcome; responsibility relates to process. Accountability must be self-described. It is owned by those who express it and is defined not by processes or activities but by the outcomes (i.e., people are accountable for achieving specific results and not for following certain routines or procedures).

Accountability demands an understanding of its contribution and the activities necessary for that contribution, and each individual in a given role has an obligation to know and to give evidence through both performance and contribution that there is value in the work.

Accountability focuses the organization and all of its resources on the purposes and the outcomes of collective activities. Accountability reflects relationship. In accountability-based systems, there is a fundamental understanding that it is the intersection of roles and functions that leads to accountability (as defined by outcomes). The relationship and interaction between the integration of action and outcome has a much larger impact on the success of the activities and the quality of results when they are viewed within the frame of clearly enumerated outcomes. Systems thinking suggests that the effectiveness of an enterprise depends on the contribution of every member of that enterprise. Brokenness in any one place in the system affects the whole system.

Accountability-based models take into account the essential relationships between the elements of the system, especially between its members. They are founded on an understanding that the results of work are strongly influenced by the intensity of the relationships of those who do it.

Accountability directly intersects with partnership. Because any partnership demands clarity of role, function, and contribution and a mutual understanding of its purpose and direction, the accountability of the players as defined previously is critical to its success and the achievement of its purpose. Dialogue, negotiation, and clarification of role and function are built on a strong core of relationship and are part of the foundation of any successful organization. In the case of accountability, clarity demands that there is nothing left to guess or assume so that all elements of a role are focused on the outcomes to which the role is directed and validated by its relationships. Evaluation of the results of partnership is evidenced in performance outcomes. Functions, activities, relationships, and experiences form the process foundations leading to good outcomes.

Accountability-based systems always demand clarity. Clarity is essential for delineating the contribution of a role to outcomes. Without clarity, processes and activities have uncertain significance and in fact have only limited value. Role definition is basically valuable because of its relationship to the outcomes to which the role contributes. The full meaning of accountability can be understood only in this context.

Accountability is a fundamental construct of shared governance. Indeed, the structures and relationships and elements articulated in a shared governance framework are evidence of the presence of accountability and its necessary foundations. The whole of the infrastructure of shared governance is built on the cornerstone of accountability. Accountability, in fact, is so important that its absence is a strong predictor of failure in any distributive decision-making model.

Ownership

In the journey into a new age of work and work design, it is simply not possible to stop the process of change. The particular journey we are on is a collective one, requiring the engagement of societies, organizations, and individuals. Regardless of how individuals respond, the journey of change will continue relentlessly and will require the ownership and investment of all players that make up a system. All players must realize that the essential characteristics of the changes occurring depend on the contribution each player makes.

> **Ownership means investment on the part of every person in the system.**

A commitment to change carries with it some risk. This risk has to do with one's sense of value in making a contribution to the journey. Individual value during a time of transformation is always driven by circumstances beyond the control of any single person. Change can never be designed to satisfy all of the needs and interests of one person. Much of the character of change is random and serendipitous at best. Adjustments and transformations in role and function are simply reflective of the perceived impact of change on the organization as a whole.

> **An organization simply cannot afford to have on board people who cannot clearly articulate their individual contribution to its purposes and outcomes.**

Context is a critical influence on the content of change. Because an organization and its people live within a larger social, political, and economic context, changes in that frame of reference have a dramatic and direct impact on who people and organizations are and what they potentially become. Because of this, it is necessary for an organization to restructure itself in a way that reflects the emerging paradigm. To do this, the organization and its members must commit to the activity of moving roles, functions, activities, processes, and structures into a new context for shaping a new framework for success. Furthermore, the collective wisdom of leaders and decisional groups must reflect the veracity and accuracy of highly effective predictive and adaptive skills.

Questions that often are raised these days include, who will survive the craziness and uncertainty associated with the journey into the new age? Who will make it and who will not? Who should go and who should not? What size should the organization be and who should be left when the organization is reconfigured (as a complex adaptive system)? These questions are examples of the kinds of issues that all complex adaptive systems confront in a time of great change. Processes of transforming can cause players to recall a naked truth that is often forgotten: One's ability to thrive depends entirely on the tightness of fit between what one has to offer and the needs of the organization. As the demand for work changes, so do worker requirements. In an era of change, the focus is no longer simply on a job or work but on goodness-of-fit. That causes pressures that, for most, are unfamiliar and requires a level of role fluidity and flexibility not traditionally expected.

The change of focus demands commitment and investment throughout the organizational system. The fit between the roles of individuals and the needs of the organization becomes crucial to its ability to sustain and thrive. The organization has an obligation to ensure a tightness of fit between what it does and what it is. The individual has an obligation to ensure that his or her skills will make a broad-based contribution to the organization and the changes it is undergoing. The level of energy and commitment demanded from everyone in the organization sometimes goes beyond basic expectations. This level of commitment is a sign of people's willingness to recognize the relationship they have to the organization and how much the organization depends on them for its success.

THE INTERDEPENDENCE OF EVERYTHING

The level of commitment demanded from everyone also shows the organization how dependent it is on all of its resources. Not only are its stock values or fiscal strength essential for organizational survival, but so are its human and knowledge resources. The balance between its objective and subjective resources creates the ebb and flow necessary to facilitate the life of the organization and ensure its ability to thrive (see Exhibit 1-6).

Exhibit 1-6   Building Interdependence

- Use single focused strategy
- Engage in planned system-wide effort
- Consistently apply organization's philosophy
- Simplify
- Support the strategic plan
- Work together, do not compete within
- Focus on the patient
- Lower costs
- Grow by design, not by accident

> **A system is always self-organizing and, given the appropriate support, will be self-sustaining and oriented toward thriving.**

In shared governance, ownership is required because it expects the stakeholders in every part of the system to participate fully in decisions that will affect the outcomes of their activities. Structures of shared governance ensure that all players have a forum and a role to play in creating a seamless system.

> **Every member of a system has both a right to membership and the obligations that brings. Both must be clear to all who contribute to the system's work.**

Fostering stakeholders and investors—people committed to the organization and its purposes—is critical work in a time of great change. The ownership and the investment of all players must be built into the fabric of the organization, not simply encouraged by the words of its leaders. It does not take staff long to find out whether true investment and commitment exist in an organization or whether expressions of commitment by its leaders constitute mere rhetoric. The language, structures, processes, and outcomes must be congruent if true ownership of an investment in the system are to be engendered. Shared governance requires the application of this principle to the work of building new structures. Shared governance by design recognizes the key role of every player in the system and facilitates the creation of a truly effective organization based on a new health system paradigm.

CREATING A REAL SYSTEM

The foundations and principles discussed in this chapter create the conditions out of which the need for a shared governance structure emerges. The coming of the new age and the changing character of organizations necessitate a shift to a new organizational format and a supporting structure.

> **Shared governance is simply a framework for whole-systems effectiveness, providing a context for partnership, equity, accountability, and ownership.**

Shared governance is an organizational model that uses systems principles (complex adaptive systems), to integrate stakeholders along a continuum of care and create an organization that exemplifies the principles of partnership, equity, accountability, and ownership. All of these principles have direct and immediate applications in a shared governance system. Together they serve as an indicator of the presence of shared governance and foster the type of implementation of processes and structures that ensure its appropriate operation.

In perusing later chapters, where the structures and elements of the model of shared governance are discussed in greater detail, remember that the principles guide the building of all structures. The principles should also be used as a template to assess the integrity of any structure and to evaluate the implementation of shared governance. Dissonance—a lack of harmony between the structure and the principles it reflects—indicates a challenge, difficulty, or incongruence and requires the leaders to be called back to the table to talk about what is missing or what has not been done to ensure integrity and effectiveness.

SUGGESTED READING

Ambrose, D. (2005). Managing self to lead others. In M. Gullatte (Ed.), *Nursing management: Principles and practices.* Pittsburgh, PA: ONS Publishing.

American Nurses Credentialing Center (ANCC). (2005). *American Nurses Credentialing Center: Best practices in today's challenging health care environment.* Washington, DC: American Nurses Publishing.

Armitage, J., Brooks, N., & Carlen, M. (2006). Remodeling leadership. *Performance Improvement, 45*(2), 40–48.

Brady-Schwartz, D. (2005). Further evidence on the Magnet Recognition Program: Implications for nursing leaders. *Journal of Nursing Administration, 35*(9), 397–403.

Collins, J. (2001). *Good to great: Why some companies make the leap... and others don't.* New York: HarperCollins.

Collins, J. (2005). Level 5 leadership. *Harvard Business Review, 83*(7), 136–146.

Collins, J., & Porras, J. (2002). *Built to last: Successful habits of visionary companies.* New York: Harper Business Essentials.

Everett, L., & Black, K. (2007). Putting the patient first: Guiding principles provide a road map for more collaborative relationships among nurses and support service groups. *Nurse Leader, 5*(3), 19–22.

Hamel, G. (2002). *Leading the revolution.* Boston: Harvard Business School Press.

Kelly, K. (2005). *Out of control: The new biology of machines, social systems, and the economic world.* New York: Perseus Books Group.

Marquis, B. L., & Huston, C. J. (2006). *Leadership roles and management functions in nursing: Theory and application* (5th ed.). Philadelphia: Lippincott Williams & Wilkins.

Pfeffer, J., & Sutton, R. (2006). Evidence-based management. *Harvard Business Review, 84*(1), 62–74.

Porter-O'Grady, T. (2006). A new age for practice: Creating the framework for evidence. In K. Malloch & T. Porter-O'Grady (Eds.), *Principles of evidence-based practice* (pp. 1–29). Sudbury, MA: Jones and Bartlett.

Porter-O'Grady, T., & Malloch, K. (2007). *Quantum leadership: A resource for healthcare innovation.* Sudbury, MA: Jones and Bartlett.

Snyder, N. T., & Duarte, D. L. (2003). *Strategic innovation: Embedding innovation as a core competency in your organization* (1st ed.). San Francisco: Jossey-Bass.

Trompenaars, A., & Hampden-Turner, C. (2002). *21 leaders for the 21st century: How innovative leaders manage in the digital age.* New York: McGraw-Hill.

Interdisciplinary Shared Governance: A Model for Integrated Professional Practice

Tim Porter-O'Grady, Marsha Parker, and Marilyn Hawkins

> *Civilization is a movement, not a condition;*
> *a voyage and not a harbor.*
>
> —ARNOLD TOYNBEE

In the industrial age, organizations, vertical structures, and command-and-control management methodologies were the predominant frames for organizational function. Globalization, however, has changed both the content and character of organizational design. No longer can typed supervisory controls, master-servant relationships, and typed superior-subordinate relationships be maintained. As we move further into the 21st century, knowledge work and the knowledge worker become critical elements of the effective organization. These workers demand a different kind of relationship with each other and with the organization. Furthermore, they also require a different organizational infrastructure to support their individual and collective contribution as a knowledge community. Building this community to facilitate professionals/knowledge workers is critical new work for leaders and requires an entirely different frame of reference for building the supportive structure and relationships.

During the industrial age, decisions were often compartmentalized based on the authority of the individual (in health care it was the physician) or the location of the service (radiology, laboratory, nursing, etc.). As discipline- and function-specific walls are broken down and interdisciplinary partnerships increasingly form the foundation for functional clinical activity, integrating decision making and structures that support it becomes a critical task for the organization (see Figure 2-1).

BUILDING ON FOUNDATIONS

In an integrated organization, it is essential to create structures that support-especially at the point of service—and sustain the work processes of the organization. As the organization builds partnerships between its providers, creates a

Figure 2-1   Point-of-Service Design

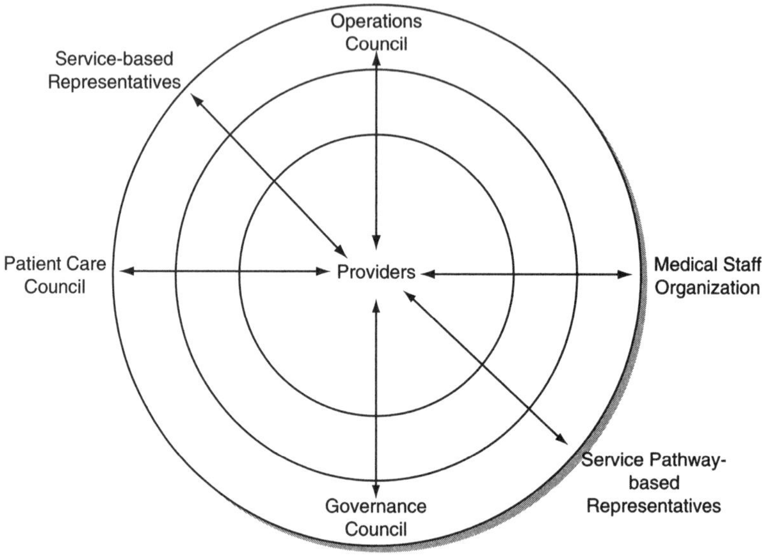

continuum of care, and integrates healthcare services along a horizontal pathway, the structures that support these processes represent a different set of beliefs than those historically present in health care.

> **Integration is evidence of the attempt to configure services around the point of care and to bring providers together in a service partnership.**

Interdisciplinary shared governance (i.e., shared governance that addresses every component of the healthcare organization) requires that some measure of integration, reconfiguring, and continuity of care be established in the organizational system. The shared governance structure reflects the processes and relationships that exist in the system, and, as Chapter 3 makes clear, the activities of transforming the organization for the knowledge worker can create conditions that will undergird the formation of a shared governance structure.

These new healthcare service constructs create a demand for a context that will support them. Shared governance structuring reflects what Collins has defined as the minimum amount of structure needed to maintain the integrity and form of the organization. Collins suggests that any more structure than the minimum often ends up serving itself in place of providing support and service to the organization's work. It is the need to find the line between sufficient structure for organizational integrity and too much structure that should motivate the leadership to look for a structural model that supports the delivery of patient services—and to be cautious in choosing one.

> **Shared governance requires a commitment to partnership to work effectively.**

> **Managing knowledge workers requires helping them to invest in decision making and express a sense of ownership over the decisions they must make.**

WHY SHARED GOVERNANCE?

There are three specific reasons why shared governance is an appropriate model for structuring professional staff in a healthcare organization. First, the sustainability of health care greatly depends on how point-of-service (point-of-care) healthcare providers will function. In a user-driven, continuum-based healthcare organization, an entirely different organizational structure is necessary. The old model of a compartmentalized, centralized, vertically integrated, unilateral institution is simply no longer workable in its current form. The organizational framework required to support health care in the new environment needs a different set of constructs. It is this set of constructs that shared governance specifically addresses (see Exhibit 2-1).

In addition, new knowledge regarding complex adaptive systems and the infrastructures necessary to support them call for a level of equity and engagement from all stakeholders in organizations in the life and change of the system. Within the context of complexity, ownership of every element of the organization's ability to adapt and thrive calls for full participation from each member and component of the system. Traditional organizational models are no longer adequate frames for supporting the kind of relational infrastructure necessary to advance full engagement. Additionally, notions of full membership from each participant in a system now require a structure that recognizes ownership processes that can tolerate multiple loci of control and points of innovation. Further, linkage of all contributors must ignore arbitrary hierarchy and position-based decisions in favor of points of contribution and sources and owners of the creative dynamic in the system.

Second, the emergence of the knowledge organization, as Peter Drucker called it, has occurred. Over the years, higher levels of knowledge have been required to provide healthcare services. As a result, dissonance between the

---

Exhibit 2-1   Complex Adaptive Systems Principles

1. The whole always defines the parts.
2. Each of the components of a system supports the whole system.
3. A problem in any one part of the system affects the whole system.
4. A system always "lives" where it provides its services or produces its products.
5. All roles either serve the customer or serve someone who does.
6. The design of a system must configure structure around its point of service or product, which always lies at its center.
7. Form must always follow function.
8. All members of a system are stakeholders. The structure of the system must facilitate the effectiveness of every stakeholder.
9. In a system, managers are facilitators, integrators, and coordinators of the processes that support the work and workers of the system.
10. Outcomes always define the value of process. Function is subordinate to its purpose.

---

needs of knowledge workers and the design of organizations has accelerated. Hospitals and other healthcare organizations have sought to revise their narrowly controlled structures to accommodate the growing need for independence of judgment on the part of the knowledge workers, the changing needs of the professions, and the increasing complexity of healthcare delivery; but although each sector has agreed to some compromises, the fundamental issues that created the conflict have been left essentially unresolved.

Knowledge workers require an entirely different framework for work and professional relationships. Because of the increased dependence of health care on the aggregated comprehensive knowledge of all the various constituencies, professions, and providers, a different kind of organizational relationship must emerge to support them. With the building of the continuum of care, the community and the patients become central components of the delivery system, and a whole new frame of reference that gives form to it, sustains and nurtures it, and allows everyone in the partnership to act in concert with each other will be essential. It is partly to meet these unique needs and to facilitate the application of the knowledge workers' skills that shared governance is arguably necessary at this point in time.

> **In a continuum of services, no one person can control all the relationships and decisions necessary to make the continuum effective.**

In addition, evidence-based health care now requires a more intensive set of collateral relationships as a part of the process of validating the value of care and service. Evidence of value, outcome, and clinical impact now requires the aggregation and integration of the data generated from each and all the related disciplines in a manner that clearly demonstrates impact on patient outcomes. This effort cannot be successful if done within the context of unilateral professional silos and with the individuated, nonaligned efforts of each of the professions. Digital data generation is required to make evidence-driven processes successful and to accurately indicate the points of intersection or interface between and among the activities of the professions most affecting patient process and outcome. An infrastructure that makes this the way of doing business is critical to the success of creating truly evidence-based clinical processes.

Third, it is vital to realize that in a continuum of care system, no healthcare organization can own, control, or unilaterally mandate all of the service linkages and connections necessary to serve a specific population. Fluidity and flexibility will be key to organizational survival in the emerging healthcare environment. Increasingly, consumer demands and payer requirements are setting the parameters for health services that will be offered. As populations shift, as services are adjusted to meet the needs of our aging populace, and as community priorities are modified, the organizational structure must make it possible to adjust to the changes quickly and efficiently.

> **Providers are partners in decision making. Ninety percent of all decisions made in a system should be made at the point of service.**

To provide a comprehensive range of necessary services, "virtual" relationships (highly fluid and flexible) must be established between players. Bringing in new services and eliminating services requires service leaders to be involved in decision making and direction setting throughout the continuum of care. Therefore, structural boundaries must be permeable to accommodate the need for flexibility of membership in those groups that make decisions, set strategy, implement processes, delineate outcomes, and evaluate results.

The three reasons presented previously constitute a good argument for implementing a shared governance structure. Regardless of whether the term *shared governance* is used to designate the type of structure, most of the principles and processes outlined in this text must be implemented to achieve organizational and service sustainability within the context of a shared governance structure. Although the term implies that all key stakeholders are involved in professional governance, it does not refer to a uniform set of rules that must be rigidly applied. Rather, the application of the principles of partnership, equity, accountability, and ownership and the related concepts is what characterizes the type of structure appropriate for service-based, community-driven health care.

BUILDING TO SUPPORT THE POINT OF CARE

The purpose of much of the current integration and clinical reformatting of healthcare organizations is to better organize services and care around the point of service. Where patient and provider meet is the place where a healthcare organization lives its life and the fundamental construct around which all structure should be built. However, organizational structures typically must be substantially revised to support point-of-care decision making and activity throughout an integrated and broad continuum of service. Among the principles to be kept in mind in the process of revision are the following:

- The primary point of decision making in the clinical delivery system is the place where patients and providers meet.
- In an integrated approach, providers are allied with each other in a noncompartmentalized way—that is, in a broad set of linked clinical relationships.
- In service-based approaches, providers and patients need much more freedom to make clinical decisions (and patients need more involvement in such decisions) than actually occurred in the past.
- A much broader range of information must be provided to the point of care to support decision making, clinical activities, and evaluation of outcomes.
- The purpose of organizational structure in health care is to help ensure that there are no impediments preventing people from making the right decisions at the point of care.
- Linkage of point-of-care activities with the system must occur in a way that engages all stakeholders and motivates them to undertake processes that will result in meaningful outcomes.
- The effective clinical organization is constructed from the point of care outward so that all structures, activities, and support systems serve the primary purpose of the organization as exemplified by what goes on at the point of care.

In the past, much lip service was given to the importance of building a structure that supported caregiving and ostensibly placed the patient at the center of the organization. However, there has been no evidence that organizational structures operated in such a way that the patient was ever at the center of anything. The traditional organization was designed to support the provider, not the patient. As a result, the patient tended to get lost. To obtain the efficiencies that come from integration, the organizational structure must reflect support for these new structures, which are patient rather than provider driven.

Some might question the importance of structure in a frame that supports a primarily relationship and behavioral process. Because it is important to create a pattern of sustainable behaviors that reflect a set of principles decided as valuable by the disciplines either individually or collectively, structure plays an important role. The primary purpose of structure in relationship to human behavior is to give a context, a frame, a vessel, if you will, within which expectations and defined patterns of behavior can be supported and sustained. Indeed, the ability to create sustainable patterns of behavior depends on the veracity and consistency of the structure in place that eliminates negative or noncontributing behaviors. Often, behaviors reflect expectations and the structures that support them. A well-defined and disciplined infrastructure provides the parameters for acceptable behavior. A loose relationship between structure and behavior allows a wide range of permissible behaviors, even from those who do not contribute to the purposes and objectives of the work. The role of structure, therefore, is to provide firm parameters around specified behavior, eliminating the option for behaving in ways not supported or sustained by the prevailing structure. This partnership between structure and behavior is an essential corollary necessary to ensure sustainability of behavioral and clinical processes.

> **Shared governance is not democracy. It is an accountability-based approach to structure in which there is a clear expectation that all members of a system participate in its work.**

THE PREMISES OF SHARED GOVERNANCE

Shared governance reflects a set of beliefs (its premises, so to speak) that have arisen from research done in the past 30 years on organizational effectiveness and human dynamics in the workplace. Applying this research to healthcare organizations attempting to create a service continuum is the current challenge of healthcare leaders. The overall goal is to respond to the changing healthcare environment by using their new understanding of effectiveness, work relationships, decision making, and human dynamics to create an organizational structure that does not replicate the limitations of past structures.

The premises of shared governance include the following:

- All structure must directly support the work of the organization. Any part of organizational structure that does not specifically support the organization's work impedes it.

- What goes on at the point of service or productivity in an organization defines the organization's life and reflects its purpose.
- The power of any profession is embedded in its practice and practitioners and organizations must be configured to support practice-driven decision-making.
- Clinical outcomes are the product of the convergence of effort requiring the confluence of disciplinary work and the synthesis of collective contribution.
- In a knowledge-based system (such as the professions in a healthcare organization), all workers contributing to the outcomes of the system have a right and an obligation to own the decisions that relate to their work. Nothing in the system should arbitrarily or capriciously moderate or remove or impede the rights and obligations of any professionals who work in the system.
- In horizontally linked organizational structures (as opposed to vertically linked structures), an emphasis is placed on relationship and integration. Consequently, a horizontally linked organization must create a structure that facilitates the establishment and flourishing of relationships among its members.
- There are three major components of an organization necessary to ensure its integrity: governance, operations, and production or service. In a systems design, each of these must be linked to the other in a seamless connection of interfaces that support the needs and accountability of the others.
- A health system's main obligation is to meet the health needs of the community it serves. It exists at its points of service, where the community need is met one person at a time. The provider-patient relationship has the same constituents as the community-system relationship. Therefore, the mandates, principles, and processes that govern the latter relationship are the same as those governing the former.
- An effective service system is an open system (complex adaptive system). This means that there is a seamless connection between the decisions and the decision makers at one point in the system (e.g., governance) and those at other points in the system (e.g., patient care). In an effective system, there are no artificial or structural barriers between the interdependent components of the system. Compartmentalization is the opposite of integration.
- Managers in a system are both stewards and servants. Their primary role is to see that the system both serves and supports what goes on at its points of service.

- Accountability (internally generated locus of control), not responsibility (delegated or externally generated locus of control), is the foundation for all performance expectations. Every member of a system (systems have members, not subordinates, superiors, employers, employees, masters, or servants) has a right and an obligation to participate fully in the activities of the system. To the extent of their ability to contribute, each member has the obligation to ensure that the system thrives.
- An effective system should provide a sustainable format for the engagement of every member of the system at every level of the organization. A system creates a framework for ensuring that the processes of empowerment operate effectively throughout the system—at every point where work, relationships, and decisions intersect.

These premises reflect the latest understanding of organizational and performance sustainability. They also reflect current systems and human relations research and are essential for any implementation of shared governance—or even for comprehending the shared governance model.

Shared governance is based on a belief about people and the nature of work in an organization: All are partners in the enterprise.

TEAMS: THE FOUNDATION OF ALL WORK

In the past decade, the understanding that relatedness is as critical as competence to achieving effective outcomes in work has revolutionized the design, structuring, and application of work across a wide variety of industries. It has also served as the foundation of the work team movement throughout the world. Team-based activities reflect a move away from the traditional system of compartmentalizing work into individuated tasks, functions, and activities in isolated and unilateral work constructs. In this approach, preserving the integrity of one's own work became the priority rather than focusing on the needs of those the organization served. As a result, there were severe incongruities between the efforts and activities of individuals, disciplines, departments, and structures in the organization and the organization's purposes and fundamental mission. Rather than a situation in which everyone worked together to meet the needs of patients and ensure the continuity of services, competition and compartmentalized, discipline-specific care brought accelerating levels of cost, created gaps in services, and fractured relationships between disciplines and between patients and providers.

Use of teams is neither new nor revolutionary. However, a full understanding of how teams work, how to apply them to the work system, and how to ensure their viability has only recently been achieved. The notion that each outcome results from the joint activity of many players rather than the efforts of—no matter how dedicated—a single player has created a critical shift in the focus of organizational design and work structuring.

> **Teams, not individuals, are the basic unit of work in a whole-systems organization.**

In a team-based approach, team members must first develop relationships with each other, and then make the decisions and undertake the activities essential to the outcomes of the team's work. Shared governance reflects the essential character of team-based approaches. It takes into account the centrality of work teams and uses team concepts and formats. Further, there is an assumption that as team-based approaches become the preeminent frame of reference for work in healthcare organizations, the shared governance structure will predominate. It will serve as a means for integrating teams within an organizational construct and linking them along the continuum of essential relationships and services in an increasingly horizontally linked system.

Any team-based approach requires a change in structure that allows teams at all levels of the organization to be given responsibility for making relevant and related broad-based systems decisions and for linking processes and providers across a wide range of services. It requires, in other words, teams to be self-organizing and self-directed and to act as the basic units of service (or work).

Building a structure, such as shared governance, that links teams and facilitates their function requires specific conclusions about the functions and activities of teams. In a team-based approach, many of the activities that were once controlled by the system in its parental role now become the responsibility of the team. The manager's role is no longer to control activities (acting as boss, superior, supervisor, administrator, or parent) but to facilitate the activities now placed in the team's hands. Some responsibilities that might devolve to the team include the following:

- Hiring, evaluating, and terminating team members
- Scheduling and assigning team members
- Determining the critical activities and flow of work of team members
- Evaluating the competence of and fit between team members

- Assigning elements of function and activity along a critical path to individual team members
- Resolving conflicts between team members and dealing with other difficulties
- Planning, organizing, and designing activities in the context of the team's accountability
- Defining standards and measures of team performance
- Aligning team behaviors and activities with performance expectations and outcome determinations
- Establishing a framework for leadership, assignment rotation, member responsibilities, and quality enhancement

Although this list is not all inclusive, it includes some of the major team responsibilities that once belonged exclusively to managers. Increasingly, organizations are recognizing that moving the majority of decisions (up to 90 percent) to the point of service and structuring work around those decisions is critical to achieving sustainable outcomes. The goal is to allow the locus of control to reside in the places where the decisions are carried out.

> **Clinical teams are the foundation for work in an integrated system and best reflect the provider relationships necessary in a continuum of care.**

The Different Kinds of Teams in a Shared Governance Context

Two kinds of teams play a role in a shared governance framework. The first kind of team focuses on specific functions and activities that constitute the work of the organization at the point of service. Its whole purpose is to work collaboratively, facilitating each patient's journey through the healthcare system.

The second kind of team focuses on system and relationship issues. It looks at the structure and framework that provides the support and context for its own activities. This team's focus is the team itself, the relationships within the team, the interactions and intersections between itself and other teams, and its relationship to the services it provides and to the system it represents and of which it is a part.

Each kind of team has a specific role in ensuring the efficacy and success of the organization. The service team (the first kind mentioned) is designed to facilitate, improve, and advance the services provided by its members. Its services constitute its fundamental focus and purpose. The second kind of team tries to ensure that the relationships between itself and the organization, between itself and other teams, and between the system and all of the teams function effectively to support the work of each team at the point of care. It is the interface and the "connectiveness" between these kinds of teams that form the core of a shared governance structure.

> **Everyone in a complex adaptive system is a stakeholder and has a right to participate fully in the life of the organization.**

Clearly, if stakeholders are located everywhere in the system, there must be a mechanism for them to intersect continuously and to ensure that their decisions are mutually supportive and facilitate the achievement of desired outcomes. In fact, it is the purpose of shared governance to create a framework for supporting effective relationships between stakeholders throughout the organization.

> **Service is the lifeblood of all healthcare systems. It is to provide service that all roles must be firmly committed.**

The Service Team

All activities in a healthcare organization center around the delivery of services to the patient population (or user group), and thus care teams are the primary units of service. These provider-based teams are the foundation for the delivery of all health care.

Because care teams are being used more in the provision of healthcare services, much is changed regarding the relationship between members and the services they provide. In a team-based format, no role is looked upon as more important than any other role. For example, although it is clear that the physician's role is to link the medical components of patient care delivery to the other essential healthcare services provided by other members of the team, in a team-based approach that role is looked at as no more important to the integrity and value of the team than any other team member's role. A team's effectiveness is directly determined by the ability of its members to work together to achieve common clinical and service-related goals. Also, it is important to note, that the role of coordinator, integrator, and facilitator of a healthcare team is fluid depending on the patient's point in the continuum of care and clinical priorities driving the professional-patient relationship. The complexities of contemporary health service now require a more integrated notion of team function with team facilitation reflecting the needs of the patient, the clinical priorities at hand, and the major source of contribution at any particular point in the patient's health-care experience.

> **All teams are configured around specific kinds of services. The population defines the work of the team.**

The organization must therefore provide a system of support that ensures the integrity and viability of its care teams. The organizational framework at the service level must be designed to ensure that the care teams are available to define, perform, and evaluate their work in an effective and meaningful way. Also, the organization must provide a mechanism for the teams to correct anything that impedes their relationships or functioning. Quite simply, they need to be able to work successfully, and the resources, structure, and operational components of the organization must support their integrity and activity.

> **A service pathway follows the trajectory of the patient through the system, not the route of the provider.**

The Population-Based Continuum

Each team functions in relationship to other teams' functioning. In the redesign of patient care along a continuum of care, an organization's structure becomes centered around either patient populations, specific subscriber groups, or clinical pathways. Further, wherever the structure is centered, an interface between teams that falls within a particular category of service is needed. Some mechanism must exist in the organization to ensure that linkage occurs and to guarantee that each team is fulfilling its obligation in a way that helps achieve the outcomes all teams are committed to achieving.

In shared governance, a collection of service or care teams centered on a specific population or service continuum is called a *service* or *patient care pathway*. These pathways can be defined in a number of ways: as departments, units, centers, processes, product lines, service lines, programs, and so on. Regardless of what they are called, they share common characteristics and require an integrated structure to support them.

> **A council is a decision-making body, not a process group. It has the power to do its work without seeking approval of other sources of power.**

In a shared governance model, the teams in a given pathway must link or interface with each other to ensure that the standards of practice, best practices (evidence-based), protocols, clinical processes, generic service requirements, system mandates, mission, purposes, and goals to which they are committed are clearly articulated and to also ensure that each team is operating in harmony with the activities of the other teams (see Figure 2-2). System linkage occurs when an individual unit of service begins to link with other units of service. The ultimate goal is linkage of all of the components of the system, and that means confronting those places in the system where lack of linkage is most evident (see Exhibit 2-2).

Everything else in the system is directed toward facilitating or supporting the work of the primary units of service, and it is at the level of the service pathway that the teams that make it up begin to converge to integrate their efforts to provide a continuum of services. The integrated service pathway is the critical point where the issues that affect both the interface of the teams and the teams' collective linkage to the system are addressed. In the shared governance model, this point of convergence creates a need for pathway-based decision making, and it is the first place where the council structure emerges. Also, as discussed in

---

Figure 2-2   Building toward the New Healthcare Paradigm

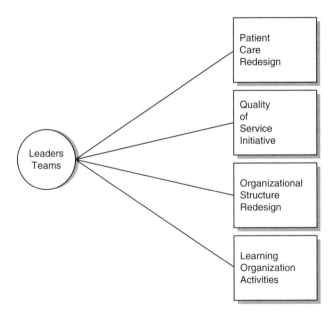

Exhibit 2-2   Outmoded Organizational Characteristics

- Separate, nonlinked institutions with their own operational processes working independently of other parts of the system
- An institutional hierarchy that maintains vertical control over the system
- A large number of senior executives and middle- and first-level management positions
- A fragmented service model where none of the providers are aware of the contribution of the others
- A centralized control structure that approves the majority of decisions made and controls most of the functions and activities of the system
- An unclear connection between health leadership and the medical staff so that decisions made by physicians and others are not linked to mutually defined outcomes
- A governance structure that does not tie the board directly to the point of service and connect providers and board leadership together in a mutually supportive decision-making process

Chapter 1, all shared governance organizations apply the principles of partnership, equity, accountability, and ownership in everything they do (see Exhibit 2-3).

Accountability is the principle that drives all shared governance structures.

All councils have the authority they need to make their own decisions. There are no external approval structures in shared governance.

COUNCILS: THE BASIC UNIT OF ORGANIZED DECISION MAKING

In a shared governance model, a council is a place where authority exists for making decisions that will affect the system in a direct way. All councils have the right to make such decisions, have accountability for the decisions that they make, and have an obligation to see that the decisions are fully implemented. There are essentially two types of councils: point-of-service (clinical pathway) councils and systems councils. The only thing that differentiates the two is the focus of their work. All councils are made up of stakeholders brought together to deal with specific kinds of issues in a way that facilitates the achievement of mutually desirable outcomes.

Exhibit 2-3   Principles of Shared Governance

Partnership

- Role expectations are negotiated.
- Equality exists between the players.
- Relationships are founded upon shared risk.
- Expectations and contributions are clear.
- Solid measure of contribution to outcomes is established.
- Horizontal linkages are well defined.

Equity

- Each player's contribution is understood.
- Payment reflects value of contribution to outcomes.
- Role is based on relationship, not status.
- Team defines service roles, relationships, and outcomes.
- Methodology is defined for team conflict and service issues.
- Evaluation assesses team's outcomes and contributions.

Accountability

- Accountability is internally defined by person in role.
- Accountability defines roles, not jobs.
- Accountability is based on outcomes, not process.
- Accountability is defined in advance of performance.
- Accountability leads to desired and defined results.
- Performance is validated by the results achieved.
- Processes are generally loud and noisy.

Ownership

- All workers are invested in the enterprise.
- Every role has a stake in the outcome.
- Rewards are directly related to outcomes.
- All members are associated with a team.
- Processes support relationships.
- Opportunity is based on competence.

Decision-making groups should be kept as small as the effectiveness of the decisions allows. The smaller, the better.

Effective decisions are ensured by the use of the right information by the right people in the right place at the right time. Access to information is essential for effective decision making.

The clinical pathway or unit council is the primary point of decision making in the shared governance model. One of the basic tenets of sound shared decision making is that 90 percent of decisions made in the organization should be made within the context of service pathways or at the unit or departmental level. This ensures the appropriate point-of-service focus of the providers and the delineation of decisions around the particular patient or service population. It is in this council that team activities converge for the making of decisions that affect all teams within the patient pathway. It is also in this council that the managers of a particular service pathway (or in the case of self-directed work teams, the leadership of the work teams) meet to make essential decisions concerning the pathway's functioning, the relationship between the teams, the clinical standards and activities that are fundamental to the work of the pathway, and other issues associated with the interface between the health system and the service pathway.

In shared governance, the councils are the convergent points of decision making for all teams at the system level and the point of service.

System councils address the relationship of the system and its internal and external communities.

SHARED GOVERNANCE AND DECISION MAKING

Shared governance is an accountability-based model. In shared governance, accountability must always be located at the place where decisions are most appropriately made. The distinctions between decisions in an organization in a shared governance model are based on the appropriate locus of control for specific areas of accountability. For example, all accountability related to patient care derives from the point of service, and therefore the majority of related decisions must be made at the point of service. Patient care decisions should not be located at any other place in the system. Placing them elsewhere contributes strongly to impeding both the ownership and the exercise of authority at the most appropriate locus of control—the patient care environment.

> **Accountability demands clarity in roles, functions, and outcomes. Accountability abhors ambiguity.**

> **Accountability implies that different decisions are made in different places and that they are carried out independently of control located anywhere other than where the accountability is expressed.**

DECISIONS AND THE LOCUS OF CONTROL

A service pathway council should not assume authority for decisions that rest specifically with the teams. The teams, on the other hand, should not assume authority for decisions best made by the service pathway or unit council. Indeed, decisions made by the service pathway council serve as checks and balances for decisions made by the individual teams (see Exhibit 2-4).

In shared governance structures, it is vital that clarity be achieved in advance regarding the kind and content of decisions and the exercise of decision-making authority. Each decision-making body must be fundamentally clear about its locus of control, authority, and responsibility for specific decisions. The parameters of decisions are defined by the content of the decisions themselves. For example, each team makes decisions specific to its clinical responsibilities, the clinical contribution of each of its members, and the relationships and intersections necessary to support and provide the team's services. Anything related to those critical functions and activities essentially belongs to the team.

> **The language of shared governance is systems language. Understanding how complex adaptive systems work is essential to making shared governance work.**

Decisions that belong to the service pathway or unit council concern the fit between the pathway and the system, in particular, the relationships between teams along the continuum of service, the problems that arise between teams, the design of an effective and efficient continuum of service, the professional standards of service that guide the teams, and the critical interface of the ser-

Exhibit 2-4   Locus of Control Decision Making

Point-of-Service Provider Teams

- Work-based clinical actions
- Functions between the team members
- Patient service problems
- Provider relationship issues
- Clinical priorities
- Application of clinical protocols
- Service/care evaluation

Service Pathways (and units or departments)

- Design of clinical protocols
- Development of clinical standards
- Definition of the content of provider relationships
- Quality improvement plan implementation
- Structural problems in the service relationship
- Conflicts and problems related to service design
- Structure, content, and processes tying together resources and service within the pathway
- Problems between providers within the pathway

Patient Care Council

- Design of delivery system
- Integration of disciplines in the system
- Service goals for the system
- Creation of continuous quality imperative
- Creation of continuous learning mechanism
- Forum for the foundations of the continuum of care
- Definition of service priorities and activities of the system

vice pathway with the mission, purposes, and objectives of the organizational system. Decisions of this kind simply cannot be made at the team level.

COUNCILS AND REPRESENTATION

The service pathway or unit council is usually a representative body. That means that, through some mechanism defined by the organization, team members are represented on the service pathway council in a way that ensures that a broad cross-section of disciplines has a say in the decision-making process. However, the council should be as small as diversity permits and the work of the council demands.

There is an inverse relationship between the size of a decision-making group and the effectiveness of its decisions. Therefore, the goal of any system is to make sure that its deliberative bodies are small enough to facilitate effective decision making and large enough to be appropriately inclusive. Although there is no hard and fast rule regarding council size, usual effective councils have membership representation between 7 and 14 persons.

SERVICE PATHWAY LEADERSHIP

In shared governance, there is a distinction between the role of the service pathway (unit or department) leader (manager) and the role of the service pathway council. The service pathway leader has a designated set of obligations derived from the system and its expectations regarding the organization, integration, facilitation, and coordination of services and generated by the service pathway members as well. The pathway members expect the leader to make available the same information and support to all of them. They also expect the structural underpinnings necessary for the provision of health services to be appropriate to their needs. The tension between resources and need essentially defines the role of the service pathway leader. Managing the support system and the resource linkages for the service providers is a critical undertaking and demands the highest level of leadership and management skills. (In fact, it has been said that in decentralized, team-based systems, point-of-service leaders require the same degree of skill and competence that once existed at the highest organizational levels in the past.)

A service pathway leader becomes the focal point for integrating and linking the activities of the pathway together in a way that ensures continuing operation of the pathway and the interface of the operational processes of the pathway and the needs of the individual teams. The service pathway leader integrates, coordinates, and facilitates the activities of the pathway. He or she makes sure that linkage and cohesion are continually resonating in the work of the organization and the pathway. Issues of concern, problems, and inefficiencies are addressed and dealt with. (Service pathway leadership roles are discussed in greater detail in Chapter 4.)

THE SYSTEM COUNCILS

The interface between a system and its patients occurs at the pathway council level. The interface between the service pathway and the system occurs at the system council level. The system councils are those decision-making bodies that render decisions that affect the system as a whole. Those decisions affect individual providers, teams, service pathways—indeed all components of the service structure.

There are primarily three foundational system councils in the shared governance model: the patient care council, the operations council, and the governance council. Each of the system councils has defined obligations for making decisions that affect the component of the system toward which the council's work is directed. In shared governance systems, other councils may be related to the broader work of the professions and of the organization. However, whichever other councils exist, they are extensions of and, therefore, build on the foundational council structures.

Although each of the components of the organizational system has accountability for specific decisions, there must be a seamless linkage between those decisions and the other components of the system. Also, each system council must also link back to the point of service through its service pathways. The linkages ensure that the decisions of each council will have a direct and clear impact on the context for decision making and foster seamlessness in decision making across the various components of the healthcare system.

DISTINGUISHING SYSTEM ACCOUNTABILITY AND SERVICE ACCOUNTABILITY

Accountability in a shared governance framework is built on the understanding that there is shared function and obligation on the part of all stakeholders in the system and that clear contributions to the system are part of the expectations of membership in the system. Accountability requires clarity of specific and unique contribution from each member of the system and from each council that reflects the decision-making authority in the system. One of the options not available to members is to behave as though they were not stakeholders. They must exhibit an acceptance of accountability for the outcomes toward which their roles and work are directed.

Accountability abhors ambiguity, and therefore clarity of accountability and contribution must be one of the attributes of every single role that makes up the system. That clarity must also be incorporated into the team framework to ensure that every individual's relationship to the team, function on the team, and obligation for the team's outcomes have been outlined and lucidly articulated.

Further, in a shared governance model, there is no one place in the organization where "ultimate" responsibility is located. Ultimate responsibility is an industrial age, linear notion—the idea that there must be some one person, one location, or one function where all responsibility aggregates. Everyone has heard the phrase, "The buck stops here." Effectiveness in an organization does not depend upon where the "ultimate" buck stops but where the best decision gets carried out most effectively. If it does not work there, it does not make any difference where the "ultimate" point of authority is. Ultimate responsibility is anathema to the notion of accountability and therefore is not a functional or structural component of a shared governance model. What often happens in organizations where there is a need to articulate an "ultimate" point of authority is that the "buck" gets passed "up" the ladder of authority until, ultimately, no one is accountable for anything over which they have any competence or personal obligation. In these kinds of systems, "buck passing" has become a ritual refined to a high art.

Accountability implies that different decisions are located in different places. Clearly, the checks and balances of the system must be strong enough to ensure that goals are achieved in the places where they need to be achieved by those who are required to achieve them. Such checks and balances must be built into the system. Accountability requires that it be clear just where those points of decision making are and just what that accountability is. Accountability only relates to decisions and actions. In fact, there is no accountability without decisions and actions. Appropriate locus of control of accountability is based on the foundational principle that the right decision will be made in the right place at the right time for the right purpose by the right person.

There are two kinds of accountability in any organizational structure: system accountability and service accountability. System accountability relates to those activities and functions that increase the effectiveness of the system as a whole and ensure systems integrity and effectiveness within every component, function, linkage, and role in the system. The primary sources of system (or manager) accountability are the resource and stewardship requirements of the organization, namely, the human, fiscal, material, support, and system resource requirements that essentially define management. Each of these has imbedded within it functional activities that provide system and leadership support to the service activities undertaken at the point of service. Indeed, they have been characterized by Mintzberg and others as the core activities of the management process.

In shared governance, decisions about human, fiscal, material, support, and system resources fall within the accountability of the system and its managers. These decisions are often referred to in systems language as *contextual decisions*.

They provide the context, the parameters, the framework, the "basket" (if you will) into which all management functions, activities, work, and roles must fit to support the outcomes toward which the organization's resources are directed.

On the other side of the accountability balance bar is service accountability. This includes accountability for the work, functions, and activities that relate to the purposes of the organization. In all healthcare systems, the main purpose is to provide clinical healthcare services. The providers of these services are called upon to undertake the shared activities intended to produce the desired clinical outcomes.

> **Service is the central role of the health system. In it you are either providing a service to a patient or serving someone who is. There is no other orientation for the service organization.**

All the activities related to providing healthcare services and achieving clinical goals are encompassed within service accountability. Service accountability demands the actual performance of the activities needed to meet the quality expectations of the healthcare system. It is a requisite for the critical interface or partnership between the providers and the system and is equally as important as system accountability.

In an effective healthcare system, there must be balance between service accountability and system accountability. Each has a direct and dramatic impact on the other. The balance between the two reflects a dynamic tension that continually ebbs and flows depending on the external and internal circumstances. This ebb and flow of influences creates the dynamic that continually defines the living interface between service capabilities and outcomes and resource availability and use. Indeed, it is this balance that advances both the service and financial viability of the organization and guarantees its ability to sustain and thrive.

In whole systems (complex adaptive) thinking, this dynamic is the fundamental core of the system-service partnership that must be continuously facilitated, defined, and refined. It is also a reflection of the foundation of the shared governance structure. In shared governance, managing the tension between service accountability and system accountability requires a seamless intersection between system and service—a connection of the partners in an inexorable and continuous relationship that is essential to the success of either partner.

> **Pathways are the routes the patient follows in accessing service from the health system. Service structures should be built around such pathways.**

THE PATIENT CARE COUNCIL

Patient care is the central activity of a healthcare system. The delivery of healthcare services provides the foundation upon which the system's purposes unfold. Therefore, at the core of effectiveness in the hospital or health system are the activities that facilitate the provision of patient care services.

In a healthcare system, there is a plethora of patient care services. In integrated organizational structures, especially within a shared governance framework, these services are often identified as units of service or service pathways. Because there is a wide variety of patient populations that may be served by any one particular health system, there may be a wide variety of patient pathways (e.g., women's health, gerontology, mental health, acute care). Each of these pathways must be designed in a way that fits the culture of the services along a service continuum that make up the pathway. This truism is expressed by the saying, "Culture always rules." Each pathway may have constructs, relationships, team members, functional activities, standards, measures, and performance expectations that differentiate it from other service pathways, and this diversity means there is a need to ensure that the culture of service tightly fits the population toward which the pathway is directed.

> **Patient care is the central activity of any health system. If you forget that, you soon forget what business you are in.**

However, in an organizational system there must be a way in which each unique service pathway is integrated and linked within the system as a whole. When a system is made up of culturally specific service pathways, it is difficult to build the system's structure in a way that does not impede the cultural specificity of each service unit or pathway and at the same time supports integration. Somewhere there must be points of convergence for service pathways so that the issues of the system as a whole can be addressed and a unified commitment to the mission and purposes of the system as a whole can be created. It is at this level that the system councils operate.

> **The patient care council is the place where staff confront model of care issues and express their partnership in making decisions that affect the entire system.**

As suggested earlier, the system councils' primary role is to provide forums for making decisions that affect the direction, functioning, and activities of

Figure 2-3   Patient Care Council Structure

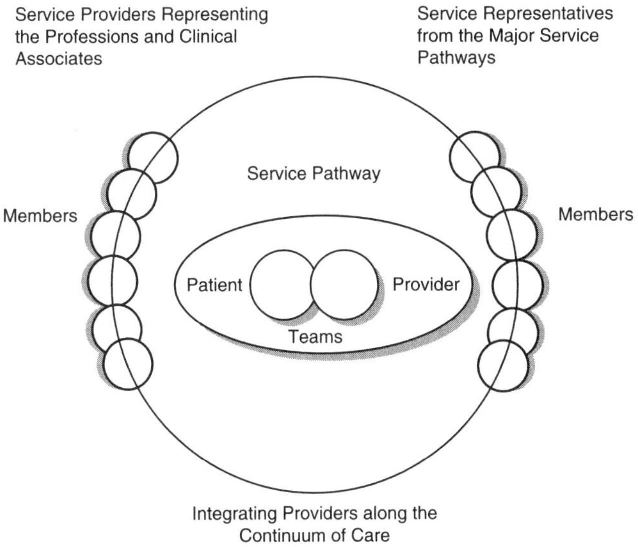

Service Providers Representing the Professions and Clinical Associates

Service Representatives from the Major Service Pathways

Members

Members

Service Pathway

Patient   Provider

Teams

Integrating Providers along the Continuum of Care

the system as a whole. The foundational patient care council serves as the system council responsible for decisions regarding patient care (see Figure 2-3). The patient care council is where the leaders from the service pathways, by bringing to bear their diverse viewpoints on issues of general concern, help to integrate the healthcare system around its main purposes—the provision of clinical services.

> **Representation on a council means taking into account the whole, not just those who sent you to the table, when making decisions. Each member represents a perspective, not a single group.**

The patient care council deals with the issues related to generic standards of practice, the relationships between the disciplines, the integration of patient care services around the community of service, the design of the patient care delivery system, all activities related to quality initiatives, and clinical performance expectations and competencies. In fact, anything related to the integrated patient care delivery process in the system as a whole falls within the ambit of authority of the patient care council.

> The leadership facilitates the council's decision making. Leaders should not make decisions that rightfully belong to someone else. Making other people's decisions for them illegitimately shifts the locus of control.

Representation from the patient care council comes from two major constituencies: the service pathways and the major provider disciplines. The partnership between the pathways and disciplines creates the linkage between the key players at the point of service and causes them to converge around the issues that affect patient care activities at the point of service. As previously indicated, councils are authorized to make specific kinds of decisions. In a shared governance model, decisions about standards of practice, critical paths, clinical service, professional relations, functions, and activities are excluded from range of authority of the patient care council and are specifically included in the decisions and actions of the unit or service pathway council.

The intent of shared governance design is to keep the majority of patient care decisions (90 percent) as close to the point of service as possible and always within the service pathways. Therefore, the patient care council is not responsible for decisions that rightly belong to and should remain within the service pathways. It is the task of the patient care council to make decisions related to the organization's patient care priorities. Adjustments in the design of service pathways as the patient population shifts; the design and construction of the model of patient care delivery; the establishment, operation, and assessment of the quality improvement initiatives throughout the organization; and the delineation and articulation of performance expectations for each of the disciplines involved in the delivery of patient care services and the principles and applications of evidence-based practice all fall within the domain of the patient care council. Other focuses of the council include clinical integration; the interface of clinical services; conflicts between clinical services; issues surrounding the service continuum; and problems associated with the provision of coordinated, comprehensive services. In doing its work, the council receives organizational and staff support from patient care services, the medical staff, quality improvement services, provider education, clinical information systems, and human resources.

> The system's councils make decisions across pathways to address issues that affect the whole. They never make decisions that belong to or within the pathways.

Because the patient care council is made up of clinical rather than management leaders (see Chapter 3), much of the control over patient- and service-related decisions remains with the providers and those who focus on the point of service. Organizational staff support is provided by those organizational functions that can best guide the work of the clinical leadership in the patient care council.

It is the responsibility of the council to deal with issues that affect the relationship between the service pathways and to provide the parameters, contexts, and foundation for the functions and activities within the service pathways. Ultimately, the council must establish some degree of consistency across pathways. It must do this in a way that fosters the investment of all of the stakeholders, keeps the system focused on the point of service, deals specifically with the issues that arise with the provision of services, links key point-of-care decision makers together in dealing with comprehensive issues as well as best practices, and provides a seamless connection between the other components of the healthcare organization.

To ensure a seamless linkage, leaders from the operations council and governance council are included in the membership of the patient care council. Decisions regarding the direction, mission, and purposes of the organization require the involvement and investment of representatives from the operations and governance decision-making forums. Also, the patient care council occasionally makes critical decisions affecting the resources of the organization. It is therefore appropriate that a linkage between leaders accountable for those decisions in patient care be provided within the shared governance structure. It is for that reason that the leaders representing operations and governance are full and active members of the patient care council.

> **Stewardship of resources is a critical part of the work of the leadership. It is one of the fundamental areas of accountability of the system's management.**

THE OPERATIONS COUNCIL

In an effective integrated system, there must always be an ongoing mechanism for the stewardship of resources and for setting direction. The operations council is the place where management decisions centered around resources and other operational issues are made and implemented. It is in this council that the management leaders of the service pathways; the system and organizational leaders; and the organizational consultants/senior leaders (in the old system, vice presidents of administrative departments or divisions) from finance, human resources, development and planning, administration, systems integration, and information services (and possibly other departments, depending on the design of the system) meet to make fundamental decisions about resource distribution, the integration of the system, and the direction of the system and engage in fiscal and capital resource planning (see Figure 2-4). The council also tries to resolve problems that arise regarding the structure and function of the system and the functional relationships between the service pathways and deals with all issues related to the contextual resource accountability of management.

The purpose of the operations function in a system is to provide a stable and safe context within which to make service decisions that are consistent with available resources and the needs of the customers who use them.

Like the patient care council, the operations council has specific goals and objectives given to it by the governance council. Also, each service pathway brings to the operations council specific resource objectives. Service pathway budget accountability, information management, and human resource requisites are examples of the issues that the service pathways present to the operations council. Although it is critical that each service pathway maintain its unique culture, the operations council's obligation must see to it that each culture does not interfere with the resource priorities and obligations of the system as a whole. Dealing with the issues and conflicts related to organizational stewardship constitutes much of the work of the operations council.

The operations council is the place where leadership translates strategies into tactics for the organization as a whole and for each service pathway in the system.

Most of the activity of the operations council concerns fiscal and capital planning and performance accountability. The operations council is where the system's financial and capital plans are constructed. It is where the system converges to resolve issues related to the application of the organization's resources to achieve its goals and objectives and to provide its essential services. Further, the council discusses and coordinates changes in the service pathway configurations, structural adjustments, design and control of the management information system, changes in the market or subscriber base, and the system's developmental plan. It also reviews the performance of the service pathways in meeting their main objectives, defines performance requisites for the service pathway leadership, articulates performance accountability, and outlines the evaluation mechanism.

Figure 2-4   Operations Council Structure

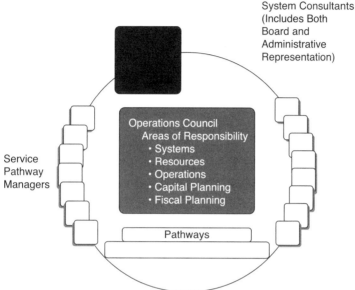

Leaders from the patient care council and the governance council are included as members of the operations council. Organizational integrity requires that the implications of decisions about patient care and the mission, purposes, and strategic direction of the organization be taken into account when decisions about resource use are made. The presence of leaders from patient care and governance on the operations council exposes them to the issues that others must confront and highlights the interdependence of all components of the system. The interface of leaders from the different components around contextual and resource issues is critical to the effectiveness and sustainability of the decisions that are made.

THE GOVERNANCE COUNCIL

In complex adaptive systems, integration is as important as function, and the ability to link the mission and activities of an entire system is critical to its effectiveness and the viability of its work. It is the purpose of the governance council to provide a locus of control whose primary focus is integration of the whole system (see Figure 2-5).

> **The governance council translates the board-defined mission, purposes, and objectives into strategies that give form to the work of the system.**

> **The governance council is the place where all designated leaders meet to link activities and integrate the whole system.**

The governance council tries to ensure that the mission, purposes, and objectives of the system are translated into practical strategies that can be carried out by all of the system's components, stakeholders, and decision makers. It is the place where all the activities of the system converge. The governance council provides a place where the designated and elected leadership of the organization can meet to (1) ensure that the mission and objectives of the system are

---

Figure 2-5   Governance Council Structure

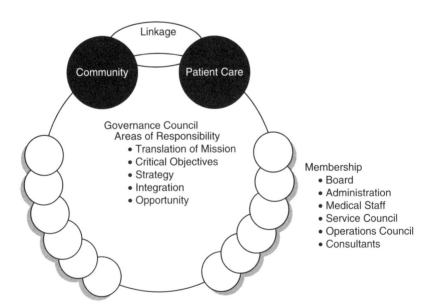

being achieved across all components of the system, (2) make the decisions necessary to connect the system to the community, and (3) ensure the integrity of the linkages between the various components of the system as they undertake their work within a shared governance framework.

> **The view from the governance council is the whole organization. The close fit of each of the components into a web of intersections and networks defines the structure as a seamless system.**

The focus of the governance council centers on the linkages between operations, practice, and governance in the system; the effectiveness of the system as a whole; system quality determinants and the measurement of their effects; and the attainment of the board-directed organizational goals. The council is accountable for the implementation of the directives for the system; the interface between the medical staff, the board, and the other disciplines and components of the system; and the development of a strategic plan for the system. The governance council deals with decisions about changes in the character, direction, and number of service pathway processes within the system and the evaluation of the interface between the strategic plan and the financial performance of the system.

> **No one council supervises the work of another. They fulfill their individual accountability, and that serves as a check on the others. The integrity of the "fit" between one council and another is their faithfulness to their own accountability.**

It is the purpose of the governance council to look at the system as a whole—its integrity, efficacy, and efficiency. Further, the governance council's facilitation of linkages to the board and to the community is critical to the creation of a healthy community and thus to the long-term viability of the system.

The governance council receives support from components involved in the strategic activities of the system, such as marketing and planning, information systems, the administrative offices that handle the relationship between the system and the board of trustees, the medical staff leadership, the finance office, and community services.

The core membership of the governance council includes selected leaders of the patient care council and operations council, the chair of the medical staff, the chair of the board of trustees, the chief executive officer, and whoever else the council deems essential to the integrity of the system and to the performance of its decision-making duties. Consultants to the system occasionally act in a supportive role.

As with the other system councils, the governance council has the right and obligation to access whatever information, resources, individuals, and supports are necessary to do its work. The non-patient-care support services of the organization are the servants of the organization's decision makers and the patient care function. Indeed, those services can be called upon for assistance wherever key decisions are made in the system. If financial information is needed in the patient care council, it should be made available to that council. If such information is needed at the point of service within a specific service pathway, the finance office has an obligation to make that information available to the appropriate players. Support must be provided wherever it is needed.

Information Support

In shared governance, the fluidity and mobility of information are critical to the success of decision making. Increasingly, as the information system becomes more amenable to the users and provides a more comprehensive range of services and data, it allows much more decentralized and localized decision making to occur. Each one of the system councils, as well as the point-of-service decision-making bodies (from team to service pathway council), should have unencumbered access to the information necessary for their activities. A seamless and fully integrated information system (see Chapter 9) is one of the essential constituents of an effective shared governance model, and there is no place where its importance is greater than in the governance council.

The governance council's role is to be able to look at the integrity of the system as a whole. The flexibility of the system depends on the fluidity and mobility of the information it has. To be able to assess the integrity of the system, the council must have ready access to critical information from finance, services, and quality improvement.

The governance council, where key decision makers sit at the same table, is accountable for creating linkages and ensuring collective effectiveness. Exposure of the representatives to each other's frame of reference, functional roles, and leadership obligations provides a common foundation for dialogue and decision making regarding strategy delineation, conflict resolution, direction setting, system integration, community issues, and other concerns. It is in fact the place where all components of the system intersect and where the evidence of whether it is performing well or not is present for all to see.

The clinical as well as the system information infrastructure is critical to the effectiveness of shared governance. A fully integrated digital information infrastructure provides the medium of communication and interaction that assures effective and appropriate decision making at each of the places in the organization where those decisions belong. Councils and other key decision makers must have access to the same system, using the same tools to ensure the efficacy and accuracy of decisions. The means of communication must be limited to the fully integrated information infrastructure, and everyone who participates in the decision process should have access to all of the elements of the same information system at any point in the system and across the system. Any truly effective and sustainable interdisciplinary shared governance approach cannot operate effectively without a truly integrated and linked information infrastructure utilized in common across the clinical system.

> **It is essential to the effectiveness of a complex adaptive system that information be easily accessed by and generously shared with every place in the system that requires it.**

> **Every integrated system requires a different insight, skill set, and behaviors to sustain it. All systems are forever learning and adapting to continuously changing realities.**

NEW CONSTRUCTS . . . NEW MINDSET

It should be clear to the reader at this stage that an interdisciplinary integrated shared governance framework calls for an entirely new mindset. It essentially revolutionizes notions of workplace design, the provision of health services, and the relationship between players. It has broad legal, organizational, governance, and relational implications for the structuring of work and the design of health care (see Figure 2-6).

> **When new structures are created, conflict always arises between old patterns of life and emerging requisites for new behaviors. Leadership means willingly confronting old frameworks and transforming them into new frameworks.**

Many readers might suggest that the current legal and organizational context for health systems does not make the structure of shared governance as outlined in this chapter possible—and they would be right. However, if one looks over the whole scope of changes in health care, much of what is currently unfolding in

Figure 2-6   Patient Care Structure in Shared Governance

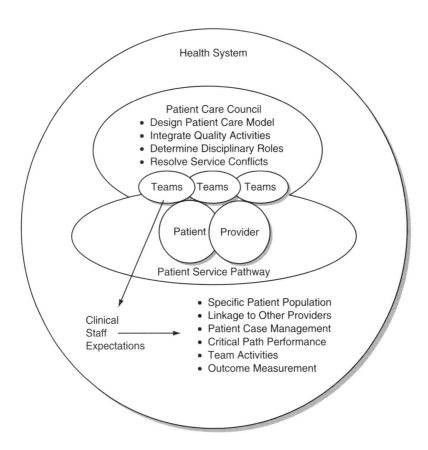

health care would not have been legally or organizationally supported even 10 years ago. All change has an impact on legal, social, and relational constructs. It can be anticipated that building a shared governance system will require changing many of the social, legal, and organizational foundations that define the relationships in health care. Certainly, movement into the digital age has transformed almost every element of healthcare delivery and technology. The organizational, relational, behavioral, and professional models that govern healthcare services in the industrial age are simply either not relevant or not applicable in 21st-century organizations. Leaders in health care, as in all organizations, now must reflect changing conditions and emerging realities as the paradigms for health service payment, provision, and delivery are transformed by the circumstances of the times.

Creating structures that challenge past mandates, prescriptions, and regulations necessitates the inclusion of new constructs and parameters that provide the kind of uniformity and consistency that usually results from a shared decision-making, shared leadership, or shared governance structure. In subsequent chapters, the components of the shared governance system are discussed in greater detail, from the individual and team relationships to the service pathway councils and the governance council.

Although its conceptual foundations are sound and reflect a growing database on work, relationships, and organizations, the constructs, models, and applications of shared governance are a work in progress. The intent of this detailed presentation is to provide a basis for continuing discussion, development, and refinement of the structural elements and intersections that will make point-of-service interdisciplinary designs efficient, effective, and viable.

Creating a whole-systems framework based on point-of-service constructs is "noisy" at best. Any organization that has already undertaken this work knows the challenges, excitement, anxieties, and noise that attend the creation of a new order of things. It is the intent of this book to challenge and to stimulate the thinking and dialogue of leaders engaged in transforming the healthcare system. Out of the process should come a variety of viewpoints, ideas, notions, and suggestions that will improve the foundations and functioning of shared governance systems. The dialogue has just begun.

SUGGESTED READING

Ackoff, R. (1999). *Ackoff's best*. New York: John Wiley.

Bradford, D. L., & Burke, W. W. (2005). *Reinventing organization development: New approaches to change in organizations*. San Francisco, CA: Pfeiffer.

Brown, J., & Duguid, P. (2002). *The social life of information*. Boston: Harvard Business School Press.

Drucker, P. F. (2001). *The essential Drucker: Selections from the management works of Peter F. Drucker* (1st ed.). New York: HarperBusiness.

Du Plessis, J. J., McConvill, J., & Bagaric, M. (2005). *Principles of contemporary corporate governance*. New York: Cambridge University Press.

Everett, L., & Black, K. (2007). Putting the patient first: Guiding principles provide a road map for more collaborative relationships among nurses and support service groups. *Nurse Leader, 5*(3), 19–22.

Gibson, C. B., & Cohen, S. G. (2003). *Virtual teams that work: Creating conditions for virtual team effectiveness* (1st ed.). San Francisco: Jossey-Bass.

Goad, T. W. (2002). *Information literacy and workplace performance*. Westport, CT: Quorum Books.

Howells, J. (2005). *The management of innovation and technology: The shaping of technology and institutions of the market economy*. Thousand Oaks, CA: Sage.

Johnson, C. E., Kralewski, J. E., Lemak, C. H., Cote, M. J., & Deane, J. (2002). The adoption of computer-based information systems by medical groups in a managed care environment. *Journal of Ambulatory Care Management, 25*, 40–51.

Kane-Urrabazo, C. (2006). Management's role in shaping organizational culture. *Journal of Nursing Management, 14*(3), 188–194.

Mintzberg, H. (1990). *Mintzberg on management*. New York: Free Press.

Morgan, H. J., Harkins, P. J., & Goldsmith, M. (2005). *The art and practice of leadership coaching: 50 top executive coaches reveal their secrets*. Hoboken, NJ: John Wiley.

Mycek, S. (2007). Under the spreading Planetree. *Trustee, 60*(3), 22–28.

Porter-O'Grady, T. (2001, January/February). 21st-century strategic thinking: Five insights for boards of trustees. *Health Progress*, 28–46.

Suh, N. P. (2005). *Complexity: Theory and applications*. Oxford, England: Oxford University Press.

CHAPTER 3

Building the Foundations: Transforming the Organization

Tim Porter-O'Grady, Marsha Parker, and Marilyn Hawkins

> *You cannot step twice into the same river;*
> *the waters are forever flowing by.*
>
> —HERACLITUS

Attempting to initiate any major change is fraught with challenges and dangers that invariably serve to complicate the possibility of seeing change to its end and achieving success. When one begins to address the entire infrastructure of an organization and attempts to dramatically alter it, the complexity and challenge multiply. Implementing shared governance and building a structure that supports it means confronting much of historic and contemporary organizational constructs, including the behaviors that relate to it. The attachment of individuals and of the whole organization to its past practices can create a significant barrier to a change of this magnitude, even if it results in a healthier and more viable organization.

THE INTEGRATING PROCESS

The implementation of any strategy should not be undertaken carelessly or unilaterally. A host of shifts and adjustments in the organization must be made in proximity to each other. Changes in the organizational structure should accompany other related changes. After all, organizational structure is meant to support the fundamental functions and activities of the organization (see Figure 3-1). Structure yields no products. Rather, the purpose of structure is to provide form and format for the work of the organization. There should only be enough structure to support the activities and functions of the organization. Any more structure than this eventually tends to serve itself and draws resources and focus away from organizational objectives.

> **Structure serves no other purpose than to give format to purpose and integrity to work.**

Figure 3-1   Point-of-Service Delivery System

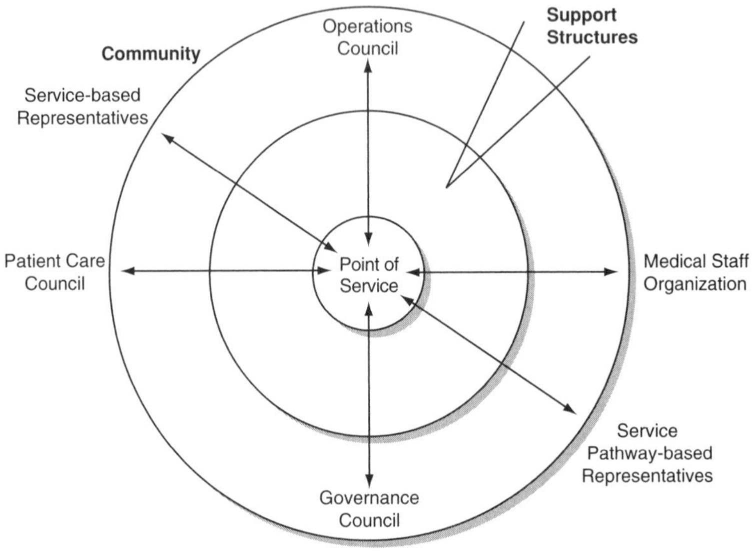

In today's healthcare organization, the main purpose of infrastructure is to support the emerging point-of-service patient care delivery system. Patient care and service are at the core of any healthcare system. Patient-centered services require a substantial reconfiguration of departmental structures. This shift integrates and facilitates the delivery of patient care over a broadening continuum of services across defined populations.

The changes in patient care design and service structure for the digital age underpin the substantial changes necessary in the design of healthcare organizations. Building organizational structures, such as interdisciplinary shared governance, helps sustain these fundamental changes. This is often why both are undertaken in a closely related time frame.

Many of the processes and teams used for service-centered patient care also can be applied to structural redesign. Shared governance is a point-of-service, accountability-based model that supports patient-focused care strategies. There is cross-referencing of work groups, task forces, and functional activities related to integrated patient care and to the building of a new organizational structure to support it. Regardless, in designing a shared governance structure, integration becomes a critical theme in the effort to provide an appropriate structure for patient-centered service arrangements.

Processes have no value in and of themselves. Structure gives them form and outcome gives them value.

THE INADEQUACY OF STRUCTURE

As hospitals and health systems begin to reconfigure themselves to create a seamless continuum of services in a cost-sensitive patient care environment, a number of conflicts with the old organizational design emerge:

- Although vertical integration is essential, the primary task of integration is horizontal or multimodal linkage across the continuum of care services. There is a natural conflict between unilateral vertical thinking and structuring and horizontal and multifocal planning and implementation. This conflict is exacerbated by the many levels of vertical hierarchy that remain in traditional organizations at a time when there is a need to reduce hierarchy and refine decision making at the point of service.
- Players and partners at the point of service must be increasingly accountable for making decisions and for owning the outcomes of those decisions. This requires a high degree of decentralization, local decision making, and fewer levels of hierarchical management.
- A central theme of the age and a function of transformation is the recognition that the information infrastructure is the emerging architecture for health services. Building decision making on an excellent information framework becomes a critical function of design in healthcare organizations.
- Relationships are the glue that holds all organizations together. Building systems to value and support essential role and decision relationships will be critical to the flexibility and fluidity of an organization as it responds to the demands of its points of service.

Shared governance changes the locus of control in the system and always favors locating power at the center of a system.

The purpose of shared governance is to fundamentally affirm local locus of control, the decision-making process, and internal relationships in an organization. Shared governance structures take into account the need to increase the amount of decisions made at the point of service (up to 90 percent) and to ensure that the decisions made there are correct, "implementable," and do not require broad organizational approval or a long decision-making process (which might reduce the efficiency and effectiveness of the clinical delivery system). Furthermore, shared governance provides a format for creating a structure that makes it less possible for decisions to move away from their appropriate locus of control to other places in the organizational system, where they will almost certainly be less effectively made or inappropriately carried out.

As the clinical and systems design of patient care services takes form, intersection with decision making in the operational and organizational components of the system becomes critical. It is at this place where implications for shared governance become more apparent. As appropriate patient care configuration pulls more decision making and accountability to the providers—at the points of service along the continuum of care—a structure must emerge that provides a supporting foundation for the changes in organizational and patient care design. Shared governance planning and decision making, therefore, interface directly with many of the functions and activities associated with user-driven service. Enumerating the impact on structure at the outset of shared governance implementation and incorporating that planning into initial patient care and service design can have an enormous facilitating effect on the fundamental activities associated with service design and patient care infrastructure.

A FOCUSED WORK GROUP

In the design process, focus on structural elements should begin at the outset of the process. If the organizational design and the supporting structures that underpin it are not revised, conflicts between the structure and the function of the organization will emerge very early on.

> **The purpose of the design team is to design and then cease to exist.**

In shared governance, every leadership role, functional activity, and decision-making process is radically altered to fit integration and point-of-service decision making (see Figure 3-2). Shared governance reflects accountability-based rather than responsibility-based processes, and therefore the new design should support the emergence of accountability at every level of the organization.

Good patient care and service design accomplish several objectives. These objectives form the framework for activities of design that affect outcome determination, process activities, service efficiencies, and quality measurement and evidence-driven outcomes. The prevailing organizational structure should support and act in harmony with the processes associated with good patient-based

Figure 3-2   Shared Governance Systems Integration

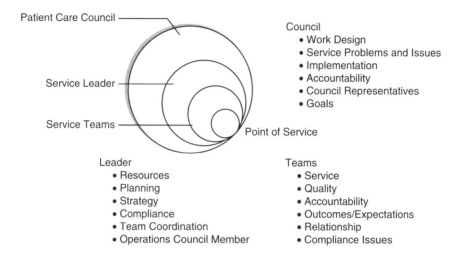

Patient Care Council

Service Leader

Service Teams

Point of Service

Council
- Work Design
- Service Problems and Issues
- Implementation
- Accountability
- Council Representatives
- Goals

Leader
- Resources
- Planning
- Strategy
- Compliance
- Team Coordination
- Operations Council Member

Teams
- Service
- Quality
- Accountability
- Outcomes/Expectations
- Relationship
- Compliance Issues

design. It should not impede the efficiencies being created in the service and patient care delivery activities of the organization. The design activities should achieve several outcomes:

- All professional and associated service providers should develop an orientation toward specific patient care populations.
- The continuum of care and the patient's journey through the healthcare experience should be facilitated by life and health processes, demand management, critical clinical pathways, continuity, evidence-based practice, outcome consistency, and quality measurement.
- The design of service should center on patient processes and bring all necessary healthcare providers into the same clinical and service context so that they will be able to offer integrated care services.
- Resource management and allocation should be focused on processes associated with the point of service. As much as possible, decision making related to resources should be located as close to the point of service as possible.
- All partnerships, clinical processes, and players (physicians, nurses, allied health professionals, etc.) are brought together to form a seamless web of interacting providers and supports configured around the patient's pathway.

This design creates the foundation for substantial patient-centered care and a configuration of the organization to support seamless care processes. A shared governance structure provides an organizational framework within which decisions can be implemented throughout the system in support of the preceding designed activities. To ensure that the organization operates effectively, structures in the system must be in congruence with the expectations for decision making, relationships, and performance at the point of service. This seamlessness in concept and design must play out in the organization's operations as well as in patient care services and provider decision making.

THE SHARED GOVERNANCE STEERING GROUP (DESIGN TEAM)

Creation of a shared governance design team focused on the type of organizational structuring and design needed to support patient care is an essential step toward interdisciplinary shared governance. This design team, the shared governance steering group (SGSG), is the place where the activities of structural design and implementation unfold. Again, it must be emphasized that the shared governance implementation is a corollary of user-driven (patient-centered) design and all service-based activities related to it. It is a part of a comprehensive strategy for organizational effectiveness. Shared governance implementation simply reflects the organizational structure portion of user-driven design (see Figure 3-3).

> **Every key role in the system, staff or management, should be represented in the steering group. The majority of planners, however, should be from the staff, not from management.**

Initiation of the activities of the SGSG should be timed to occur simultaneously with the implementation of key components of the design activities. For example, when the service pathways are created, the structures that support decision making at the level of the service pathways must also be created. Therefore, cross-linkage between the membership of the SGSG and the clinical systems implementation process is essential. Not only are timing issues important for cross-referencing the work of the two processes (work design and shared governance implementation), but elements of fit between the two processes must be considered by both. The SGSG will want to ensure that the stages of structural change match closely the stages of the clinical design process. Each level of redesign, from the patient care pathways to the management structure, the support system, the administrative configuration, and the board-organization

Figure 3-3   The Shared Governance Steering Group

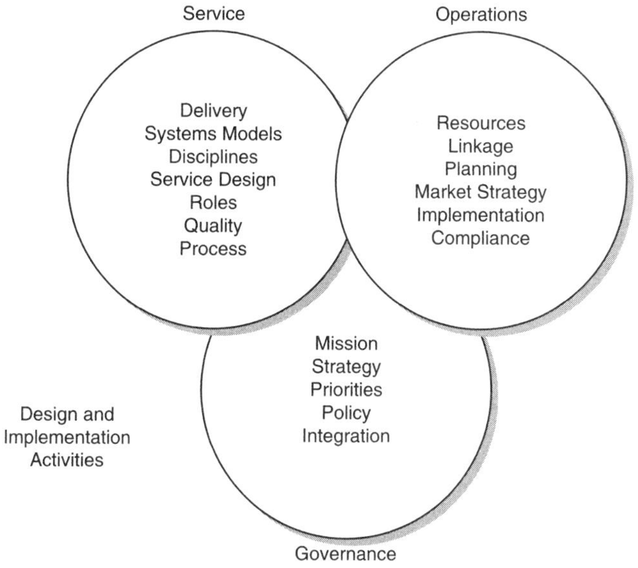

interface, has implications related to successful construction of a good organizational structure.

The tasks of the SGSG should include the following:

- Review of the existing organizational structure and its interface with current patient care system design activities
- Identification of the key elements of structural change supporting process shifts at the point of service
- Enumeration of the structural supports necessary to underpin the patient care design at the point of service in the organization
- Delineation of the essential characteristics and accountability of emerging roles in the new structure and the articulation of those roles in position descriptions or role charters
- Outlining of the team, service pathway, and system council format for decision making throughout the health system from the point of service to the policy and governance levels
- Definition and implementation of the activities and change events necessary for formally reshaping the organizational structure

- Institution of developmental and learning processes appropriate for the leadership changes, role shifts, performance expectations, service adjustments, and leadership outcomes associated with a shared governance design
- Evaluation of the effectiveness of staged implementation of the shared governance design and the effectiveness of decision making at the various loci of control within the organization

Creating a service-based infrastructure in the organization and modifying the structures demand a concerted effort on the part of the leadership. The shared governance structure changes the role of leaders, alters the character and number of leaders, and shifts the locus of control for decision making to the point of service. Revising the leadership roles and functions while simultaneously implementing a shared governance approach is critical to the success of both design and shared governance implementation. It must be remembered that the purpose of the shared governance structure is to support the point-of-service design and to ensure sufficient structure to sustain its activities and create linkages and efficiencies in the system, especially in decision-making arenas.

As with everything in life, timing is everything.

Shared Governance Steering Group Membership

The criteria for selecting the SGSG members should include not only breadth of representation but also linkage of the representatives to other parts of the system. Clearly, included in the SGSG should be individuals involved in the reengineering process-to ensure cross-referencing and appropriate timing of changes.

However membership for the steering group is selected, it should draw in the best and the brightest. They will be needed to do good design.

A decisional group like the SGSG should be as small as possible and as large as the breadth of representation requires. The preferred number of members is between 7 and 14. A group any smaller usually lacks representativeness, and a group any larger might not be able to reach decisions efficiently. Because every major constituency in the organization is going to be affected by the decisions of the SGSG, it is critical that each component have someone serving as a member of the group.

Following is a list of staff members who could be considered for SGSG membership. The importance of empowerment and stakeholder accountability requires that a broad range of organizational leaders be involved in the SGSG's processes. Not surprisingly, the majority of members in the group may represent staff rather than management. Role representation is critical, but distributing representation to favor management leadership is not. Ensuring breadth and diversity of representation is far more important than ensuring that most of the representatives come from management. For one thing, effective decision making depends on the diversity of the members. Therefore, the following should receive due consideration when the SGSG is formed:

- Service pathway/unit staff
- Service pathway/unit management leaders
- Support systems leaders
- Quality control staff
- Departmental management leaders
- Information systems staff
- Medical staff leaders
- Senior administrative staff
- Trustees

The process of selecting team members depends on the dynamics of the organization. Clearly, the SGSG should include the best and the brightest but at the same time include those who play key roles in the organization. Selection of steering group members should be based on the following criteria. Each member should

- Hold a key position in the organization
- Have good group skills
- Demonstrate a commitment to design work, good group process, and the implementation of shared governance
- Demonstrate a commitment to self-development
- Have the ability to engage in dialogue with diverse individuals and to participate fully in the work of the steering group
- Have the administrative or leadership support of those the person will represent
- Have the ability and willingness to remain with the process through its completion
- Have the time and the energy to commit to the level of intensity of activities associated with implementing shared governance

The character of the interface between members is a critical issue. Nothing is more disheartening than to have the wrong mix of players involved in as serious an undertaking as implementing a new structure. The more diverse the behavior, leadership styles, and gifts of the members of the steering group, the more effective the process of deliberating and decision making. Also, a clear commitment on the part of the members to the process they are undertaking is essential for the "sustainability" of that process. High turnover and short tenure of members can be very disruptive. It should be clear to all members what the time frame expectations are, why a strong commitment is necessary, and what the expectations are for each role.

The Initial Developmental Process for the Shared Governance Steering Group

Once the steering group members have been selected, nominated, or elected, their frame of reference, knowledge base, and other foundations for deliberation should be equalized as much as possible. Clearly, there will be different levels of understanding and application of shared governance principles at the outset of the SGSG's work. There must be a mechanism in the organization that makes it possible for the knowledge base and understanding of the members of the steering group to be developed and their learning cycle to be accelerated.

Obviously, the organization wants to ensure that good and sound decisions are made. The activities related to designing shared governance implementation must be correlated with the developmental framework of those who will lead the process. As participants are obtained for the pathway- or unit-based design process (including members of the SGSG), integration of their activities and the activities associated with implementing shared governance will need to be a focus of SGSG deliberations. Education and development sessions and creation of a schedule for establishing a common frame of reference constitute an essential first step. This step can be accomplished in any number of ways, but the following topics need to be covered:

- The mission, purposes, and goals of the design process
- The principles of point-of-service organizational design
- The principles of decentralized management and accountability-based work systems
- The principles of shared governance and the use of the concept of a seamless organization as a foundation for structuring organizations
- The characteristics of effective organizational change processes and their application to interdisciplinary shared governance

In creating a learning organization, there is no better place to start than the steering group. Its development and skill building will be essential to the quality and thoroughness of the restructuring.

The developmental cycle is critical to obtaining the breadth of knowledge the members will need to undertake the activities of design. Although development is by definition a work in progress, the implementation process teaches the members about the application of interdisciplinary shared governance to the organization. Therefore, there should be opportunities to take risks and to experiment with the application of new concepts. The spirit of experimentation can create a frame of reference that allows decisions to be implemented without the kind of confidence that is based on previous experience. Because new structures are being created to respond to a new age and changing demands, it should be expected that some of the processes implemented will reflect different ways of thinking. Staff are applying elements that have never been applied before in a framework for decision making that is relatively untested. Each of these elements should be anticipated and incorporated into the process of implementation and the work of the steering group.

> **There is no one model of structure that must be implemented. A system's culture drives the development of models. It is principle that is constant, not the process.**

The membership of the SGSG should be reminded that there is a certain amount of serendipity and uncertainty in any change process. The dynamics of the environment, the shifting social context, the design of change, and other components of the change process (e.g., user-driven care, performance and evidence-driven processes) all create new demands in the organization. Each of these has an influence on the character and content of shared governance design. The steering group members should take into account all of the factors that can influence the rate and timing of change (see Figure 3-4). The group's response must evidence a commitment to fluid and flexible processing that shifts and adjusts as the demand for it is altered. Flexibility in membership work and function keeps the members from creating rigid structures that are as unchangeable or impermeable as the structures they are attempting to remove and replace.

CONCEPTUAL DESIGN FOR SHARED GOVERNANCE IMPLEMENTATION

> **Development of a work group is as essential as the work it does. Failure often results from what a group did not know rather than what it did not do.**

Figure 3-4   Shared Governance Steering Group Membership

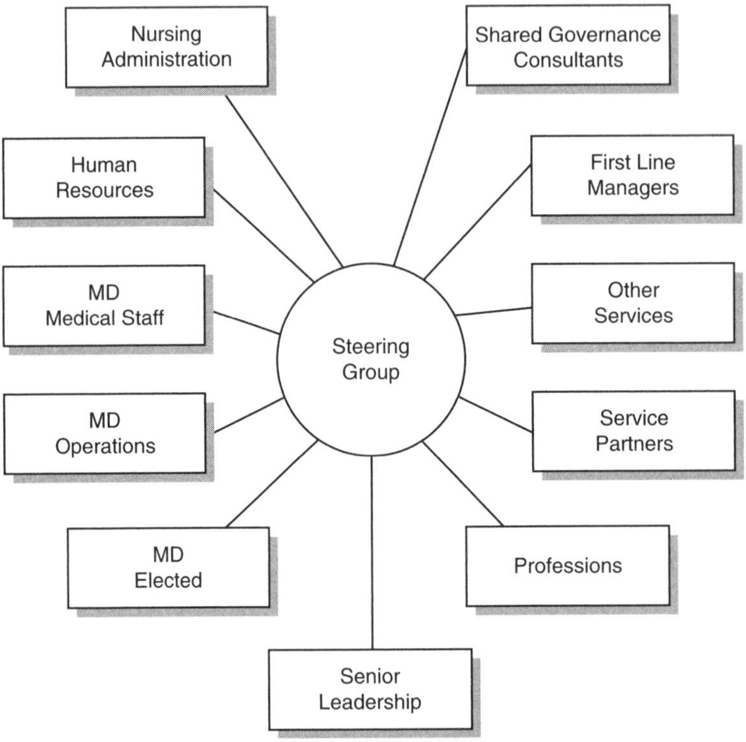

Before the SGSG can fully begin the implementation, it must be aware of two principles of change: All sustainable change is comprehensive, and change that occurs in one place in a system affects every other place in the system. Therefore, it is important for the SGSG to be well informed about the design and other structural changes going on in the organization. It will be important to link unit and other departmental activities of shared decision making with the formal processes of shared governance design. Most pathway, service line, or unit-based shared governance developmental activities need to reflect the parameters established by the steering group and the principles that ground shared governance wherever it is developed in the system. Information and connection to this group are critical to the ongoing work of the SGSG. Harmonizing the strategies and timing of the bilateral efforts will increase the effectiveness of both.

It is a further obligation of the SGSG to be fully aware of organizational constructs, theory, and function. As the organization is retooled, there will be broad implications for the entire system. Therefore, it is important that solid principles and good conceptual foundations be established. Members of the group should know about the complexities of systems and be able to apply organizational principles to their own system to ensure that the new structure is reared on solid foundations. Much has been written about shared governance, but perhaps the most significant models of implementation are those that have been used in highly complex nursing organizations.

NURSING SHARED GOVERNANCE

Nurses make up 60 percent of point-of-service providers. If they do not change, it does not matter who else does.

In many hospitals and organizations, the nursing service has used principles of shared governance as a foundation for implementing point-of-service empowerment processes (see Figure 3-5). As a result, many organizations assume that shared governance is strictly a nursing concept. Nothing could be further from the truth. Although many of the shared governance models that exist in health care operate within the nursing service, the conceptual foundations come from a much broader theoretical and research frame of reference. Shared governance is most common among nursing services for two main reasons. First, the large aggregate of diverse members that make up a nursing service has a major impact on services. Second, most nursing services encompass a range of differentiated functions that need to be integrated to deliver patient care services efficiently. In addition, nursing services have implemented empowerment point-of-service processes for 10 to 15 years—processes that provide a strong foundation for shared leadership, shared decision making, and shared governance.

Shared governance is a systems concept, not a nursing model. It began with nursing because it could and because nurses are the largest group of providers closest to the point of service.

It has always been understood by those promulgating the concept of shared governance that it could not be limited to a single discipline in any system. In a healthcare system, the integration, coordination, and facilitation of disciplinary

Figure 3-5   Nursing Council Model

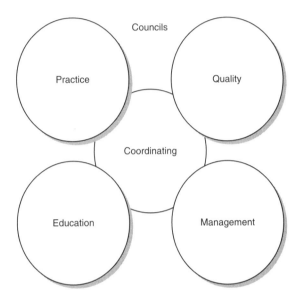

relationships among the various members of the healthcare team are critical to the effectiveness of service provision and the continuum of care. In an age of evidence-based practice, the need for a connection between the disciplines will become increasingly important, and thus, the principles of broad-based shared governance will continue to grow in value. Time and circumstances have created a situation in which shared governance can be expanded from use in single disciplines to the entire organization (see Figure 3-6).

Nursing shared governance does not disappear in whole-systems approaches. It does expand to accommodate all the partners that make a system work.

In many organizations, the nursing shared governance may be the natural beginning point for the application of shared governance principles to the broader organization. As outlined in Chapter 2, different considerations arise when implementing shared governance in an entire organization instead of a single component (e.g., nursing services). Therefore, nursing-specific design and application of shared governance are essentially nontransferable to the whole system. The principles are unchanging, but the approach is highly variable. Culture always provides the final framework for the implementation of any con-

Figure 3-6   Moving from a Nursing Model toward a Whole-Systems Model

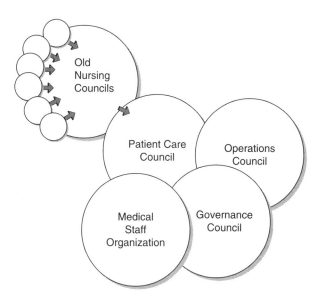

cept or process. Each healthcare discipline has created its own framework influencing the implementation of shared governance. Organizations will also need to create their own framework for expanding shared governance to the whole system.

> **Nursing representation now expands to the system. If nurses are to have the impact on decision making they should, they must expand their frame of reference.**

In an organization in which nursing shared governance exists, the organization is not obligated to adapt to the nursing shared governance framework. Instead, the nursing shared governance component must fit itself within the broader framework of a multiple-discipline approach to implementing shared governance. The benefit of having begun shared governance within the nursing service is that the largest group of point-of-service providers in the organization is already operating within the appropriate framework. That increases the chance of a successful organization-wide implementation of shared governance. In particular, it creates an opportunity to extend the necessary patterns of behavior, styles of leadership, and characteristics of point-of-service decision making to the remaining components of the organization, building on what is already present in the nursing service.

INTERDISCIPLINARY SHARED GOVERNANCE

> Shared governance represents the partnership between all who provide service and support in a system. It requires their engagement in decisions and actions that support their work and relationships.

Inviting others in the organizational system to become involved in shared governance does not guarantee that there will be an increased level of interest. In many instances, other disciplines and work groups in the organization may see shared governance simply as an externalization of the nursing service and another opportunity for nursing to influence or control its relationships with the rest of the system. This viewpoint is inadequate and woefully incomplete. It is reasonable to assume that if empowerment, shared leadership, and shared decision making are to occur in an organization, all members must ultimately participate. When clearly half or more of the point-of-service providers are nurses, it is also reasonable to assume that implementation of empowerment processes, shared leadership, and shared decision making should begin with that large group.

Regardless of when other groups might be willing to engage in the change process, if the largest professional group in the organization has not moved a significant distance toward acquiring the behaviors associated with shared governance, it will not matter who else has. Simply by virtue of its volume, location, and diversity, the nursing service will require additional time, effort, and energy to acquire such behaviors, and allowing it to have a head start is not a bad idea— in fact, it reflects the better part of wisdom. In many instances, it is for this reason alone that shared governance begins with the nursing service—although of course it should not end there.

Following the collection and dissemination of information on the theory, principles, and foundations of shared governance activities, the SGSG must begin to assess the activities it will undertake to facilitate the translation of theory and concept into practice. In doing this, the SGSG should follow a particular pattern of deliberation and decision making.

SHARED GOVERNANCE STEERING GROUP BASICS

> Teams are the future of work.

The initial activities of the SGSG concern its own functions and activities. Setting up the rules of engagement and defining the issues associated with undertaking its work are the first step in the SGSG's design and construction of a shared governance structure. This step encompasses the following tasks:

- Creating a clear statement of purpose and direction as a foundation for its work
- Designing a charter for change that clearly enumerates the commitment of the most senior levels of the organization and of the steering group and assuring the organization that the process will be sustainable and participation will be faithful through the completion of the shared governance process (and posting publicly for all to see)
- Outlining the obligations of membership, the commitment expected, the meeting schedule, the work to be done, and the shared obligation for that work
- Delineating the decision-making processes and tools that are available and will be used for stimulating dialogue, seeking direction, defining work content, resolving conflicts, and seeking solutions to problems
- Devising a timeline to guide the SGSG's work and the evaluation of the team's processes
- Enumerating the mechanisms of linkage with the other change processes going on in the organization
- Defining the mechanism for communicating and intersecting with other leadership groups in the organization to ensure that each is informed and involved to the extent necessary
- Defining the specific accountability of the SGSG in light of its obligation to implement shared governance throughout the organization
- Outlining the evaluation activities that will be used to measure, evaluate, and validate the stages of implementation and their impact on the organization

These first rules of engagement are an essential foundation for the work of the SGSG. Like all teams, it requires a clear understanding of its mandate, the tools that it will use to undertake its work, the expectations of those who are members, the time frame for accomplishing its objectives, and the outcomes required. Also, it must establish linkages with components to key parts of the organization—those that depend upon its work or that the SGSG depends on for completing its work successfully.

Membership requires commitment, which in turn requires presence. You cannot commit to anything when you are not present.

A number of stakeholders in the organization are going to be very interested in the work of the SGSG. Whoever these stakeholders are (e.g., administrators, service pathway, unit, departmental leaders, support services staff, board members, medical staff), a mechanism should exist for either incorporating or communicating with them so that they understand the developmental process and the activities related to it. In shared governance implementation, there are no hidden agendas, no secret meetings, and no closed-door processes. It is assumed in shared governance that investment, engagement, and ownership operate across the board. Initially, any member of the organization who has the time and interest has the option to either observe or be involved in decision making.

UNDERSTANDING THE LIMITS

Commitment always demands personal ownership. No responsibility, no rewards.

The SGSG must also understand the expectations and limitations that exist. No group can successfully undertake its work free of the constraints imposed by limited resources, limited time, and competing demands. All areas of activity must be balanced in a meaningful way to provide appropriate support for the work of the SGSG, and several issues must be addressed to ensure that the realities of the organization are fully taken into account.

Budgetary Availability

Don't ever attempt to produce what you can't pay for.

There should be a delineation of the costs associated with the work of the SGSG. The budgetary allocation for this work should be clarified in advance so that, when the SGSG undertakes its activities, it knows the financial parameters within which it must operate. No decision group that gathers key players together operates without having a cost impact on the organization, and the time, energy, commitment, and results of the deliberations of the group all affect the viability of the organization. Thus, the financial impact of the SGSG's work should be anticipated to the fullest extent possible before the group begins its activities and should be incorporated into its deliberations. Furthermore, the SGSG should make a commitment to help generate whole-systems budget enhancements, revenue reductions, cost reductions, and performance improvements that total more than the costs associated with its work. This helps build an understanding up front that decisions and activities unfolding within the context of shared governance must demonstrate value-added to the organization as an explication of the viability and veracity of shared governance to have a positive impact on organizational functioning.

Deadlines

No group can insulate itself from demands made by the organization to accomplish its ends. Deadlines are a requisite for motivating and guiding work in any system. They should be clear and outlined in advance of the undertaking of activities. The time frames for associated activities, such as budgetary activities, should be communicated to the leadership of the SGSG so that it can incorporate them into its planning.

Workload

Time is as much a resource as money. Neither should be wasted.

Obviously, the work of the SGSG is affected by the availability of the team members. The workload of the members in their regular work setting must be moderate enough to allow them to fulfill the duties of the SGSG. If the workload requirements make it impossible for members to commit their energies to the SGSG, then the SGSG's performance will be seriously impaired.

A discussion of the workload, time, availability, and obligations of each of the members is essential during the formation of the SGSG. Membership and participation in these activities should be reflected in the work scheduling and assignment of SGSG members far enough in advance to plan for activities associated with participating in the SGSG work. Workload adjustments can easily be justified, by the importance of the work of building a new structure.

INDIVIDUAL DIFFERENCES

People in a work group are different. They bring a variety of skills and talents to the work group. Some are assertive and creative, innovative and energized, and able to verbalize their thoughts with great ease. Others are reflective and cautious and will need to be coaxed into making a contribution. Knowing the various characteristics of the members of the group, understanding their unique talents, and utilizing strategies that capture most of what each has to offer will be the job of the leadership. Use of techniques and tactics that allow every member of the group to contribute is essential, as is careful planning and a sensitive awareness of the ever-changing balance of participation.

OTHER RESOURCES

Any work group should have available to it whatever resources it needs to do its work. No support, no outcome.

The SGSG should not assume that its membership possesses all of the expertise and insight it needs. There will be times when other players will have to be involved and incorporated into the SGSG's decision making. If a nonmember has required information, expertise, leadership abilities, or insight, that person will need to be brought in as an adjunct. In any work group there are essentially three kinds of members: core members, expert members (members by right), and ad hoc members. Core members are those that have been appointed, and they make up the continuing membership of the group. Expert members are individuals who are included in the deliberations of the group because they have a requisite set of insights and skills. Ad hoc members are individuals who are positioned either by location, power, or role to have useful information, insights, and relationships. At varying times expert and ad hoc members must be joined with the core members to ensure effective deliberation. Such fluidity in its membership allows the SGSG to focus on the proper issues and perform its work successfully.

DEVELOPMENT AND TRAINING

You cannot do what you do not know how to do. Learning is as important as the work that it enables.

As mentioned previously, development is important. There will be points in the implementation process where the SGSG membership may need to stop to assess what it knows and what it needs to know to advance its work. A constant commitment to development, growth, and advancement is critical to the ongoing competence of the work group.

AUTHORITY AND DECISION MAKING

The group must be clear at the outset as to which decisions it is accountable for making, what authority it has for making those decisions, and the extent of its ability to implement the decisions made. Clear support from the leadership of the organization and enumeration of the authority and decision-making power of the group are essential to the group's ability to accomplish its work. Clarity of authority at the outset is essential to its accountability and its ability to implement its recommendations. It would be unfortunate if those who have been given the task of spreading empowerment throughout an organization did not themselves have the necessary power to accomplish this task. Clarification as to what SGSG can do and cannot do will help form the framework and parameters for its deliberations and decision making.

INFORMATION ACCESS

Every work group must have access to whatever information it needs to make decisions. The major reason for inadequate decisions is lack of the right information at the right time.

In performing its work, the SGSG must have access to all the information it requires. Without access to the tools that it needs, including appropriate information, the SGSG will achieve only limited success; the organization, therefore, must ensure that it always has what it needs.

DETERMINATION OF BOUNDARIES

As important as it is to know what the group can do, it is also important to know what lies beyond the scope of the group. Increasingly, in an integrated organizational system there are different loci of control and decision making. In the design process, different groups responsible for varying components may have authority to make decisions within their appropriate context. Their authority and the boundaries that define it must be clear also to the SGSG. On the other hand, the boundaries of the functions and activities of the SGSG must be made known as early as possible so that when those boundaries are reached and the involvement of other components of the organizational system are necessary to continue the work of the SGSG, that will be clear to the members and incorporated into their deliberations.

THE PLANNING PROCESS

Every team must know what it can and cannot do. There is nothing more destructive than assigning a team its work and not giving it the authority necessary to do it.

The preceding are important issues for any steering group involved in implementing shared governance. Again, clear accountability is the foundation of any team's efforts to accomplish its work successfully. If this and other basic components are in place, the SGSG can begin to undertake the design and implementation of an interdisciplinary shared governance structure. Clearly, the first step is the delineation of a plan that sets out the SGSG's goals and objectives and the creation of a timeline that sets their time of accomplishment.

The planning process appropriate for this kind of a work group is not the incremental, long-range planning process so familiar to healthcare organizations in the past. The planning activities need to be directed toward delineating expectations, outcomes, and design components for a shared governance structure. The following three elements of the planning phase are critical to the initial work.

Expectations

The design and implementation of a shared governance structure depend on what processes and structure are anticipated. It is important that the shared governance principles be enumerated clearly so that they can be used as a database for implementation and later as a tool for evaluating the stages of implementation and the ultimate success of the design. The expectations, presented in a bulleted format, should be stated in such a way that they can be used to measure the functional components of the design and implementation. For example, the statement that there will be no more than two levels of management leadership and the statement that 90 percent of all decision making will occur at the service pathway or unit level each indicate a principle and a device for measuring the effectiveness and appropriateness of any structure based on that principle.

It is suggested that an accountability grid be developed that delineates the locus of control for specific decisions in the current organization as opposed to the shift of the locus of control in the shared governance organization. Because shared governance is an accountability-based design, it is important to be clear about where decisions are made and who is accountable for those decisions. Because shared governance is constructed based on the locus of control for decisions, not on positions or roles, it is important to be clear about current locus of control for decisions as opposed to the legitimate locus of control for those decisions within the context of shared governance. An accountability grid identifies the decision-making roles or positions on the vertical axis and the specific and relevant decisions that are made on the horizontal axis. This process is undertaken for both current structure and proposed shared governance structure. Through undertaking this comparison and clarifying legitimate and appropriate locus of control for decisions the location of accountability can be more clearly enumerated and the restructuring of that accountability can be more specifically delineated.

Functional Components

The second task is to identify functional components of the new structure. For example, if the word *council* is used to refer to a deliberative body, the SGSG must define what this particular council does and what its decision-making authority is. For example, the SGSG might need to define what a team is and what its authority, functions, activities, membership, and accountability are.

Roles and Positions

The steering function requires sufficient time to do its work. However, the timelines for this work must be established at the outset, and they must be clear to everyone in the system.

Once the principles and structural and functional components of the organization are clearly articulated, the next step is to delineate the new roles and positions. In the change to shared governance, a number of roles will have to be modified and others will have to be eliminated. For example, in the switch to an interdisciplinary design, vice president and other senior management positions may change and the content, functions, obligations, and relationships associated with these positions will of course change as well. Each of the functional shifts should be identified in the planning process so that every member of the organization is clear about the implications of the move to shared governance for his or her position and role in the organization.

In addition to the three elements described, the SGSG needs to develop a vision of how the organization will look. This vision should be "expressed" graphically and it should include the basic elements of the organization; the relationship of the functions and structures to each other; the interface between the individual structures; and the work, accountability, and decision-making authority of each of the components of the organization. A shared governance design cannot be described using a line and box chart. Because shared governance depends essentially on the interfaces between as well as the accountability and relationships of the various players and components of the organization, intersecting circles and cycles of relationship are often used to indicate authority, position, relationship, and accountability in a shared governance organizational chart.

> The steering group must know that designing is merely the beginning of its work. Implementation of the design will change where it takes the system.

Two types of models are important in the design of a shared governance organization. The first consists of the linkages and intersecting lines of functional accountability, relationship, and position in the organization. The second consists of the management and leadership intersections along a continuum of decision making from the point of service to the system level. These two models, although closely related, display different categories of accountability. The first identifies the accountability of groups within the system, and the second identifies the accountability of individuals within the groupings in the system. Constructing these models is one of the main tasks of the SGSG's planning phase.

Through use of these tools and the design processes, a better picture of the implementation process begins to emerge within the group. It is important to note that the beginning design is not permanent. It is simply a demarcation point, a place for the dialogue to begin. No structure is permanent. The parameters and design of a structure are forever shifting in response to the surrounding realities. This must be understood and accepted by everyone in the steering group. If the steering group does not recognize the need for fluidity, its efforts may result in the building of a permanent, rigid structure—the very thing the design process was intended to do away with.

THE WORK OF THE STEERING GROUP

Design is like art—necessary to human experience but subject to the tastes and judgments of others. You will never satisfy everyone.

Over the life of the SGSG, there will be many activities related to the implementation process for which it will have summary accountability. Anything related to the design and implementation of the shared governance structure falls within the auspices of this group. It therefore is critical to make sure that all of the phases of implementation, stages of development, and components of the structure fall within the purview and range of accountability of the SGSG.

In doing its work, the SGSG has many diverse mechanisms and options available. Clearly, control of all of the elements of the shared governance implementation process should rest in the hands of the SGSG leadership. However, work groups, task forces, implementation groups, and various other tools can be used to delineate the steps in the implementation process. In many cases, implementation around the point of service or along the service pathway in the continuum of care will require the creation of culturally based work groups that fall within the auspices of the individual service pathways. Also, as teams are better defined and more thoroughly developed, leadership for team development will become a service pathway/unit responsibility. Although the SGSG may be accountable for application of the principles of shared governance, the framework for decision making, and the range of accountability and authority of teams and other decision-making bodies within the units of service or service pathways, the actual functions and activities related to the implementation of shared governance will unfold in the cultural context of each pathway/department/unit.

The steering group must be free to do its work. Its accountability must be clear up front, and the support it needs must be articulated before it makes critical decisions. Countering decisions after they are made destroys the credibility of both the group and its work.

The primary goal of the SGSG is to facilitate the implementation of shared governance and to ensure that it proceeds basically uniformly throughout the system. A secondary goal is to ensure that, where possible, the principles of shared governance are applied with enough flexibility to allow important unique characteristics of the individual service pathways to survive the initial design.

In undertaking its work, the SGSG must address the following:

- The fit of the shared governance implementation schedule and the patient care and systems design schedule
- The design of a shared governance structure that integrates the whole organization
- The linkage of the medical staff organization and the point-of-service, empowered shared governance structure
- The design and creation of the patient care council and the design of its relationship to the service pathways/departments/units and the teams of which they consist
- The design and creation of the operations council (the design should integrate management and resource decision making throughout the system and within each component of the system)
- The design and creation of the governance council (the council's main role is to integrate the shared governance structure so that it functions like a seamless decision-making network)
- The participation of the board of trustees in the conception, design, and implementation of whole-systems/interdisciplinary shared governance within and across the components of the organization
- The definition of the roles, functions, levels of management and leadership, and administrative relationships at the support and systems level of the organization
- The development and implementation of a learning and development model for the clinical and resource leadership
- The enumeration of learning organization characteristics and tools operating at different levels of the organization (e.g., team-based learning; support service roles; consultation roles; and revised administrative, governance, and medical staff relationships)
- The delineation and appointment of work groups, task forces, and other activity groups directed toward the implementation of components of the shared governance structure
- The delineation of accountability and authority at every decision-making point in the organization
- The evaluation of the effectiveness of the implementation of shared governance for the whole system through assessment of
  - The consistency of application of the shared governance concept
  - The effectiveness of decision making by individual providers, individual leaders, department/unit/team service councils, and system councils
  - The impact of empowerment on the efficiency and effectiveness of decision making (taking into account decision timelines, appropriateness of decisions, and decision outcomes)

- Staff investment in system-level decisions and staff compliance and satisfaction with the empowerment resulting from point-of-service decision making
- The effectiveness of the new roles for administrative officers and the impact those roles have on council decision making, service pathway decision making, and leadership development
- The critical flow of decision making and communication throughout the organization (the focus is on effectiveness, efficiency, flow problems, and inadequacies in the communication system)

Each of the preceding items encompasses functions that will be essential to effective implementation of interdisciplinary shared governance. In subsequent chapters, each of the elements of the implementation for which the SGSG is responsible will be discussed in relation to the development of the main components of the shared governance organization. What should be clear already is that fundamental accountability for the success of the implementation of interdisciplinary shared governance rests with the SGSG.

THE CHANGE PROCESS

The steering group must be flexible and fluid. The conditions present at the beginning of its work will not likely be the same as those later in the process. The possibility of change of course must always be built into planning.

It should be clear by now how time bound and transitional each element of the implementation of shared governance is. External and internal variables affect the rate of change, the intensity of change, and the time frame for change. Further, there are definite stages of change, and these must be understood by the SGSG and incorporated into its implementation plan. These stages include the following:

- Planning and preparation
- Design and movement
- Creativity and application
- Testing the value of the application
- Integrating the components of change
- Evaluating the effectiveness of the change over the long term

The SGSG should be aware that these stages are highly variable. Certain pathways and teams will develop at a faster rate and in a different way than other pathways and teams, and this fact must be taken into account in devising the timeline and the evaluation process.

> Whole-systems shared governance has few precedents—it is a new application of systems principles. The designers are living the script as they write it. Adherence to the principles will help ensure the integrity of the process.

Often, adjustments in what was planned will have to be made to respond to unexpected internal developments. Chaos and complexity theory states that the serendipitous often has an influence on the formal and controlled part of change. Room for the serendipitous (and for anticipated problems) will need to be incorporated into the strategy and planning of the steering group. As it moves through the implementation process, challenges will inevitably arise, and it must be prepared to react efficiently. "Gridding out" or flowcharting (using a Gantt chart, for example) the stages of shared governance implementation can provide a tool for measuring progress and handling the variability embedded in the implementation of a comprehensive restructuring.

The SGSG should always keep in mind that it is undertaking an activity that has few precedents. Redesigning an organization using shared governance principles is a relatively new type of undertaking. Few tools and models can be replicated by the organization as it begins to alter its structure to fit the emerging service and care delivery system. Undoubtedly, there will be many times the organization will need to redirect activities, alter plans, and adjust the implementation process.

Flexibility and a good understanding of the elements of change within a whole-systems context will serve the SGSG well as it facilitates the implementation of shared governance. The task will require insight, patience, and determination. However, if the key elements of the change process, as outlined in this chapter, are incorporated into the functional components of design and implementation, the tools necessary for success will be available to the SGSG. It should be remembered by the SGSG leadership that the application of the principles of shared governance is critical to the sustainability of any shared governance design. Using the principles as a template and applying them consistently throughout the implementation process ensure that a meaningful relationship exists between the organization's services and the structures in place to support them.

SUGGESTED READING

Albrecht, K. (2003). *The power of minds at work; Organizational intelligence in action.* New York: AMACOM.

Antonakis, J., Cianciolo, A. T., & Sternberg, R. J. (2004). *The nature of leadership.* Thousand Oaks, CA: Sage Publications.

Cornforth, C. (2003). *The governance of public and non-profit organisations: What do boards do?* London: Routledge.

Dow, G. K. (2003). *Governing the firm: Workers' control in theory and practice.* Cambridge, England: Cambridge University Press.

Everett, L., & Black, K. (2007). Putting the patient first: Guiding principles provide a road map for more collaborative relationships among nurses and support service groups. *Nurse Leader, 5*(3), 19–22.

Gandossy, R. P., & Sonnenfeld, J. A. (2004). *Leadership and governance from the inside out.* Hoboken, NJ: John Wiley.

Goldsmith, M. (2004). *Challenged up: A key to organizational integrity.* Unpublished manuscript, New York.

Hamson, N., & Holder, R. (2002). *Global innovation.* Oxford, England: Capstone.

Harland, L., Harrison, W., Jones, J., & Reiter-Palmon, R. (2005). Leadership behaviors and subordinate resilience. *Journal of Leadership and Organizational Studies, 11*(2), 2–14.

Oliver, R. W. (2004). *What is transparency?* New York: McGraw-Hill.

Pointer, D. D., & Orlikoff, J. E. (2002). *Getting to great: Principles of health care organization governance.* San Francisco: Jossey-Bass.

Salas, E., Bowers, C. A., & Edens, E. (2001). *Improving teamwork in organizations: Applications of resource management training.* Mahwah, NJ: Erlbaum.

Thomson, S. (2007). Nurse-physician collaboration: A comparison of the attitudes of nurses and physicians. *Med-Surg Nursing, 16*(2), 87–93.

Vardi, Y. A., & Weitz, E. (2004). *Misbehavior in organizations: Theory, research, and management.* Mahwah, NJ: Erlbaum.

Wilson, T. B. (2003). *Innovative reward systems for the changing workplace* (2nd ed.). New York: McGraw-Hill.

CHAPTER 4

Constructing Integrated Care Delivery: Building a Service Continuum

Tim Porter-O'Grady and Marsha Parker

> *Life can only be understood looking backward,*
> *but can only be lived looking forward.*
>
> —Sören Kierkegaard

Creating integrated care delivery requires planners to seek care delivery from a systems perspective. True systems are nonhierarchical and are built in a way that reflects the intersecting relationships that advance the system and continue to ensure their viability. What has become especially important in today's health system, influenced by high levels of clinical technology and information infrastructure, is an organizational and system structure that provides the appropriate frame for true integration. Building systems on intersections and relationships is the critical dynamic that best reflects the operation of true systems. The linkage sets that will be necessary across the system must represent the key interface between persons, processes, and practices. In fact, user-driven systems in health care must establish a continuous and dynamic relationship with patients, reflect a script for the life process, and reflect value and cost in delivering the service (Figure 4-1).

The concepts in this chapter reflect a whole-systems view of the clinical organization. New concepts and language are utilized to better reflect a more systems orientation to the implementation of an interdisciplinary shared decision-making infrastructure. The challenge here is that the concepts reflect a more linked and integrated model representing flow, mobility, and the interface of structure, system, provider, and patient in a more relational than functional design.

Interdisciplinary shared governance can be implemented in more traditional organizational constructs, although with some difficulty. In fact, interdisciplinary shared governance may actually create the foundations or the urge for the organization to shift its mental model from a static vertical and departmental structural design to an infrastructure that better represents contemporary systems thinking. Still, regardless of whether traditional constructs are maintained, true interdisciplinary shared governance can drive the organization toward addressing serious questions of systems effectiveness and efficacy. Challenges

Figure 4-1   User-Driven Approaches

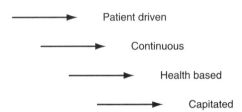

arise regarding current organizational constructions, calling leadership to confront the inadequacies of traditional structure, unbundle the attachment to it, and challenge clinical and management leadership to reconfigure the clinical and operational infrastructure. This chapter serves to advance that challenge and makes some initial suggestions for stimulating effective systems redesign within an integrated interdisciplinary shared decision-making format.

In user systems, comprehensiveness is critical to success. The buyers of services are looking for a composite of services that addresses their prevailing concern, which is cost-effectiveness, and users are looking for breadth of relevant services and satisfaction with care.

Certainly, linkage of all the components of service is critical to the effectiveness of the organization. Internal alignment serves to facilitate the formation of seamless integration along the continuum of care. The design of the internal structure follows the patient flow and advances patients along the clinical pathway that most effectively meets the patients' needs and operates least expensively.

THE PATIENT PATHWAY

All service structures should follow some pathway that represents the demand for service along the continuum. Patients are not simply looking for good illness services. Given a choice, they would not seek to become ill at all. Few, with the exception of those with severe mental illness, consciously seek to be ill. Illness is frequently caused by lifestyle choices—the way one works, interacts, eats, exercises, thinks, and lives. Many of the illnesses experienced in American society result from excess and not living a balanced, active life.

Much of what constitutes health care today relates to sickness care services. The focus of the system on providing sickness services inherently advances sickness unless there is some offsetting factor that reduces dependency on such services. Historically, there has been no interest in or economic benefit from health-driven services. However, in user-based approaches, where cost is always a central factor, not wasting dollars is increasingly important. There is an over-riding need to be judicious in the use of services and the expenditure of dollars, and profits are directly related to the ability to keep as many dollars as possible and to reduce the use of services that consume a large number of dollars. That ultimately means reducing the use of services solely directed to sickness care, where the highest amount of cost is located.

> **Much of what is offered as health care in America is really sickness care. Health has never been the issue, and that is the core of the problem in American health care.**

It is in this frame of reference that the need to build new linkages unfolds. As comprehensiveness becomes the critical factor in the delivery of service, linkage to necessary services is accelerated (see Figure 4-2). The ease of access to and use of such services by the user become important to both the provider and the patient. The low cost and the effectiveness of these services become everyone's concerns. Anything that does not improve the individual's health and reduce dependency on the services of the system adds demand and cost to the system. Thus, the new focus is on creating health.

NEW REALITIES

The new focus on health has many implications for the service system, and strategies such as these are becoming necessary:

- Constructing services that center around managing lives rather than managing disease
- Reducing institutional services that require the consumer to come to the provider rather than the provider going to the consumer
- Recognizing providers as partners in the provision of service rather than as customers of the health system
- Identifying and minimizing need rather than intervening and treating after a condition is present
- Creating linkages that advance the health status of consumers rather than aid in illness identification and response

Figure 4-2   Patient Pathway

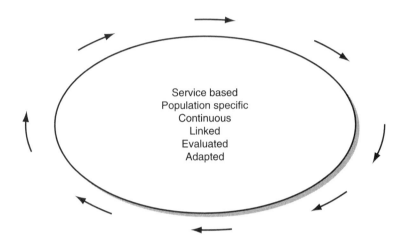

- Engaging employers in efforts to improve health and thus reducing the health services costs and intensity costs
- Decentralizing services to the user's locations, thus making it easier to meet demand early than to simply provide services at the supplier location

Each of these strategies radically changes the approach to the delivery of services, and the traditional physician- and hospital-centered framework must be replaced by a broader community-based framework. In this new framework, the following occurs:

- Providers focus on assisting individuals to delineate risk factors and influences on health status over their lifetime.
- Health screening becomes a fundamental focus of health care rather than an adjunct to treatment.
- Clinical sites are created where users live and work to make access to services as convenient as possible.
- Healthy behaviors and the costs and risks of nonperformance are identified.
- Providers create partnerships with certain members of the user group, who then assume responsibility for the health relationships in the workplace or community setting.
- Primary care networks and providers are linked to ensure quick and convenient access to essential information and services.
- The information system network is used to support information sharing and consumer linkage at all points along the service continuum.

- Focus on excellence of the user experience and the application of evidence-driven protocols as a driver for practice and care.

BUILDING THE CONTINUUM OF CARE

The movement toward value-driven care forces the health system toward linkage along the continuum of care. Payers and buyers of health services simply cannot sustain a focus on price for very long and ensure that viable services are provided to users. The ability to manipulate prices carries the relationship only so far. Currently, pressure exists to drive prices downward without affecting the character of the services or the willingness of health providers to negotiate prices. The suicide level is reached when services promised cannot be delivered at the price promised, and the users do not get what their agents contracted for.

> **Focusing on the price of services alone is not a sustainable strategy. The buyer and user eventually need to get the outcomes paid for.**

It is early in the price-service cycle. Therefore, providers and buyers are still at some distance from dialogue regarding the balance between cost and appropriate service. In fact, a new language on the horizon with regard to payer-provider relationships driven by the increased demand for a national health system is better integrated, more accessible, and available to all. Two factors will occur to create this situation, and neither is far off. First, the price parameters will be stretched to the limit beyond which no health system can go and survive. Second, there will be a demand to know what is happening at the service end of the arrangement and whether users are getting what they need and that it represents both patient and payer value. It will be necessary to achieve evidence-based service outcomes that will themselves affect the future generation of costs and expansion of interventions.

Long-term success will not depend on the price-service relationship. The value equation shows the importance of three factors: cost, quality, and time (or activity). No one of those factors can be applied without an equal effort being directed to the others. This is a hard-learned lesson, but the long-term viability of any value-based care approach depends on its mastery.

It is incumbent upon the leadership in any health organization to be cognizant of this reality and to structure services in a way that anticipates the requisites of the value equation. In the long run, the organization's competitiveness will depend on how well the balance between price sensitivity and service effectiveness has been maintained and how sustainable that balance is.

RELATIONAL SERVICE DESIGN

Providers increasingly need to configure around populations rather than patients. This changes the focus from treating illness to creating health.

An increasingly important goal in health care is to integrate around specific patient populations. These populations are composed of users who represent a specific set of needs. The kind of services offered depends entirely upon the complexion of the user base. If service viability is to be maintained over the long term, there must be a tight fit between the kind of services offered and the needs of the user population.

Therefore, the healthcare organization must be fluid and flexible, portable and mobile, in its service structure. For every population served and problem addressed, the organization must have a service framework available to satisfy the demands of patients and populations. It is in this context that the continuum of care and appropriate linkages become central to the structure of the healthcare organization.

User satisfaction does not result simply from excellence in any one component of the delivery system. Also necessary is a strong connection between providers within the full range of services the user expects. Furthermore, users will not remain satisfied if the services obtained do not match their expectations or their genuine needs. An inexpensive price tag will not long interest any user whose wants are not met.

Health providers need to ensure that the fit between the services provided and the population served is clearly defined.

Ultimately, it is important to be able to enumerate clearly what is obtained for the price paid. It is equally important to look at what users are getting in other buyer-provider arrangements. If the data show that superior services are being offered at the same or a better price elsewhere, it should come as no surprise that buyers will be interested in switching contracts. Over the long term, the fixation on price will give way to interest in the components of the service framework and the context for service the provider has constructed (see Exhibit 4-1). There are a number of areas buyers will become increasingly interested in knowing more about:

Exhibit 4-1   New Payment Requisites

- Flat sum
- No pay categories
- Defined service limits
- Evidence-based quality outcomes
- Seeking/achieving excellence
- Continuous contract renegotiation

- What are the measures of care that determine the relationship between what is done and the outcomes that are achieved?
- How does the cost per unit of service compare with the cost for like services offered by other providers?
- What is the range of services provided to specific populations?
- How does the provider know the appropriate fit between the character of the user population and the provider's service configuration?
- What are administrative and support costs per user in the provider organization?
- How are evidence-based best practices maintained and improved as a foundation for the clinical routines and activities of the key providers of health services?
- What are the focused service activities that address the health concerns of users and keep them from using more expensive intervention services?

These questions form a framework for considering the interests of buyers and users. Increasingly, the ability to keep people from expending resources is as critical as the kind of resources used. The current focus on lowering the levels of intervention creates a dynamic that is threatening to existing service patterns. It makes many of them obsolete and forces the provider organization to match what it does to the health needs of those it serves and what the buyers are willing (or should be willing) to pay for.

LINKAGE DEFINES THE SYSTEM

Linkage between components of the delivery system will become increasingly critical to the viability of service provision. Some new thinking about what service provision should look like will be required. Some changes in existing relationships will have to occur. Practice arrangements will need to reflect the different character of clinical connections in the delivery system:

- Gatekeeping roles will be assumed by primary care providers (nurses and physicians), who will manage entry to the system and direct people along the clinical pathway.
- Many primary care providers will not be physicians simply because not enough physicians will be prepared to meet the demands of the role and the transition to primary care roles will be primarily assumed by DNP (Doctor of Nursing Practice) nurses.
- An increasing number of patients will need life management skills rather than illness services, requiring them to acknowledge their risk factors and to deal with them.
- Required but nonowned services will have to be provided under shared risk agreements to ensure all the services needed are available to users.
- Ownership of health activities will be taken over by the users, who will have increasing responsibility for making decisions about what services will and will not be used.
- Nonallopathic methods of treatment that produce significant outcomes will become fully accepted.
- Services will be brought to the workplace so that factors influencing the degree of health risk experienced by users can be quickly and adequately addressed.
- There will be significant cost sharing for health programs, especially those that relate to the reduction of existing health risks over which the users have direct behavioral control.

Horizontal Linkage

Horizontal linkage requires virtually every provider to gain the ability to negotiate relationships along the continuum of care. In the past, the marketing or development office would provide most of the services needed to make and finalize the connections and contracts between service entities. It is now necessary for connections and contracts to be fashioned by the point-of-service leadership, with the support of marketing and development. Ownership and stakeholder requirements encourage the parties to any relationship to play the major role in defining it and in building the specifics that will act as a foundation for the relationship. Some specific activities will have to be considered:

- Articulating a mutual purpose so that the parties are clear about the reason for the relationship
- Clarifying the expectations each has of the relationship and the benefits that will accrue to both

- Knowing what real barriers to the relationship exist and making it safe to put them on the table for the parties to address jointly
- Identifying the quid pro quo for each party and the outcomes anticipated from the relationship
- Negotiating the roles of the two parties so that accountability can be clearly defined and duplication and cross-referencing activities can be kept to a minimum
- Addressing the financial obligations associated with each role and the way those will be managed and distributed over the course of the relationship
- Developing a continuous evaluation mechanism (including periodic group review) that looks at the character of the relationship and the outcomes of work over the course of the relationship.

Provider Linkage

Linking the providers along the continuum of health care is the critical work of the system's leadership today.

Internal linkage throughout the service system will be vital to the success of the organization. Building a seamless system of services means that the essential relationships are always supporting the purposes of the services. Therefore, a mechanism must exist to ensure the resolution of conflict and service flow over the life of the relationship. The consumers have a right to expect that the service providers have a mechanism for building their relationships, solving problems, and advancing the work of the health system to the benefit of the consumers.

History, however, tells a different story. The silo approach to organizational structure created functional and departmental barriers between people and did not foster the development of meaningful and functional relationships between the disciplines. Often one part of the clinical system would work in conflict with other parts of the system. The issues at stake were not always clear, and the problems associated with the immaturity of the relationships began to spill over into the patient-provider relationship. Now, to ensure effectiveness, it is critical that the stakeholders form clearly defined relationships that allow them to progress toward mutually defined goals. The process of creating the necessary type of relationships should be guided by the following rules, among others:

- Physicians are not outside the relationships necessary to the obtaining of desired outcomes and, therefore, as partners, should no longer be treated as customers of the system.
- Physicians and the other disciplines must establish new relationships configured around the contribution of each to the attainment of patient service outcomes.
- The medical staff organization must be formally reconstructed to remove all barriers to the development of relationships and shared decision making with point-of-service providers and problem-solving mechanisms strictly within the point of service.
- The independent entrepreneurial physician practice will no longer be able to thrive unilaterally in the emerging marketplace. Increasingly, multidisciplinary practice arrangements will be necessary for success.
- Nurses will play an increasingly large role in building and maintaining the continuum of care and fostering the linkages necessary to fully serve the needs of the users.
- Multidisciplinary group practice arrangements centered around particular patient populations will require equity in decision making and resource sharing.

ORGANIZING AROUND POPULATIONS

Patient populations will form the core of service configurations. As indicated in this book, organizations will configure around the point of patient care and provide services to specified patient populations. The continuum of care will serve as the template for the services provided. Meeting the need for clearly enumerated protocols and cost-moderated activities will demand the investment of all who have a stake in the relationship. Time and energy must be committed to discovering the activities and evidence-based practices that demonstrate the greatest impact upon the users' health. Identifying those activities and building on them will be the main work of the clinical leadership for some time.

DEFINING LINKAGES

Service organizations are no longer built from the top down or from the bottom up. Rather, they are constructed in a dynamic from the inside out and the outside in.

Building a more horizontal organization requires starting from the top down and the bottom up at the same time. The disciplines of visioning and mental modeling are crucial in helping the organization move forward as a whole. Progress depends on breaking down linkages and building them back up. No less important is the context within which processing occurs. The leadership must learn to create overview templates with the necessary flexibility to allow people at the point of service to re-create linkages. It is a noisy, messy enterprise and demands continuous leadership skill and group competence.

One of the most important things to learn about radical change is that it is more important to build something based on principles and shared goals than to simply eradicate the old barriers. Unfortunately, once the old barriers come tumbling down, so do all the old linkages. All those influences and feelings that give workers some sense of where they stand in the organization, what their value is to the whole, are suddenly gone. Bereft of those guideposts and attachments, workers feel abandoned and "outside the information loop." It is of paramount importance that the vision for the new structure be very widely shared so that workers have the choice to enroll in the new paradigm. In the absence of a vision, informal parallel structures will be built.

BUILDING THE VISION

The propagation of a shared vision is not accomplished by the mere construction of the vision, nor by communicating it a dozen times or so. Constructing a sustainable vision requires commitment and engagement from all who will participate in its execution and will be expected to play a key role leading to its successful application in the system.

> **Complex Adaptive Systems thinking is essential to outlining how the organization functions. From a whole-systems perspective, the contribution and constraints found in any part of the system are clearer to all.**

If the vision entails the implementation of interdisciplinary shared governance, most players will not have a clue what that means. Even after years of implementation, not all the definitions will be clear to everyone. What is crystal clear, however, is the need to view health and health care from an entirely different perspective than has been used in the past. The value of using systems thinking is that it offers a much more complete context for observing, learning, and designing for sustainable change.

The learning that happens along the way continuously alters people's viewpoints. As is true with all evidence-based approaches, what is thought to be true may change radically from one day to the next, depending on what new information or insights have occurred in the meantime. Although some may feel the previously held views are invalidated, experience is indicating that each new level of learning refines the old views rather than nullifies them. It is just that the evolution is so rapid that it can appear chaotic. Developing comfort with that chaos is one of the challenges of the new environment. In fact, it is very difficult because so many of the old linkages are gone, whereas the new ones are not yet fully in place.

So what is a linkage? No doubt everyone involved will be struggling with that question for many years to come, but progress is being made. In our view, a linkage consists of the following characteristics:

- A set of interrelationships that control behavior and connect elements of a system
- The influences on the dynamics at work in any given situation that are the living parts of the interrelationships
- The drive of the structure itself to develop certain types of interrelationships
- The feelings each individual has in trying to be aware of his or her own personal needs and what the whole organization needs at the same time ("Are my thoughts and actions in tune with the whole?")

At innovative hospitals and health systems, the learning goes on, but linkages are felt, and their absence is noted very quickly when shared governance-oriented reorganizing and restructuring has occurred. As soon as the dismantling of old structure begins, the breakdown in linkage is often revealed by the increasing number of complaints and the feelings of being outside the loop, even among those who were heavily involved in designing the changes.

What is observable in shared governance is the representation of the various perspectives. For example, policies and procedures, memos and minutes, plans and conceptual drawings are all tangible. What may be more important, though, is what can be felt. One feels linkage when there is a pressure to behave in some way defined through one's relationships. There is an energy that flows along the linkage that creates a sense of urgency to act. This is often evidenced in the revealing of the distance between where one is and the location of the agreed goal. Reinforcing and balancing influences have their effect through these linkages. There can never be a change in one element of the system without some exchange of energy with other elements through the linkages.

A change in any one part of a system means a shift in every part of the system.

STRUCTURAL LINKAGES

A typical hospital system in the United States used to be made up of hundreds of cost centers supervised by hundreds of supervisors and managed by 10 or more layers of expert managers and administrators (see Exhibit 4-2). As indicated in other chapters of this text, there were dozens of vice presidents and senior vice presidents, many assistant administrators and directors, several presidents (one of whom was also a chief operating officer [COO]), and the chief executive officer (CEO). Decisions were made in a hierarchy of management groups and committees, such as the CEO cabinet, the CEO council, the administrative staff committees, and specialty-specific management groups. It frequently took months to get capital requests through the system. Any major policy change or tactical plan change took even longer. No one manager or director in the system had a picture of the whole, nor was anyone accountable for the success of the whole. Indeed, the senior leader had an incentive to make his or her own facility succeed even if at the cost of harming one of the other facilities in the system. It is not easy to understand what the benefits of this structure were, but there was and still is significant bemoaning of its loss.

In one hospital system, restructuring in an interdisciplinary shared governance approach reduced 214 management positions to a total of 34 management positions and 6 consultant positions. The position of only one person was not touched, and that was the CEO, who was the unswerving champion of the changes then and since. The 34 managers included 30 service leaders (pathway), 2 facility integrators (physical plant), and 2 service integrators (administrators). The two service integrators and the consultants answered to the CEO, and the facility integrators answered to the service integrators. The principles used in creating the structure and creating new linkages were these:

- The continuum of care across an individual's lifetime should be the backbone of the living system.
- The shared governance principles of accountability, equity, partnership, and ownership should be the behavioral ideals.
- A shared vision incorporating these principles should be the center of all design efforts.
- The congruence of the structure with all the preceding must be ensured.
- Support systems need to be designed around the shared goal of "managing the health of the community to a value standard."

Guiding ideas were then spun off of these principles. These ideas have become more and more the rules of action followed by staff working on any problem or project.

Exhibit 4-2   Management Layers

- Service or team coordinators
- Assistant supervisors
- Supervisors
- Assistant managers
- Managers
- Assistant directors
- Directors
- Assistant administrators
- Associate administrators
- Administrators
- Vice presidents
- Senior vice presidents
- President
- COO
- CEO

NEW VALUES

The range of options can be made congruent with the theme by asking the question, "What evidence of value does this add to managing a patient to a value standard?" Value standards fall into four categories: localness, openness, quality (service), and flexibility. Examples of possible value standards include these:

- Localness. Ninety percent of all decisions should be made at the point of service.
- Openness. Resources such as information belong to everyone. Everyone can be trusted with the information they need to make their decisions.
- Quality. Everyone is accountable for ideal patient flows (experiences and outcomes).
- Flexibility. None of our structures, systems, policies, or procedures is perfect. All can be changed in the light of new information or ideas.

The gestation period for instilling guiding ideas is not short. It often takes years, not months. One of the service integrators in a transforming hospital carries around a verse from Longfellow's "Psalm of Life":

> Let us, then, be up and doing,
> With a heart for any fate;
> Still achieving, still pursuing,
> Learn to labor and to wait.

The labor spent in instilling guiding ideas and designing the structure based on these ideas is an investment in the future, and although it always has some short-term benefits almost immediately, the larger benefits will take a longer time to arrive.

DELINEATING THE PATHWAYS

Functions are sorted into two categories along the continuum: member service pathways and support service pathways. The pathways function as illustrated in Figure 4-3.

At the outset, the focus of the change leadership is on the corporate organization and does not expand to include the full integrated health network and the service community until later in the process. The pathway design drives the management structure, and the number of service leaders (pathway managers) is determined through agreement to a span-of-control target of more than 100 to 150 workers per manager.

Decisions regarding the practice, quality, and education issues for the pathways fall within the accountability of the pathway councils. Decisions across pathways are the accountability of the corporate councils (service, operations, and governance). Figures 4-4 and 4-5 show the linkages to the medical staff

---

Figure 4-3   Service Pathways

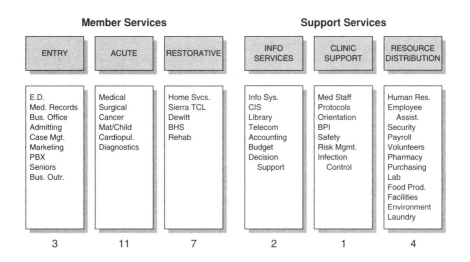

Member Services			Support Services		
ENTRY	ACUTE	RESTORATIVE	INFO SERVICES	CLINIC SUPPORT	RESOURCE DISTRIBUTION

E.D.
Med. Records
Bus. Office
Admitting
Case Mgt.
Marketing
PBX
Seniors
Bus. Outr.
	Medical
	Surgical
	Cancer
	Mat/Child
	Cardiopul.
	Diagnostics
		Home Svcs.
		Sierra TCL
		Dewitt
		BHS
		Rehab
			Info Sys.
			CIS
			Library
			Telecom
			Accounting
			Budget
			Decision
			  Support
				Med Staff
				Protocols
				Orientation
				BPI
				Safety
				Risk Mgmt.
				Infection
				  Control
					Human Res.
					Employee
					  Assist.
					Security
					Payroll
					Volunteers
					Pharmacy
					Purchasing
					Lab
					Food Prod.
					Facilities
					Environment
					Laundry

3	11	7	2	1	4

Figure 4-4   Integrated Pathways

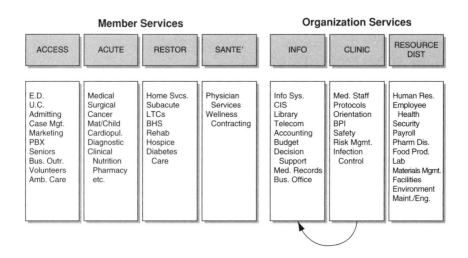

Figure 4-5   The Patient Care Leadership After Integration

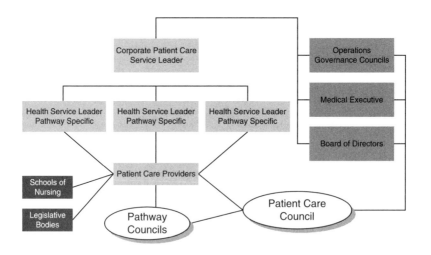

structure as well as the linkages between councils and provider teams (within each pathway).

The provider team is the core of the service system because it lies at the heart of the point of service. All linkages are designed to directly or indirectly support the functional service areas. The provider is now empowered to make point-of-service decisions and is supported by the structure. The accountability of each of the decision centers of the structure flows from the work needed to sustain and preserve the relationships between the team members and those they serve. In some integrated models, for example, the patient is also a team member and has the same goal—achieving the best outcome possible.

The support area teams (engineering, laundry, grounds, etc.) are called *service teams*. Early in the development of the new system, the support pathways are often a step removed from the point of service and are therefore viewed as less critical to the outcomes. This perception of them is at odds with the notion of whole-systems integration, in which each element is of value to the whole. Such thinking also begins to create pathway boundaries that, although fewer in number, are no less debilitating than the department barriers of the old model. At the inception of shared governance, the focus is on changing the support pathways into process teams that are more fully integrated into the continuum of care activities. In time, what were once identified as separate support structures will disappear.

SYSTEMS LINKAGES

A continuum of care cannot be maintained without tools. The information system becomes the center around which the health system revolves. Indeed, information forms the foundation of the sustainability of the future health system (see Figure 4-6). The ability to link professions and information together becomes critical to speed, portability, and technology application. Without an adequate information infrastructure, none of the current teletechnologies can be implemented. There is a need to identify the contributing factors increasing the cost of health care and control them. In a user-based approach, the only way to ensure control is to build an information system that provides immediate and accurate data to those who need it.

THE NEED FOR INFORMATION

Information, to be effective, must be in a format that meets the needs of those who receive and use it. Most information systems reflect the perceptions

Figure 4-6   The Future Shared Governance Community Health System

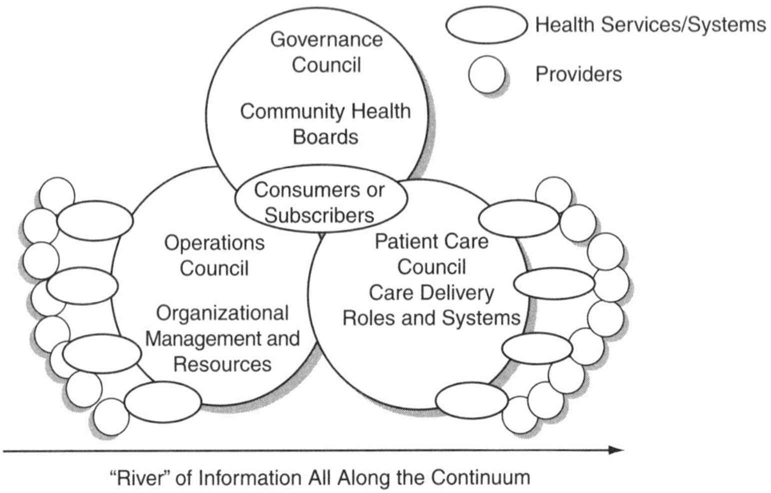

"River" of Information All Along the Continuum

of the information experts, not necessarily the needs of the users. In the future, user-friendly and provider-driven information structures must be built that tie all the components of the system together in a meaningful way.

> **Information is the lifeblood of the shared governance organization. Indeed, it is the central variable that will determine the organization's sustainability.**

The multimodal linkages related to building a clinical continuum demand support constructed so as to interface with the clinical process. Further, whatever information systems are built, they must intersect in a way that addresses the organizational system's comprehensive information needs. Some considerations that will have to be addressed are as follows:

- The information system must reflect the patient's health journey or pathway and must track the patient through all the intersections needed in the system.
- The information that is available must be comprehensive. It should include financial, resource, and clinical data in a format that makes service delivery effective and resource issues clear to all the providers.

- Everyone who needs information should have easy access to it, and it should be in a form that allows it to be understood and used.
- The information system is expected to link the various service settings, such as the physician's office, the clinic, the outpatient center, the patient's home, and acute services.
- Clinical performance evaluation along the care continuum is essential to determine clinical effectiveness at all levels of the service system.
- The ability to evaluate and change the parameters of service when the data suggest they need to be changed is increasingly necessary as clinical protocols become more precise and more fully inculcated into the delivery of patient care services.
- Information systems operate at the point of service so that the clinical users can access what is needed and document the activities of clinical work in a way that interfaces well with the other parameters' guiding action.

Perhaps nothing will have as great an impact on the design of health services as the development of an integrated, portable, and decentralized information system. The major capital project for most forward-thinking health systems will be a well-designed and integrated health information infrastructure.

PATHWAYS AND INFORMATION

Building service-specific pathways that are clinically focused and user driven is an essential task, and structuring them within the context of a well-defined and functioning information system will be critical to long-term success. It is also important for users to be computer literate, because any provider's work life will be influenced by what the information system provides in the way of support and information about outcomes. Therefore, the development programs of the health system of the future must provide a thorough understanding of computer and information systems.

> **Systems linkage tells the members of the organization where the key intersections are and how the system maintains its integrity.**

To begin to understand why some of the system linkages were built, one must keep in mind four system levels at once: events, patterns of behavior, systems, and mental models. All four are interrelated, and a change in one causes change in the others. Systems thinking was in its infancy during the initial development of information systems, and at that time the goal was simply to make sure that the weight of the old manual and paper systems did not impede the burgeoning new systems. That meant that, in each case, the kinds of things influencing workers' beliefs and actions should "look" like the new system, leaving as little of the old system as possible to break the workers' dependence upon it. Performance evaluation, competency testing, compensation policies and procedures, style of communication, informal rewards, and access to resources (purchase requisitions, etc.) all had to change to reflect the new information infrastructure principles and models.

The effort to incorporate complex adaptive systems notions should begin when the shared governance process is initiated. The implementation process associated with information system development will lag behind the full understanding of the principles and guiding ideas underpinning interdisciplinary shared governance. For example, compensation management changes will require abundant education of human resource and information management personnel as well as other members of the health system. At the outset, many of the staff will still see the old system operating, which will delay the generation of evidence demonstrating the viability of the new approach to compensation management. Leadership forbearance is especially important during this period of change. Even senior managers can experience this developmental lag and might long for the old system because of its familiarity and stability while they are struggling with the application of a better but uncharted compensation information system.

In the first year, as more of the information infrastructure is implemented within the shared governance model, the new system begins to work better and eventually becomes the accepted means of performance measurement and compensation management.

COMMUNICATION LINKAGES

In contemporary systems, it is no longer optional to unfold a continuum of clinical processes without linking it tightly with the operating information infrastructure. The movement to a digital system from a paper system is fraught with all kinds of difficulties. Organizational leaders will recognize early on how powerful the addiction to paper processes has become and how revolutionary and transformational the construction of a paper-free approach to the management of organizational and clinical information is. Building a digital information infrastructure calls not only for new systems, but also radically transformed mental models that call people to new conceptualizations of communication and information in a way radically different from that most providers have experienced.

> **The major problems in implementing any change can be most frequently attributed to failures in the communication process.**

Deep in the struggle to redesign the shared governance structure, both staff and management come to feel they are on a roller coaster ride while living the changes. No matter how comprehensive, the changes themselves seem to be only superficial evidence of the organization's real shift. The real changes are much deeper—at the heart of the organization. The interdependence of individuals, one relying on another, in times of "noise" is incredibly energizing, whether the consequences are positive or negative. Everyone feels the energy of transformation but no one can pin it down or define what it is. Yet, at the heart of it is the significant reconfiguration of the entire information infrastructure that supports contemporary clinical practice.

> **Before it can become a learning organization, any healthcare organization must ensure that its members engage in systems learning.**

All kinds of lessons are learned about communication while implementing new organizational structures. According to systems thinking, dialogue lies at the foundation of every human enterprise. Without it, little agreement in the organization will be possible. Ruffles of change may appear around the edges, but a critical mass is never attained unless it has been preceded with vast amounts of focused, intense dialogue. New communication linkages must be built and tested against the new patterns of behavior and events unfolding every day. There must also be coherence between what is "talked" and what is "walked" before dialogue gains momentum.

One thing that is learned once communication becomes formalized in the infrastructure is that sensitivity to linkages pays big dividends. For example, one learning lab process that can be helpful in building commitment to learning and achieving positive outcomes is called *whole-system templating*. This process can also be used to help change agents consider linkages and impacts of change while in the design and redesign phases of their work. Whole-system templates are brainstormed with mixed groups of stakeholders as a means of helping novice and advanced beginner systems thinkers to look at the broader implications of changes they might be considering.

Templating is not flowcharting or model building but rather the practicing of new disciplines together with colleagues in a defined practice field. All templates result from a walkthrough of some of the linkages identified in health delivery organizations that create general parameters for the practice field. The process itself must be loose, drawing more from the right side of the brain that houses our capacity to comprehend wholes, patterns, and synthesis. It requires integration rather than analysis and therefore concentrates more on relationships and context than a tally of neatly ordered parts.

Often, visualizing a change helps translate it into a plan that can be implemented.

The desired outcome of a templating session is greater awareness of the whole. Only a few basic assumptions are used in all templating sessions. One is that all open systems are constantly exchanging energy with their environments and that the exchanges are highly organized but in constant change—a constantly flowing or moving exchange of energy. The principal task is to establish a new cycle of learning that connects practice and performance (note that synthesis is an important method for the whole). The goals are the following:

- To achieve breakthroughs in learning infrastructure
- To help everyone imagine the whole
- To help everyone rethink and recognize his or her own relationship to the whole
- To strive for alignment of vision and mental models

The technique of templating grows through application and is different for every group that attempts it, but the results are usually very positive.

Another helpful exercise is based on an old technique called *focusing*, which grew out of Eugene Gendlin's (1998) work at the University of Chicago. Roughly, it requires people to sit quietly, focus on an image or idea, and allow feelings to well up. They then ask that feeling to identify itself and judge whether the answer is correct by whether it "feels" right. A feeling-based consensus can sometimes result when a group tries to visualize linkages and their relationships to the whole. The group outcomes are amazingly easy to translate into the practical and concrete designs for new processes and systems. It is as if a road map is laid out in front of a traveler who has been trying to create it one mile at a time.

THE PROCESS OF BUILDING LINKAGES AND TEAMS

The building of linkages is an ideal place to use the template approach. The first step is to select a group of empowered, energetic workers who represent a variety of perspectives. They must be willing to take risks and withstand some noise from their co-workers to do the right thing for the patient population and community they serve. Once that group is organized, some basics must be agreed upon:

- Rules of engagement
- Rules of brainstorming
- Use of the five disciplines of a learning organization
- Common problem-solving steps
- Definitions of template elements

The rules of engagement are meant to define how the individuals interact within the group setting to maximize the ability of the group to accomplish its work. The group determines what those rules are going to be, but the rules generally include both the rules of polite society (e.g., do not interrupt others and be on time) as well as rules for handling issues (e.g., be willing to confront issues and be honest and truthful).

The brainstorming rules are intended to create an environment conducive to creative thinking, especially the sort in which one member's thoughts inspire others to have even more creative thoughts. The rules consist of such items as these:

- Have fun.
- All ideas have merit.
- Allow no one person to dominate.
- Encourage all members to participate.
- Try to build on one another's creativity.
- No pagers!

The five disciplines of a learning organization—shared vision, mental models, systems thinking, personal mastery, and team learning—form the foundation for linkage design. They are used to "see" the system and the implications of changes. They channel the group's thinking so that it is productive and the linkages are congruent with the needs the new system is designed to meet.

Common problem-solving steps are discussed to develop a common language for talking about change. Unless change terminology is discussed early with the team, it will be difficult to flowchart the "as is" in language the team can understand and to which they can respond.

Defining template elements is the way the group begins to narrow the universe of work possible in linkage design. Examples of template elements include the following:

- Vision, values, guiding ideas
- Structure
- Governance
- Decision-making loci
- Information flows in and out of decision-making loci
- Cultural dynamics, such as
  - Informal leaders
  - Linguistic interpretation
  - Traditions or customs
  - How ideas flow through the informal networks
  - Changing roles and status
- Formal information flows
  - Expectations of council and team members regarding verbal communication
  - Written communication flows
  - Access to information systems
  - Design of information systems
- Observable signals of empowerment
- Culturally determined systems of competence (the understanding of the differences in linkage required by populations of various cultures)

INTERACTIONS IN THE SYSTEM

Anything that influences the relationships between the system components (or any place where there is an exchange of energy) can be used as a template element. These things become the pieces of a jigsaw puzzle. The outside border, like the jigsaw pieces with the straight edge, is made up of the vision and mental models that are shared.

> **All systems support what goes on at their center. The purpose of the structure is to support the service.**

The vision and mental models grow out of the need to do more than deliver inpatient care. The mission of most facilities includes the goal of "improving the health status of the community." This cannot be effectively achieved using the old department structure. The natural barriers to stretching care across the continuum of care are often too tough to break. For example, unit managers usually possess accountability for a unit budget and will rarely risk dealing with issues related to the care of whole patient populations. CEOs and finance officers whose bonuses are based on annual hospital profits are reticent to spend precious dollars on things with no clear short-term benefit.

ORGANIZING AROUND THE PATIENT

For the mission of improving health status to be fulfilled, a new "model of response to patient need" is required as the first step. Health is a continuum from birth to death, whereas an illness lasts from onset to cure or death. Old-style hospital systems are built around segmented functions (departments) designed to deliver repetitious tasks within a specialty to all the patients for whom services are ordered in a given day. In a more user-driven health system, the services are designed around the movement of each person along their continuum toward the best health status possible. Systems are then organized around the patient (patient-focused or -centered care), and the organization is designed around patient populations. Support functions are created as process teams organized around a set of outcomes that support the delivery of services to those populations. As an example, in the master path diagram (Figure 4-7), the continuum displays parallel paths toward the best health status possible for individuals and populations. At the system level, this means that the primary care provider (PCP), in partnership with the member, is the manager or facilitator of the master path. The goal is to maintain maximum health, and only a failure of that pathway results in illness or a detour from the pathway.

When a member has some episode that requires more intensive application of resources, the result is a detour from the master path. Detours may require that the member become an inpatient in an acute facility, have surgery in an outpatient surgery center, spend a few weeks in a convalescent facility, or have some other less intensive intervention. In the case of any detour, the goal is to get the person back on the healthy master path as soon as possible.

The patient populations or users are broadly described and are basically healthy. Those requiring closer focus are the chronically but not acutely ill population and the acutely ill or injured population, and of course these populations can be further divided. Operational pathways are designed to create an operational organization to support the various identified patient populations and to make it easier to manage each population (or individual patient) across the continuum, as shown in Figure 4-8. These pathways initially are just acute care related but expand to include physicians' offices and clinics. Integrating efforts

Figure 4-7   Master Path Diagram

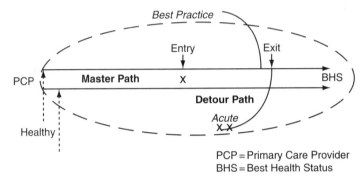

Purpose: to manage the health of the community to a value standard

Figure 4-8   Integrated Health Network Core System Components, Phase One

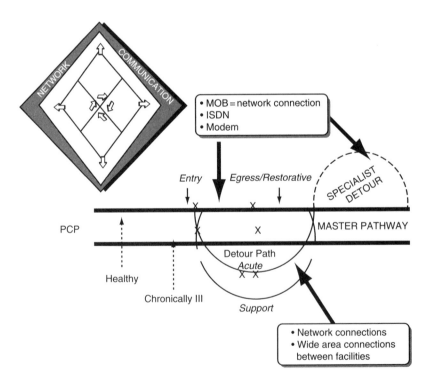

across all points of service is the responsibility of leadership. It is leadership's obligation to see clinical pathways in the same way that we conceive neural pathways, systems linkages, and information systems. This "systems" context provides the framework for a narrative that better articulates the clinical system with the flow realities associated with population or patient characteristics.

Ultimately, interdisciplinary shared governance reflects these broader whole-systems conceptualizations and brings them into the life of a healthcare organization and structures it based on the realities of processes associated with such systems. Without conceiving out of this systems context, whole-systems activities such as interdisciplinary shared governance cannot be fully realized. In the translation of systems concepts into reality, each pathway covers all related facilities and services and has one management and governance structure. Corporate service and operations councils with members from all pathways deal with issues affecting all the pathways (see Chapters 4 and 5).

MAKING THE SYSTEM FUNCTIONAL

In keeping with a systems construct, service elements within the pathway are organized into a pathway council and point-of-service provider teams. These pathways are a refinement and a more systems-reflective transition from the traditional service or product line structural models. The pathway council has staff members representing perspectives from all the service areas within the pathway. Managers often sit as advisors and bring the requisite resource perspective, but the chairs are providers. Physicians are strongly encouraged to be members of these councils and provider teams rather than critics or distant advisors. The meetings are held at times that make it as convenient as possible for physicians to attend. The groups are multidisciplinary and make all the decisions about how the work is to be done. The one exception to the rule is the "best practices" process. It should be a part of a support pathway, and its council is made up of best practices physicians and providers from other disciplines. The work of this subpathway is to generate a best practices environment for the whole system and is heavily focused on providing the physicians in the system with the things they need to manage patient populations successfully.

Physician membership on councils builds partnerships between stakeholders and ensures that all stakeholders are involved in the making of decisions that will affect them.

Exhibit 4-3   Continuum of Care Services

Everything must integrate across the system for the purpose of building a seamless continuum of care.

Continuum
- Primary and Family Health
- Cancer Services
- Rehabilitation
- Behavioral Health
- Home Services
- Women's Health
- Community Services
- Acute Services
- Trauma Level 1
- Burn Unit

The linkages between the points of service are complex and critical. Not only must the pathways work across facility lines, the provider teams must work and have support across pathway lines (see Exhibit 4-3). Decision making is moved increasingly to the point of service, requiring point-of-service access to the information needed to make informed decisions.

There is no way to put together new provider teams across a whole system and have them all be competent on the first day. Everyone starts out as a novice and must stumble a little on the way to competence. It is very important to provide an environment in which the standards are clarified and reclarified and in which the stumbling is viewed as positive learning instead of a reason for termination.

> All transformation requires learning from everyone in the system. Indeed, the system becomes a learning organization.

In the pathway design, the template elements are considered one at a time and then expanded as all try to see the way these influences might operate on the components of the system. For instance, the way physicians used to make things happen when they were unhappy was to go to the CEO or to the board of directors. The new linkage requires them to go to the point-of-service team if the issue is a patient care, clinical, or relational issue. The team member who deals with the issue then discusses with the physician how to directly address it. They come to an agreement about how to proceed and put in measures to ensure successful follow-up. If the concern cuts across pathways, the team member brings the physician to the pathway or corporate council to further refine the solution. Whatever solution is agreed to here is final.

Should the problem require immediate action, the team member and physician can act on the spot or include an empowered chair of the unit or pathway council in the decision making. This allows the "management by committee" barriers to be sidestepped when speed is important. All quick-response decisions are reviewed by the appropriate group to make sure any needed communication linkages are constructed and any education requirements met. The CEO should always refer complaining physicians back to the point of service. Such a response, made in a supportive way, begins the slow and inexorable culture shift. Physicians must always be actively involved in making collaborative decisions in most, if not all, of the pathway councils and provider teams.

All members of the system experience role changes. For the acute facility caregiver, the old role was to complete all assigned tasks according to productivity targets without any untoward patient events. Accomplishment of tasks over a long period usually meant a salary increase, and working occasional extra shifts, mentoring new workers, or taking on special assignments would likely result in an outstanding performance review rating. Historically, there was little or no requirement to fully collaborate with other disciplines, and the outcomes of cases were not carefully tracked. The goal was simply to get tasks done while avoiding unpleasant incidents.

In the new environment, the requirements are significantly different. Now care providers are accountable for moving each patient through the episode of illness or injury to the best value outcome (meaning the best clinical outcome at the least cost). Not only must a caregiver do the kinds of things necessary to achieve the desired outcome whether they are on a traditional work list or not, the provider must also marshal other resources to expedite recuperation. The new environment has standards for value outcomes that must be met or exceeded, and any variance from these standards must be reviewed by the team so that any problems can be solved. Instead of the traditional approach to the performance of individual providers being evaluated, the systems construct now reflects individual accountability such that it becomes the obligation of each participant in the membership community to demonstrate the effectiveness of performance using definitive evidence-based measures and targets.

> **Shared governance is not management by committee; if it is, it simply does not work. It is, instead, an accountability-based approach to obtaining effective decisions.**

A number of linkages are required to enable providers to operate effectively in their new role. Information must be complete and easily accessible. It must include not only the clinical data and the standards but the financial data and the targets. Real-time glimpses of how providers are doing on a given case would be the ideal. Other linkages include connections to the evaluation, compensation, and competency processes, which must all be redesigned to support the new role. The providers must have a loose relationship with the pathway council and feel supported by that council when evidence-based practices lead them to a better way to deliver care.

The availability of resources is critical to the success of the providers. Providers must have the ability to purchase what they need when they need it to improve outcomes without having to go through a long or convoluted approval process. At some hospitals, for example, a checking account containing $10,000 is disbursed to each care area for staff to spend as they see fit. This is a commitment to empowerment that might average a minimum of $200,000 over a 6-month period. The fear initially was that the workers would spend indiscriminately. The opposite has actually occurred. Many provider teams spent less than the allotted amount; they all tracked what they spent, and wonderful, thoughtful things were done to help patients and their families, with no manager intervention or approval required. The results were so encouraging that the same amounts have again been allotted to the staff. There are now more people understanding budget and purchasing in the organization than ever before and making independent decisions at the point of service to help patients reach their best health status.

Manager roles also change significantly. In the old paradigm, the manager directed activities, and all significant decisions had to be made by or approved by the person in control of a department. The managers, in turn, were restricted by the department structure and by facility boundaries. In shared governance, the manager is coach, mentor, teacher, and resource manager. The boundaries between facilities or institutions are gone because the structure does away with departments, and the service or pathway manager is accountable for providing whatever the providers need in any pathway across all facilities.

Managers may budget dollars, but they rarely spend them; their staff does!

The management group is the hardest group to get to accept their new role because it represents a shift of individual power to the point-of-service teams. The linkages required for this group to move have to do with core values and lots of dialogue. Eventually managers learn to value helping the teams find their own way to the best outcomes instead of making them follow the steps the managers think will lead to the best outcomes.

The issue for whole-systems shared governance leaders very quickly becomes; how big is the whole? With large corporate concerns currently swallowing up health care-related organizations, there is little doubt that building an organization that is fast, fluid, flexible, and horizontal is a good survival tactic. Understanding the linkages within one's own system and the linkages to the global system requires a new awareness. As Kenichi Ohmae (2002) points out in his book *Triad Power*, "However managers do it, however they get there, building a value system that emphasizes seeing and thinking globally is the bottom line price of admission to today's borderless economy."

The next step after integrating across organizational boundaries may be integrating across zonal (regional) boundaries on a much grander scale. Regardless of the requisites for inclusion, there must be a format, a structure, through which relationships can be obtained, facilitated, and sustained. This structure must bring the stakeholders together and provide a format for the work they do. Its parameters must be flexible and fluid in a way that allows for adaptation and dramatic change. In shared governance, a framework is established that moves an organization from vertical to systems linkages, fosters inclusive relationships, and provides the parameters for changing the organization's configuration to one that supports a systems view and the intersection of all the elements that make a system successful and sustainable.

REFERENCES

Gendlin, E. (1998). *Experiencing and the creation of meaning.* Chicago: Northwestern University Press.

Ohmae, K. (2002). *Triad power.* New York: Free Press.

SUGGESTED READING

Ball, M. J. (2000). *Nursing informatics: Where caring and technology meet* (3rd ed.). New York: Springer.

Caldwell, J. T. (2000). *Electronic media and technoculture.* New Brunswick, NJ: Rutgers University Press.

Cloke, K., & Goldsmith, J. (2002). *The end of management and the rise of organizational democracy* (1st ed.). San Francisco: Jossey-Bass.

Cook, D., & Das, S. K. (2005). *Smart environments: Technologies, protocols, and applications.* Hoboken, NJ: John Wiley.

Gueutal, H. G., & Stone, D. L. (2005). *The brave new world of eHR: Human resources management in the digital age* (1st ed.). San Francisco, CA: Jossey-Bass.

Johnson, C. E., Kralewski, J. E., Lemak, C. H., Cote, M. J., & Deane, J. (2002). The adoption of computer-based information systems by medical groups in a managed care environment. *Journal of Ambulatory Care Management, 25*, 40–51.

Kelly, K. (2005). *Out of control: The new biology of machines, social systems, and the economic world.* New York: Perseus.

O'Neil, E., Dluhy, N., Fortier, P., & Michel, H. (2004). Knowledge acquisition, synthesis and validation: A model for decision support systems. *Journal of Advanced Nursing, 47*(2), 134–142.

Oostendorp, H. v. (2003). *Cognition in a digital world.* Mahwah, NJ: Erlbaum.

Shi, L., & Singh, D. A. (2004). *Delivering health care in America: A systems approach* (3rd ed.). Sudbury, MA: Jones and Bartlett.

Trompenaars, A., & Hampden-Turner, C. (2002). *21 leaders for the 21st century: How innovative leaders manage in the digital age.* New York: McGraw-Hill.

U.S. President's Information Technology Advisory Committee & U.S. National Coordination Office for Information Technology Research and Development. (2004). *Revolutionizing health care through information technology: Report to the President.* Retrieved July 22, 2008, from http://purl.access.gpo.gov/GPO/LPS52723

Wilson, T. B. (2003). *Innovative reward systems for the changing workplace* (2nd ed.). New York: McGraw-Hill.

Wingate, G. (2004). *Computer systems validation: Quality assurance, risk management, and regulatory compliance for pharmaceutical and healthcare companies.* Boca Raton, FL: Interpharm/CRC.

Decisions from the Center: Building a Sustainable Interdisciplinary Microsystem at the Point of Service

Kami English, Curtis Takamoto, and Tim Porter-O'Grady

> *The first order of business is to build a group of people who, under the influence of the institution, grow taller and become healthier, stronger, more autonomous.*
>
> —ROBERT K. GREENLEAF

Obtaining the commitment of each player in the system is a fundamental expectation of any distributive decision-making system. In fact, professional organizations are considered to be membership communities (as are all social-clinical microsystems). These kinds of communities have a specific set of expectations upon which membership depends. Membership in the professional community (microsystem) expects a certain kind of preparation and education, standards of performance, behavior, and outcomes. In membership communities these expectations should be clarified and clearly enumerated in advance of membership. This level of clarity makes certain that the accountability for performance is clearly defined, the measures of that performance are clearly outlined, and the behaviors associated with that performance are clearly evidenced by the member. The need for clarity of accountability is critical to performance against the expectations of membership. Accountability abhors ambiguity. And because shared governance is built on accountability as its cornerstone, clarity with regard to what accountability means and how it is applied within disciplines and between them is critical to the success of this structure (see Exhibit 5-1).

Accountability is the foundation for good systems design. It is not participation that defines a good organization; it is, instead, sustainable results.

Shared governance is intended to provide a framework for ensuring that an accountability-based approach can be sustained over an extended period of time. The effectiveness of a shared governance system is dependent upon the full

Exhibit 5-1   Key Principles of Shared Governance

1. Always build both decisions and structure on a point-of-service foundation.
2. Stakeholders are always involved in their own decisions.
3. Shared governance is an accountability-based approach, not a participative management model.
4. Team-based strategies are always basic to any shared governance structural design.
5. The locus of control in a system is placed wherever appropriate for the decision required.
6. There are no approval structures in shared governance.
7. Managers focus on context; staff focus on content.
8. Partnership, equity, accountability, and ownership are the principles that undergird shared governance.
9. Shared governance reflects the relatedness between people and systems, not their status within the system.

and complete engagement and ownership of those who make it up. A system that creates barriers to the engagement of workers or uses parental strategies to control and manage workers, creates the basis for its own undoing. New organizational constructs, the emergence of the knowledge worker culture, and point-of-service-driven work arrangements have changed the relationship between the participants in the workplace and created a basis for the design of a shared governance structure. In fact, this notion of full engagement, partnership, and ownership of one's work is fundamental to shared governance and critical to the successful performance of all professional organizations.

PATIENT CARE: THE FOUNDATIONS OF HEALTH SERVICE

The ultimate aim of the healthcare system is to improve the health of the general public. Although this purpose may have been obscured over the years by the focus on treatment of illness rather than the much broader goal of building healthy communities, there is a growing new emphasis on healthcare service driven by the need to determine value, the demand for sustainable outcomes, and the growing focus on the continuum of services.

The primary aim of healthcare systems is to improve the health of the general public. Many healthcare professionals have forgotten their mission and have instead become self-serving.

The design and structure of the healthcare system is being radically altered. The demand is growing for a shift in focus from illness and intervention to user-driven primary care and community health. This shift in focus creates an essential shift in the design, structuring, and integration of the point-of-service delivery of health care.

Newer notions of work and how it is organized have changed some of the constructs and contexts for the delivery of healthcare services. Organizing around patient pathways, a seamless continuum of service, and the use of product or service lines are examples of these changes. In all of them, integration, interdisciplinary interaction, care management, demand management, evidence-based practice, and advancing the continuum of care serve as a foundation for the design and structuring of the future of health care.

Always, in any design and delivery approach, the focus is on appropriate use of resources. During the first stage of healthcare reform in the United States, cost has been the driving force, but ultimately it will not be sufficient as a factor motivating increased effectiveness. The issues of culture, quality, and sustainability must become a focus for building a comprehensive approach to managing and delivering healthcare services. Again, to ensure the viability of an organization, all stakeholders must at some level be involved in activities that address price, quality, and service. Within the shared governance context, it is believed most of those activities must occur at the point of service, requiring the involvement and investment of stakeholders whose work it is to deliver cost-effective and evidence-based services and to evaluate the value of the services provided.

> **Although cost may be the portal through which we enter a period of significant change, it is not sufficient alone to sustain either effective service or viable outcomes.**

It is no longer an option for those at the point of service to have a limited responsibility for ensuring the value and effectiveness of the work they do. Increasingly, knowledge of the outcomes of work activities is used to delineate and assess the delivery of healthcare services individually and collectively. Through the use of tools such as clinical protocols, best practices, service algorithms, evidence-based dynamics, and care maps, the appropriateness and value of point-of-service activities are gradually becoming better understood.

The information infrastructure of an organization can supply meaningful data on the efficacy of the services provided. The availability of this information, its locus of control at the point of service, and the necessity of knowing the outcomes of one's work converge to create the conditions that require ownership, investment, evaluation, and response to what the data show about clinical practice and its impact. In healthcare systems, as has been learned in the business community, real value-driven decision making should be located at the point of service, and thus effective healthcare systems increasingly must develop relevant information services and systems to support the decision making and activities of those at the point of service.

> **It doesn't pay to live in the past. . . . There's no future in it!**

One major purpose of a shared governance structure is to create a configuration that not only allows but requires those at the point of service to fully participate in decision making, planning, and evaluation of their efforts. In particular, a shared governance structure is designed to limit any other process, position, or location for making decisions anywhere else in the system that properly belong at the point of service and as well provide a legitimate context supporting point-of-service decision making.

THE FUNDAMENTALS OF THE PATIENT CARE COUNCIL

> **Achieving value is more than simply controlling costs and providing a service. It is the "tight" balance between what is done, what it costs, and the results obtained that forms the foundation for real value.**

The structure of the organization should provide just enough format to ensure that decisions that belong at the point of service are not made elsewhere. Therefore, it is important to determine what kind of decisions are made at what places in the organization (see Figure 5-1).

Clearly, critical decision making and supportive interfaces require a sharp delineation of the appropriate location for each kind of decision. Summary authority (i.e., the right to make increasingly broader based decisions as one moves up the hierarchy of control) is not a valid principle of decision making within shared governance. Instead, in shared governance organizations, decision making is based on the recognition that competence to make decisions does not necessarily increase as one climbs upward. In a truly effective organizational system, it would be known who the best person to make a decision is—and that person would indeed make the decision.

Figure 5-1   Linkage of Shared Governance Councils

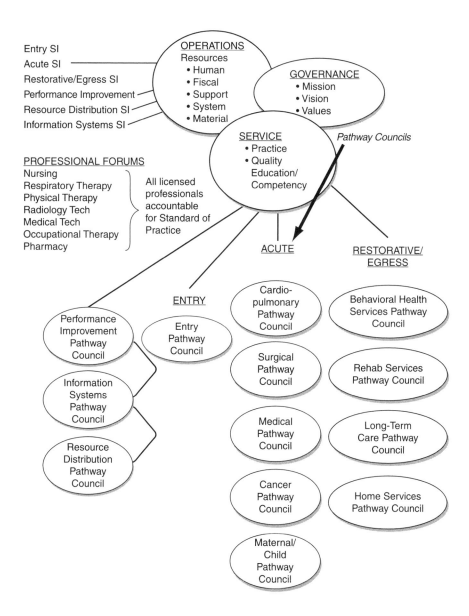

> It can no longer be assumed that one's competence increases as one climbs the organizational ladder. Competence does not necessarily change, but access to information is enhanced.

As noted in Chapter 3, decisions related to team functions and clinical activities must be made at the point of service. The structure of the system should prevent those decisions from being made any other place, and it should provide the decision maker whatever supports and tools are necessary for evaluating the options and choosing the one most likely to lead to a positive outcome.

At the unit/department/service pathway level, a different set of decisions—those related to the integration of relationships, critical paths, and best practices—are located. Here the focus is on linking the various teams along a particular clinical continuum. The service pathway devotes all of its resources and activities to the task of providing services to a specified group of patients.

The service pathway leadership is interested in the linkage and viability of the activities of each team. It does not have the obligation to define the activities and functions that belong to a team. It only looks at the interface between teams and the integration of their activities from a truly systems perspective.

> It does an organization no good to have the right competencies located in the wrong place.

The unit/department/service pathway council, which includes representatives from all pathway teams, deals with the broad issues of integration, intersection, continuity, effectiveness, efficiency, cost, relationship between services, and outcome. In fact, the service pathway council's role is to view the pathway as a whole in relationship to the population that it serves.

> A service pathway organizes work around the patient, not the provider. It depends on a good fit between the nature of the service provided and the demand of the consumer.

The notions of integrity and fit are at the center of the work of the service pathway council. Its focus on integrity and fit keeps the council from making decisions about functions and activities that fall within the authority of the individual teams. It is only when a relationship between teams becomes problematic, when clinical protocols or pathways are incomplete, or when a team's activities are clearly inconsistent with the service pathway's purposes and work, that the council pays close attention to specific activities. Further, because the service pathway council is made up of team leaders, it is the place in the system where their issues are pursued.

> **All services are now organized around the patient, not the provider. The tightness of fit between the population needs and the services provided creates the conditions for sustainability.**

The service pathway council and the pathway teams (unit/department/service) make up the core of the governance structure in a healthcare organization. More than 90 percent of the decisions are made and implemented within the pathway, and it is here where the critical work of building effectiveness, efficiency, integration, and relationship as well as evaluating the outcomes and service components of patient care delivery is undertaken. It is rational, therefore, to structure the organization in such a way that information and evaluation tools are available within the service pathway (unit/department/service).

> **The service pathway is focused on the specific culture of the services. The system is focused on the support of the services and their fit with the system's purposes and goals.**

The Purpose of the Patient Care Council

> **The patient care council integrates the service pathways in a decision-making process that addresses their relationship across the system.**

Any system must have a mechanism for maintaining its integrity. As mentioned previously, much of the structure of a shared governance organization is designed to support its point-of-service activities. The critical framework for those activities consists of the various service pathways that cater to the different populations served. Because each pathway is unique, a mechanism must exist to link the pathways and represent the purposes and principles of the organization as a whole. It is, after all, the organization that has an obligation to meet the full range of community healthcare needs.

While each of the service pathways looks at the functions and activities for a defined culture or patient population, the patient care council articulates the mission and objectives of the organization in light of the patient care processes devoted to providing appropriate and meaningful services to its community of consumers. The patient care council is also a place where the provider leadership can deal with issues of relationship, integrity, effectiveness, competence, and quality. Because the primary obligation of providers is to look after the interests of patients as both advocates and suppliers of care, it is important to ensure that conflicts between providers are addressed expeditiously. Resolving conflicts is one of the key functions of the patient care council.

The Patient Care Council Membership

The patient care council is not a management council and is therefore not made up of management leaders. Most of the members are clinical leaders, selected from the various service pathways, units, and departments in a way that provides linkage between the pathways and the council (see Figure 5-2). Because the responsibility for clinical decision making rests with the clinical providers, it is logical that the responsibility for decisions concerning the delineation and delivery of healthcare services also rests directly with the providers. Within a shared governance context, they have the obligation to maintain control and have accountability for these kinds of decisions.

In organizations, as in all structures, the system is not simply the sum of its parts. A system is exemplified by the seamless linkage of all the elements that define it.

Other members who help integrate the system, such as support service personnel and administrative personnel (e.g., the information services staff and the finance office), should also be linked to the patient care council in a way that provides the council with the essential information it needs to make effective decisions.

The patient care council is driven by clinical decision making. Therefore, it is made up of providers from the variety of pathways in the system.

It is recommended that half the members of the patient care council represent the licensed disciplines and the other half represent the service pathway (Exhibit 5-2). This ensures that the two groups get an equal hearing.

Figure 5-2   Patient Care Council Membership

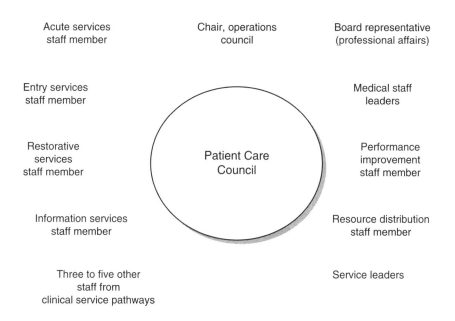

Acute services
staff member

Chair, operations
council

Board representative
(professional affairs)

Entry services
staff member

Medical staff
leaders

Restorative
services
staff member

Patient Care
Council

Performance
improvement
staff member

Information services
staff member

Resource distribution
staff member

Three to five other
staff from
clinical service pathways

Service leaders

The patient care council must not assume authority for decisions that belong elsewhere in the system. Decisions are accountability based, not authority driven. The notion of summary control is anathema to shared governance.

Exhibit 5-2   Principles of Council Membership Selection

- Each pathway should be represented.
- All members should be practicing staff or point-of-service workers.
- Tenure of service should be defined in advance.
- Expectations of service should be outlined in advance.
- All time spent doing council work should be compensated for.
- All councils should have access to any resource needed for decision making.
- Required qualifications should be published in advance.
- Work schedules should accommodate council work.
- Council accountability for decisions should be clear to members.
- Requirements of member roles should be understood prior to service.

Authority for decision making is invested in different bodies of the organization, and each decision-making group must have available to it the necessary competencies, support systems, and decision-making tools. Likewise, in the framework of shared governance, point-of-service decision-making supports must be available to ensure that appropriate decisions are made at the point of service (within teams and the service pathways).

To enhance organizational integrity, the patient care council should include representatives from the board of trustees, the medical staff, the administration, and the operations council. This notion usually creates some challenges in the organization because of the history of the separation of the board governance from the operations of the organization. Because shared governance is based on decision-making integrity, the notion of distinct roles and contributions is important to its success. Shared governance in no way diminishes the unique character and contribution of specified roles within the context of the system. Governance functions are just that, governance. However, membership on the patient care council by a member of the board brings to the table the unique governance perspective that only board representation can bring. Indeed, in shared governance, members at the table are expected to fully engage their unique role, not step out of it, but instead, bring it to the deliberation with the contribution that unique role provides to advance the quality, veracity, and efficacy of the decisions made. The inclusion of these representatives creates an interface between key decision makers and increases the probability that appropriate information and support will be available to facilitate sound decision making within the patient care council. It also ensures that the patient care council has access to persons who are accountable for the effectiveness of decision making, the provision of services, and the quality of the outcomes. (See Exhibit 5-3 for a list of basic council member responsibilities.)

Exhibit 5-3   Council Member Responsibilities

Council members are expected to
- agree to fully participate in council decision making
- ensure availability in work schedules
- become informed regarding organizational issues
- accept key decision task assignments
- communicate effectively with the point of service
- represent the council in other forums
- support the decisions of the council in dealings with others

In shared governance, a seamless linkage between the decision-making components of the organization is a basic expectation.

In shared governance, an important consideration with regard to decision making is the recognition that accountability and clarity regarding the decision should remain at the table where the accountability for that decision resides. The conceptual requisite here is embedded in the recognition that the decision never leaves its legitimate locus of control as a way of ensuring that it will be made in the place and by the appropriate decision makers that can most effectively make that decision, serve it, apply it, and evaluate its effectiveness. Rather than moving decisions from their appropriate locus of control, individuals who can inform them, influence them, challenge them, or guide them should be brought to their legitimate "table" for appropriate deliberation, decision making, and resolution.

Defining the Work of the Patient Care Council

The patient care council is accountable for ensuring the following:

- The appropriate delivery of patient care services according to the standards and expectations set by the board of trustees and the patient care council
- The appropriate delineation, measurement, and evaluation of the outcomes of service delivery
- The continuing competence and development of the professional and support staff

Although the council's accountability for service, quality, and competence is one focus of its activities, it also has an obligation to look at the practice accountabilities in the whole organization and the relationship of the parts to the whole. Its tasks include defining, implementing, evaluating, and controlling the broad-based *principles*, *priorities*, *plans*, and *programs* the organization commits to for the achievement of its patient service goals. By focusing on these four Ps, the patient care council keeps its attention focused on the decisions over which it has authority and away from those decisions that belong to the service pathways.

Although it is the obligation of the service pathways to deal with clinical standards, protocols, and practices, the patient care council provides the framework for those activities. The system councils (including the patient care council) operate at the system level (the level of principles, priorities, plans, and programs) with the goal of creating a foundation and the frame for the pathway councils and teams to operate at the service level (the level of standards, protocols, critical paths, team processes, quality measures, and outcome determinations). This division of labor builds checks and balances into the system and helps to ensure that decisions are made in the appropriate places (see Figure 5-3).

> The patient care council focuses on those issues that give direction to clinical decision making. It does not make clinical decisions.

SERVICE PATHWAY COUNCIL AND TEAM ACCOUNTABILITY

The presence of checks and balances creates in a horizontal, nonhierarchical organization an opportunity to ensure that decisions are implemented, outcomes are obtained, and confusion regarding locus of control and decision making is reduced or eliminated. Use of the accountability grid helps allocate most clearly the specific and appropriate legitimate locus of control for specific decisions whether that be in the patient care council or within the service pathways/units/departments. The delineation of accountability provides a vehicle for determining expectations and performance measures within the context of each category of decision making. It is critical, therefore, that the delineation occur early on in the shared governance design process. Because shared governance is an accountability-based system, the delineation of accountability is essential to the effectiveness of the organization. Further, it must be remembered that a continuum of horizontally linked decision-making and service processes is being constructed to better configure patient services (see Figure 5-4).

> The councils are a locus of control, with the authority to make the decisions for which they are accountable. Their authority should not be located anywhere else in the system.

The role of an interdisciplinary team within a service pathway is to configure itself around the specific patient population it serves. To function effectively, it must have accountability and authority for all decisions concerning its relationship to other teams and the services it provides to patients.

As already indicated, all groups possessing accountability have a defined range of authority sufficient to meet their accountability. A team is no different. In shared governance, the team, not the individual, is the basic unit of service. The accountability for desired outcomes belongs to the team. Indeed, sustainable outcomes of a comprehensive nature along a pathway can never be achieved

Figure 5-3   Patient Care Council Tasks and Performance Indicators

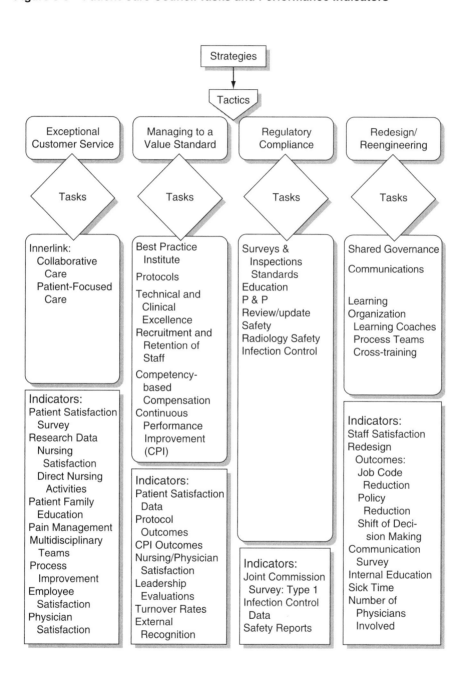

Figure 5-4   Service Pathway Linkages: Building the Continuum

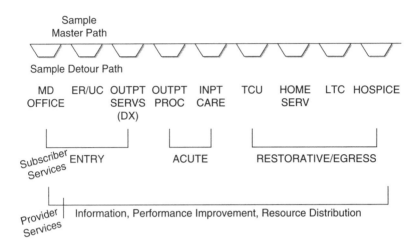

unilaterally. Team member accountability is always directed to fulfilling the accountability of the team through the aggregation and integration of the differentiated contributions of each individual. It is through the congruence of the activities of team members that outcomes are sustained. Therefore, individual accountability is defined specifically within the context of team accountability.

> **Parallel decision-making processes constitute a major obstacle to empowerment. They indicate a lack of trust by the leadership and a lack of commitment to the empowerment process.**

Obviously, the construction of teams is a major organizational task. Because teams are the basic units of service in the organization, they demand the strategic, planning, and developmental resources necessary for success. In addition, considerable energy should be devoted to educating staff about team functions.

> **It is as important to know the results of a team's work as to know its processes. Work has no value if there is no desired outcome.**

Typically, the core areas of team accountability in shared governance are as follows:

- Identification and delineation of the expectations, functions, performance, and accountability of team members
- Development, approval, and implementation of team-based clinical practices, activities, roles, and functions along a clinical pathway
- Discussion of all issues related to the development of team activities and review, approval, and application of team standards concerning the clinical delivery of patient care services
- Determination and articulation of the roles and responsibilities of team members and their relationships
- Assessment and resolution of conflicts, controversies, and interpersonal issues
- Review, revision, and application of quality improvement activities and value-driven processes
- Determination of performance compliance, evaluation of individual and collective performance, assurance of team discipline, determination of recommendations for disciplinary action, and assessment of individual and team competency and development needs
- Determination of service pathway council and/or the patient care council membership eligibility and participation in service pathway-related decision making
- Acceptance and implementation of council decisions within the context of the team's specific service requirements

Each area of accountability has many functional components. Clearly, as teams develop and refine their ability to perform, interact, and meet accountability demands, a broader framework for their activities will emerge. It should be clear in reviewing the preceding areas of accountability that, increasingly, teams have a high level of accountability for the functions and activities that constitute the content of their work. The development and use of a team "playbook" help individual team members identify the demands of membership, role obligations, and relationship factors that contribute to the success of the team's activities. This playbook then becomes the predominant terms of engagement regarding the roles and expectations of team members against which they can be evaluated and with which their performance can be validated or challenged.

Teams are free to attempt to meet their obligations in any number of ways. Obviously, along with this authority come the consequences of its application. Both the service pathway council and the service leadership have a right to expect each team to perform the duties it has accepted in a manner consistent with the standards they have set. In addition, it should be clear that the consequences of performance (both rewards and disciplinary actions) are also part of the obligations of the team.

The team, having accountability for specific functions, including the assignment of tasks to individuals, needs to identify the appropriate consequences for an individual's performance of his or her tasks. Because an individual's performance at the team level is critical to the system's effectiveness, clarity and applicability of accountability are also critical. It is to be remembered, however, that there is no accountability without consequence. The consequences of both performance and nonperformance must be clear in advance of expectation so that all parties are aware of the demands related to their action and of the impact of both performance and nonperformance.

By specifying performance requirements, evaluating performance, and rewarding good performance (and addressing poor performance), the team can help an individual member develop the skills necessary to act as a representative on the service pathway council or the patient care council. As well, these clear delineations of performance expectation, accountability, and consequence also help the team and the individual know when the relationship is not working, leading to decisions regarding how that relationship might need to be changed.

The Accountability of the Service Pathway Council

Accountability creates its own set of checks and balances. That is precisely why it is not located in just one role or place in the organization.

Just as the team is accountable for the focus, functions, and activities related to the delivery of patient care services and the relationship between the team members at the point of service, the service pathway council is accountable for the integration, facilitation, and coordination of the various team functions along a service pathway continuum of care. The role of the service pathway leadership is to bring together the components of the service pathway in a way that links the teams and the support structure, ensuring continuity along the continuum of care (see Figures 5-5 and 5-6).

Because the service pathway council is made up of representatives of the teams in the pathway, it is a place where issues related to performance; the fit between team activities, coordination, and comprehensiveness can be dealt with in a realistic way and where guidance and direction can be obtained. Therefore, the specific areas of accountability of the service pathway council are as follows:

- Integration of discipline-specific activities with the activities of other related disciplines throughout the continuum of care

Figure 5-5   Point-of-Service Team

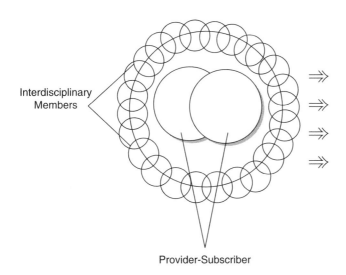

Figure 5-6   Point-of-Service Pathway

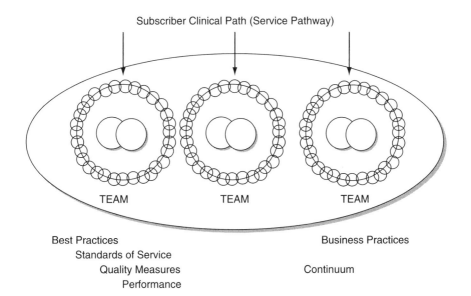

- Design, initiation, and evaluation of critical processes, clinical paths, best practices, protocols, and other processes or devices that help define the integrated, interdisciplinary complex of care services
- Establishment of evidence-based standards, protocols, policies, and practices that facilitate team functions, decision making, problem solving, performance evaluation, and clinical services evaluation across teams and along the continuum of care
- Establishment of service pathway policies regarding the design, implementation, and evaluation of performance standards for the various roles within the teams that make up the service pathway
- Design and development processes for evaluating individual performance as well as team performance
- Delineation and articulation of quality criteria for evaluating the protocols, practices, pathway activities, and team-based activities
- Creation of a novice-to-expert development program for the various disciplines and the associated mechanisms for measuring progress and ensuring individual advancement
- Design and implementation of an educational program specific to the service pathway as well as mechanisms for the educational advancement of teams and individuals
- Collaboration with other pathways and with the patient care council directed toward integrating the service pathway within the system as a whole and linking it with other components for the purpose of facilitating its clinical activities
- Definition of generic team performance standards for the purpose of creating a framework for team functions, resolving conflicts between teams, evaluating the effectiveness of team functions and team interfaces, establishing performance criteria for team leaders, and comparing team performance data against service performance outcome data for the service pathway as a whole
- Implementation of the service pathway principles, priorities, plans, and programs defined by the patient care council

The service pathway council's two main obligations are as follows:

1. To facilitate the decisions and work of the teams along the service pathway's continuum of care
2. To link the service pathway with the activities of the system as a whole

The service pathway council provides an interface between the system and services in a way that links the decisions of the system and the decisions of the services. Conflicts, challenges, and opportunities arising from the interface are the focus of the council's work. The council also has an obligation to refine the activities of the teams and help the teams to mature and become more effective.

The newer concepts related to clinical microsystems have tremendous implications with regard to service pathway council activities and the development of the point of service. Clinical microsystems locate decision making at the point of service and include the relationship between patient and provider within that dynamic. Also, it is expected that support systems such as the information infrastructure tightly connect the elements of the microsystem in a way that ensures a seamless integration between professional choices, practices, value, applications, and evaluation. The creation of the shared governance structure both broadly and specifically facilitates and sustains effectiveness of the clinical microsystem within a construct that ensures its continuance and provides a framework within which it can be further developed and refined.

The Work of the Service Pathway Council and the Pathway Teams

The delineation and distribution of the activities associated with decision making and the establishment of a framework for designing, implementing, and assessing the activities of the service pathways and their teams are critical organizational tasks. Clearly, they take time—and they also require the investment of all players in the organization. At the team level, it is expected that team-based obligations and team decision making are rotated among and assigned equitably to the members of the team. The skills and abilities of each member of the team determine what contribution the member can make to the performance of the clinical and relational activities of the team. The delivery of effective services is impossible if there is not sufficient time for defining what effectiveness is, how it is obtained, and how it is to be evaluated.

> **In an accountability-based approach, nonparticipation and nonownership of the process have no place. If you are a member of the organization, you are expected to be invested in its processes. If not, why are you there?**

> **At the pathway level, it is expected that all staff will play some role in decision making, either through representation or through implementation.**

This also holds true at the service pathway level. Here, however, more formalization occurs. Selection or election of team members who will represent the teams on the service pathway council (remember, what applies to the service pathway council can also be used in those organizations that have unit or departmental structures instead of service or product lines) may help rotate the responsibility for pathway council (unit/department) activities among the members. Regardless, it should be the expectation of all members that they will participate in the making of decisions that will influence the efficacy of the service pathway and its teams. Meeting times, agendas, tools, processes, mechanisms, activities, and evaluations are all part of the work of the service pathway council (unit/departmental councils) and of team decision making. Each of these will be affected by the culture of the particular service pathway. The various approaches may address the issues differently, but one underlying assumption of shared governance is that all members of a team have something to contribute to the team's activities and its fundamental work—and potentially to the work of the service pathway council as well.

A rotating leadership member must be selected or assigned, depending on the mechanism used by the service pathway, to provide linkage and to represent the service pathway council on the patient care council. Because the patient care council makes system-level decisions that have a direct impact on the service pathway, representation on the patient care council is important to the viability of the service pathway and its integration into the system. The representative also, in a sense, represents the patient care council in dealings with the service pathway and the teams that compose it. This type of dual representation is an inherent characteristic of shared governance decision making. Also, embedded in the disciplines associated with the establishment of standards, expectations, and decision-making practices are the checks and balances necessary to ensure that each decision is made in the appropriate place and that the individuals who have a stake in the outcome of the decision participate in the making of the decision as well as its implementation.

The Accountability of the Patient Care Council

System councils focus on integration, not operation. They must not usurp the role or authority that rests within each service pathway.

Good decisions require good data. All councils should have access to whatever information they need to make the right decision at the right time.

The patient care council does not have the authority to make decisions that are carried out at the service pathway or team level of the organization. Each service pathway and each team has its own unique range of accountability. It is the duty of the patient care council to make sure that no decision that properly belongs to a team or service pathway is usurped by the patient care council. The development of staff accountability is the most significant work of the organization (see Figure 5-7).

The only need for a system council to deal directly with a service pathway arises when the service pathway's activities and functions are not congruent with the principles, priorities, plans, and programs of the system council or with the organization's mission and objectives as defined by the board. In such a case, the system council has the authority to delve into the service pathway council's activities (or unit/department councils for those organizations that have them), but only to the extent of facilitating the service pathway's revision of its activities and functions. It is the role of the system council not to make decisions for the service pathway, but to see to it that the service pathway and its teams are functioning at the level their accountability demands. It does not act as a surrogate for the service pathway or its teams or take on the task of making their decisions. It simply ensures that they are capable of fulfilling their obligations.

This issue of accountability and locus of control is important in shared governance because of the tendency of individuals and groups to "turf" decisions up the traditional hierarchy. Because of this tendency for accountability to be shifted away from its legitimate locus of control, the organization must work diligently to make sure that decision and action accountability is clearly enumerated with regard to the places where it is both decided and exercised. Other components of the organization should work diligently to fulfill their own accountabilities and to prevent the generation of accountabilities that are not legitimate to either individual or council.

The patient care council, as a system council, is oriented toward the whole. It is the duty of the patient care council to ensure that a comprehensive approach to the delivery and evaluation of patient-based care is undertaken across the service pathways. The patient care council provides the consistencies and commonalities necessary to ensure that there is appropriate system integrity.

The patient care council focuses on those areas that give guidance or provide a frame of reference or a set of principles that can be utilized by the leadership at the service pathway level and throughout the system. Therefore, the patient care council has accountability for the following:

- Design, implementation, and evaluation of an integrated, coordinated patient care delivery system that operates cohesively and seamlessly

Figure 5-7   Steps to Accountability

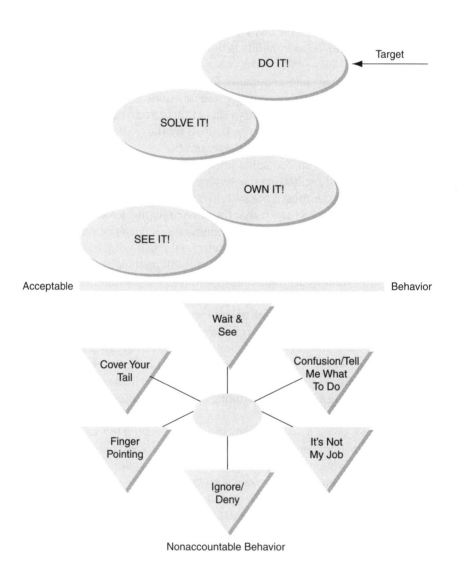

- Design and application of standards for and normative approaches to clinical delineation, the planning and implementing of care services, and the designing and structuring of team activities

- Development of a framework for and a systematic approach to the quality review of clinical practices within and between disciplines and across service pathways
- Creation of an organizational framework for a learning system directed toward continuous staff development and advancement
- Outline of an accountability delineation framework to help guide the consistent delineation of accountability within each service pathway
- Outline of a performance criteria development framework to help guide the consistent development of performance criteria
- Development and maintenance of an intra- and interdisciplinary set of mechanisms for dealing with standards, licensure, regulations, competence requirements, and service requirements within each discipline and across disciplines
- Maintenance of a system of continuous team development and maturation within the various service pathways
- Development of a comprehensive continuum-based community clinical services plan that reflects the needs of the community of subscribers
- Identification and delineation of a team-based disciplinary and corrective action program or model that is adaptable to the individual culture of each service pathway and possesses a uniform set of action criteria and a flexible implementation framework
- Development of a mechanism for translating the board-mandated mission and objectives into the priorities, plans, programs, and specific service pathway objectives as a mechanism for their full implementation

Although the preceding tasks do not exhaust the patient care council's accountability, they are central to its role as a decision-making body oriented toward addressing patient care issues across the whole system. The patient care council has system-wide accountability for defining consistent, organizationally driven constructs that either provide a generic framework for clinical processes or a context for the management and application of teamwork within each service pathway. The council also provides tools that can be modified to fit each service pathway's culture. Here again the system perspective keeps the council's work broadly focused so that it does not impede service pathway accountability or create barriers to ownership of that accountability at the team and service pathway levels.

An example of the work of the patient care council is the design and implementation of an evidence-based approach to the development of clinical practice standards and outcomes of valuation.

THE TRANSITION FROM NURSING SHARED GOVERNANCE TO WHOLE-SYSTEMS SHARED GOVERNANCE

As indicated earlier, many healthcare organizations have already instituted nursing shared governance. As the next level of organizational maturity emerges—the linking together of the disciplines in a whole-systems approach— many of the nursing shared governance models are placed in a critical position. A transition to the next stage of development needs to be undertaken to ensure the viability of shared governance and the practical application of its principles across the entire system.

> **A good nursing shared governance model can serve as the underpinning for the whole-systems approach. One does not preclude the other.**

The move from nursing shared governance to interdisciplinary shared governance can be challenging. Although the same set of principles applies, the shared governance structure developed in the nursing department is not necessarily transferable to the system as a whole. This does not mean, however, that the nursing department must dismantle its shared governance structure. Indeed, the nursing model may be an appropriate shared governance model for dealing with discipline-specific issues and requirements as the organization becomes more interdisciplinary and multifocal.

> **Each discipline will have to have a specific shared governance function that deals with the discipline-specific issues that only it can address.**

Each discipline should have a shared governance mechanism for undertaking accreditation, legislative, licensure, regulatory, and standards development work. It should also have a shared leadership, shared decision-making model as a prerequisite for working within the interdisciplinary structures of shared governance. It is expected that as each discipline uses its own shared decision-making model, it will take care of its discipline-specific issues itself and refrain from bringing those issues unresolved to the interdisciplinary forums (service pathway/unit/department council, patient care council, operations council, governance council, and team-based decision making).

In building an integrated approach to interdisciplinary shared governance, the nursing model can be used as a guide for the development of the patient care council, the service pathway council, and team decision making. At the team level, the nursing-driven team functions can now expand to become an inter-disciplinary frame of reference so that other partners and players are included in decisions about patient care. This should also happen at the service pathway level in the organization. All disciplines that make up the key decision-making team have a right to representation and partnership at the service pathway council level, and all disciplines that play a key role in patient care planning and delivery should be involved at the patient pathway council level and on the teams (i.e., the medical staff and the therapeutic disciplines as well as nursing).

It is not the obligation of the organization to attend to the requirements of each discipline. The organization expects that each discipline has a mechanism for attending to its own affairs.

Expanding the Nursing Practice Council

In some organizations, nursing's practice council has been expanded to become the organization's patient care council. Although challenging, this strategy does facilitate the linking of the nursing service's shared decision-making structures with the organization as a whole. However, in most organizations a new patient care council is formed at the outset, and all of the appropriate representatives from nursing's patient care council, education council, and quality council are included as initial members of the patient care council as a way of connecting the nursing shared governance structure and the integrated whole-systems shared governance structure. Here again, the discipline-specific shared decision-making model remains intact and is linked to the interdisciplinary shared governance model through representation. These or any number of amenable approaches can be used to build toward integration.

Perhaps the most significant challenge in creating an interdisciplinary model is some of the sentiment of proprietary ownership of shared governance that may come from the nursing service. It is hoped that this feeling or sense will dissipate quickly as effective integrative models for shared decision making and shared leadership emerge in a whole-systems frame of reference. It should have been clear and continue to be clear to the nursing service that although initiating the model in nursing provided a firm foundation for nursing's involvement in shared decision making, it simply served as a pretext or template for the inevitable implementation of much broader whole-systems approaches. As mentioned in Chapter 1, it has been the author's experience that those organizations with an existing nursing shared governance model find it much easier, faster, and more facilitating to move toward interdisciplinary approaches than those organizations that have no shared decision-making models.

> **Connecting with the medical staff early in the process of structural change gets at their issues sooner. There will be plenty of work to do with the doctors; delaying the work will not make it any easier.**

Interfacing with the Medical Staff

In traditional healthcare organizations, the organized medical staff has always been viewed as an entity separate from but correlated with the hospital organizational structure. In integrated healthcare systems and integrated service structures, a compartmentalized approach to the relationship between physicians and the organizational structure is no longer appropriate. Increasingly, methods of integration, participation, investment, and ownership in the clinical process and clinical decision making are emerging as preferable models. Shared governance is nonexclusive. All stakeholders are expected to be invested in the design and implementation of the shared governance model—including the medical staff. Physicians are members of teams and sit on service pathway councils and the patient care council (see Exhibit 5-4).

Integrating the current organized medical staff structure and the emerging interdisciplinary shared governance structure is usually no easy task because of the opposing points of view regarding leadership, organization, and role. However, activities can be undertaken to begin linking physicians to the decision-making process as the organized medical staff constructs shift toward becoming more partnership and ownership oriented. Following are some suggestions for ensuring that occurs:

Exhibit 5-4   Key Principles of Physician Involvement in Shared Governance

- Physicians are always engaged at the point of service.
- Physician membership on service-oriented bodies is not optional.
- It is more important to link physicians at the point of service than anywhere else in the system.
- The physician is a partner in deliberation, not a control point. Interface is necessary, hierarchy is not.
- Physician practice is evaluated within the continuum of service, not separate from it.

- Representatives from the medical executive committee should sit on the patient care council as it establishes the protocols and framework for the delineation of evidence and performance-driven clinical practice for the system.
- Service chiefs, associates, chief residents, or other physicians should sit at the service pathway council to participate in making decisions related to standards, clinical protocols, the interface between disciplines, the evaluation of team-based activities, and the delineation of continuum-based performance expectations.
- Teams should be designed around specific patient populations in a way that includes attending physicians, residents, and interns as full partners. Because the teams are clinically driven and implement and refine clinical protocols, care maps, best practices, and clinical pathways, the presence of physicians on the teams should be unquestioned. Difficulties related to the appropriate role of the physicians must be resolved in a way that takes into account the nature of the teams, the role and potential contribution of the physicians, the character of the teams' work, and the teams' approach to collective decision making.
- As the medical staff increasingly are tied to point-of-service decision making and operate within the patient care council and services structure, the system and the medical staff leadership will have to modify current medical staff decision making and problem solving.
- Increasingly, the locus of control and authority for implementing clinical process and resolving clinical difficulties are at the point of service, and thus there is a decreasing need for physician problem solving at what were once considered the higher echelons of the organizational system.

Because point-of-service accountability brings critical decisions regarding clinical practice and relationships to the point of service, the role of the physician in decision making is increasingly moving there as well. The design and implementation of physician-based decision making and problem solving at the point of service is crucial for the inclusion of physicians in interdisciplinary decision making (see Exhibit 5-5).

Involving physicians more fully in the shared governance structure increases their ownership of protocol development, evidence-based practice, quality determination, performance evaluation, and outcomes determination. Moving decision making to the point of service facilitates their inclusion and investment in all clinically driven decision processes and the evaluation of the outcomes of these processes.

Exhibit 5-5   The Role of Physicians on the Patient Care Council

- Medical staff problem solving as it relates to the continuum of care
- Critical pathing the standards of care across the continuum of care
- Integrating the physician's role and the roles of other clinical providers
- Modifying the delivery system to strengthen the links between the providers of care
- Establishing a strategy for harmonizing the service priorities and the priorities of the system

---

The centerpiece of all activity within the healthcare system is health services delivery. Nothing should impede the delivery of services.

PATIENT CARE INTEGRATION

In shared governance, facilitating the development of the continuum of care is a fundamental activity of patient care professionals. The patient care council and its relationship to the service pathway council and teams provide the framework for increased practitioner involvement in delineating the continuum of care (see Figure 5-8) and ensuring the attainment of outcomes and the evaluation of variance. Because the point of service is the fundamental place of decision making in the organization, it is critical that patient care design facilitates decision making at that point of service (see Figure 5-9).

As the patient care council carries out its work, it inexorably fulfills the purpose of linking and integrating patient care with the other operations and the governance activities of the system.

A great deal of development must happen at the point of service before interdependent and independent decision making can occur there. Historically, it was the role of providers at the point of service to undertake actions that had been defined and planned at other places in the organization. In shared governance, those places are eliminated, which means that the providers can no longer expect others to offer guidance and information and make decisions on their behalf. Increasingly, the goal is to ensure that providers have the support, tools, and structure necessary for clinical decision making.

Figure 5-8   Patient Service Path

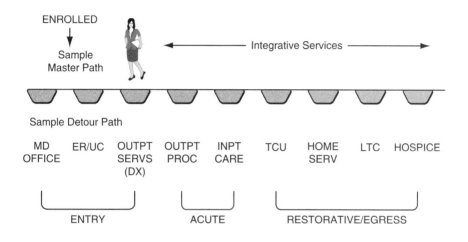

Figure 5-9   Pathway Structure: Conceptual Basis

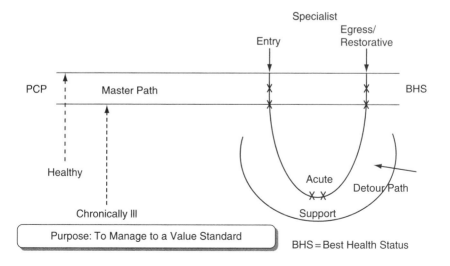

Supporting clinical management at the divisional, departmental, and unit levels used to be the primary role of the system. As health care has become more decentralized and moves more fluidly along a continuum of service, the supporting structures and services must move accordingly. Building the information infrastructure in a way that supports its use by providers in the making of judgments about cost, effectiveness, process, and outcome becomes an important developmental task for the system (see Figure 5-10), as is the task of creating direct relationships between financial, information, marketing, systems, and human resources and leadership at the point of service.

What is especially important to emphasize here is that the legitimate locus of control for the vast majority of decisions that affect clinical providers is at the point of service. Within the context of shared governance, it is vital to configure operations and relationships at the point of service in a way that ensures competence and effectiveness in deciding and acting. Good management at this level ensures that problem-solving, good process, innovation, and solutions seeking can occur at the point of service without significant constraint. Engaging and empowering professionals and workers at the point of service effectively minimizes the cascade of potential and real problems occurring across the system and better ensures effective decision making in the places where it has the greatest impact.

Figure 5-10   Point-of-Service Design

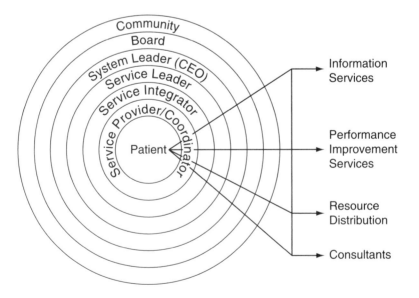

Providing a supportive decision-making structure, facilitating the appropriate locus of control and accountability, and ensuring the creation of tools to support the achievement of defined outcomes constitute the central work of the systems councils. The patient care council simply serves as the primary interface between clinical providers, the system, and the community. The patient care council and the service pathway councils, along with the service pathway teams, form the composite of relationships necessary to ensure the effective integration of decision makers and the provision of services along the continuum of care. Such integration is not only an empowering process for the participants and members in the organizational system but reflects the growing dependence on point-of-service accountability and the expectation that each member of the system is included in the activities of decision making, is committed to building a sound process, and recognizes an obligation to achieve excellent clinical outcomes. Each member, playing his or her role, exercising the accountability that is the extension of the rights of that role, helps ensure the effectiveness of the system and the quality of the services it provides to the community and to each patient it serves.

SUGGESTED READING

Batson, V. (2004). Shared governance in an integrated health care network. *Association of Operating Room Nurses. AORN Journal*, *80*(3), 493–512.

Carroll, L., & Ameson, P. (2003). Communication in a shared governance hospital: Managing emergent paradoxes. *Communication Studies*, *54*(1), 35.

Erickson, J., Hamilton, G., Jones, D., & Ditomassi, M. (2003). The value of collaborative governance/staff empowerment. *Journal of Nursing Administration*, *33*(2), 96–104.

Hosmer, L. T. (2006). *The ethics of management* (5th ed.). Boston: McGraw-Hill/Irwin.

Malloch, K., & Porter-O'Grady, T. (2005). *The Quantum leader: Applications for the new world of work*. Sudbury, MA: Jones and Bartlett.

Miller, E. (2002). Shared governance and performance improvement: A new opportunity to build trust in a restructured health care system. *Nursing Administration Quarterly*, *26*(3), 60–66.

Pfeffer, J., & Sutton, R. (2006). *Hard facts, dangerous half-truths, and total nonsense*. Boston: Harvard Business Books.

Porter-O'Grady, T. (2001). Is shared governance still relevant? *Journal of Nursing Administration*, *31*(10), 468-473.

Porter-O'Grady, T. (2006). A new age for practice: Creating the framework for evidence. In K. Malloch & T. Porter-O'Grady (Eds.), *Principles of evidence-based practice* (pp. 1-29). Sudbury, MA: Jones and Bartlett.

Rondeau, K. (2007). The adoption of high involvement work practices and Canadian nursing homes. *Leadership in Health Services*, *20*(1), 16.

Smith, P. (2004). *Shaping the facts: Evidence-based nursing and health care*. New York: Churchill Livingstone.

Styer, K. (2007). Development of a unit-based practice committee: A form of shared governance. *Association of Operating Room Nurses. AORN Journal, 86*(1), 85.

Surowiecki, J. (2004). *The wisdom of crowds*. New York: Doubleday.

U.S. Congress House Committee on Education and the Workforce, Subcommittee on Employer-Employee Relations. (2005). *Examining pay-for-performance measures and other trends in employer-sponsored healthcare: Hearing before the Subcommittee on Employer-Employee Relations of the Committee on Education and the Workforce, U.S. House of Representatives, One Hundred Ninth Congress, first session, May 17, 2005*. Washington, DC: U.S. GPO.

The Operations (Management) Council: Leading Engagement, Making Shared Governance Work

Jeff LeFors and Tim Porter-O'Grady

Judge a tree by its fruit, not by its leaves.

—EURIPIDES

Although shared governance demands full engagement from everyone in the organization, it cannot achieve any level of success without strong and effective leadership. Contrary to common belief, management and leadership do not diminish or decrease in both function and impact in the shared governance organization. In fact, the reverse is true: The role of management and good leadership actually accelerates in effective shared governance organizations. However, the skill sets and competencies related to the leadership role become more specific and focused and require stronger components of facilitation, coordination, and integration of decisions and actions across disciplines, between units of service, and within the entire system.

In old models of organization, the management structure was more vertically defined, reflecting Newtonian concepts of compartmentalization and distinctions between categories of work and the functional organization of work activities. In this newer model of organization, which reflects more quantum principles of human dynamics, the structure of the organization is multifocal and multilateral, representing a stronger relational and competency-based approach to organizing and structuring professional work. Both models represent a way of thinking of work and workers that represents a fundamentally different core or foundation in values. Quantum leadership reflects more contemporary notions of relationship, decision making, and action in knowledge-based organizations. This creates a need to change the role of management, redefine the function of manager, and establish new relationships between all players in the organization.

In a point-of-service and professional organization, it is critical to view the role of management in a different context. In the old organization, management had summary authority for the direction and decisions of the organization. Managers delegated those decisions down the chain of command and implemented them as expected at the point of service. In a whole-systems organization, the recognition of the partnership between those who do the work and those who link and integrate the system changes the format of the relationship

169

between the players. In fact, partnership is driven by the realization that the future sustainability of the organization is dependent upon the linkage and integration of the activities of all of its members.

Workplaces are membership communities. Expectations of membership suggest the requirement that everyone participate and express their contribution to the organization with which they have voluntarily become associated. One of the foundational expectations of shared governance within the context of the notion of membership community is that every member plays a role that makes a difference, has an impact on the organization, advances the mission and purpose of the system, and demonstrates a definitive impact on the results of work effort. Because most of the members in a work community operate at its point of service, that becomes the critical locus of control for both decisions and actions. Many of the decisions that affect the viability of the system are made at its point of service, and it is critical that those decisions be effective and that the stakeholders implement those decisions in a way that creates ownership of and commitment to the purposes and outcomes of the work of the organization.

> **The world of work is being radically altered, changing relationships and interactions forever.**

ENSURING EFFECTIVE DECISION MAKING

> **In the old organization, the manager predominated and had summary control over decision making.**

The only way to ensure good decision making at every point in the system is to foster the committed involvement of all players in decision making and implementation throughout the organization. This requires a shift in mindset and in action. First, everyone must be brought around to accept the following principles, which articulate the specific management and workplace changes within the new paradigm:

- Managing knowledge workers is different from managing assembly line workers. Knowledge workers own the inputs of their work and therefore have a direct and dramatic influence on its outputs or outcomes.
- The organization is essentially a membership community, a gathering of adults, and adult-to-adult interchange requires a different communication and relationship dynamic than the parent–child, superior–subordinate, and master–servant interactions common in the past.

- The results of service and production depend almost entirely on the efficiencies and effectiveness of the interactions and intersections at the place services are provided and products are produced. It is increasingly apparent that sustainable quality is caused by the effectiveness of decisions and functions at the point of service more than by any other single factor.
- The role of the manager increasingly encompasses functions associated with linkage, integration, fit, and information.
- The manager is servant to the system and those who do its work. The primary role of the manager is to integrate the system activities design to fulfill its mission and achieve its objectives. A subsidiary goal is to build a foundation of empowerment throughout the organization, ensuring that appropriate decisions are made by the right people in the right place at the right time.
- An organization should have the number of managers that organizational integrity and functioning require—but no more. One of the key roles of the manager is to develop the leadership skills of others to improve their decision making and increase the level of their interdependence.

Empowerment

Empowerment is widespread in an organization when the following are true:

- Workers possess accountability for their own destiny.
- Workers exercise the right to define their own purposes and develop their own vision within the context of the mission and purpose of the organization.
- Staff emotionally invest in their work environment.
- Workers recognize that they have an obligation to partner with those historically located above them, not to simply wait for direction from leaders.

CHANGING CONCEPTS OF MANAGEMENT

Many of the old notions of management developed during the industrial age are no longer valid. Managers were led to believe that an organization was essentially an entity independent of those who composed it. Management represented the board and the senior level of the organization and made certain that the desires and wishes articulated by those at the top were carried out by the workers. It was assumed that there was an ownership relationship generated from the board through senior-level management to line management that

Exhibit 6-1   Mentor or Coach Behaviors

- Stimulating enthusiasm
- Maintaining high expectations
- Giving credit for performance
- Being approachable
- Listening to new ideas
- Encouraging risk taking
- Helping people learn from their mistakes
- Showing sensitivity to feelings of others
- Believing people can be more effective

ensured that the work performed at the point of productivity or service was consistent with the desires of the owners.

The board and senior-level managers were looked at as the stakeholders in the organization. They essentially represented those who invested in the organization—in some cases, the stockholders; in other cases, the public; and in still others, private entities. In the old model, it was assumed that it was the exclusive obligation of those who represented the owners to make decisions about the mission, purposes, and the direction of the organization and to ensure that the activities of workers were consistent with these decisions. The line management role was essentially to operate as a link between the board and those at the point of productivity or service (see Exhibit 6-1).

> **Empowerment is recognizing the power already present in a role and allowing it to be expressed.**

This notion of the relationship between owners and workers goes back a long way. It represents a particular set of economic realities and builds organizational behavior on those realities. In the traditional corporate mindset, owners were assumed to be those who invested financial resources and thus placed their financial resources at risk, in return, of course, for a portion of the profits generated by the organization's productivity. Financial investment was viewed as the significant critical measure of the value of the organization, and those who invested and managed the financial resources were viewed as producing or creating future financial advantage for the organization and for those who invested in it. On the other hand, those who simply did the work of the organization and were paid for it were primarily seen as users of its resources. The main obligation of managers was to improve productivity and maintain the organization's financial viability, and they thus were required to keep costs and inflationary factors (including the size of the employee pool) to a minimum.

The traditional corporate mindset, while modified, is still the underlying construct of the economic enterprise that is health care in America. This mindset, itself based on the belief that those who own the means of productivity also own the rewards of that productivity, is threaded through all the work activities in almost every organization in a traditional free enterprise system.

TECHNOLOGY-DRIVEN SYSTEMS AND WORK

In the late 20th century, changes have occurred that have altered work relationships dramatically. As technology and knowledge have exploded, and globalization continues to expand as the networked construct for the future of work, they have changed the economic conditions and the very nature of work. The variables affecting the production of profits, the sustainability of systems, and the future growth of businesses in a growing and transforming global community have been radically altered.

Organizations are increasingly dependent on knowledge and technology. Their dependence on knowledge and technology has changed the locus of control and affected how systems operate. Those individuals who have the knowledge to create technology, utilize it, and manage it have become the new stakeholders in the process of technical application. Indeed, organizations are becoming more, if not completely, dependent on individuals who have specialized technological knowledge and less dependent on individuals who "control" the organizations. This is increasingly so in health care.

The interdependence of multiple knowledges and technologies creates a different relationship between providers than existed previously. Health care today is essentially highly specialized knowledge work and requires a high level of education and a firm foundation in particular technologies. Much of the foundation, learning, and expansion of skills occurs outside of the work setting. Knowledge, now one of the major prerequisites of work, is no longer under the control of the organizations that must have it to thrive. Knowledge is now mobile, portable, fluid, and increasingly owned by those who access it and process it. The portability and mobility of knowledge and technology alter the locus of control for work and the character of work relationships, and these factors also affect the various organizational roles.

The Knowledge Worker

Managers today, at the outset of the 21st century, coordinate the resources and facilitate the work of knowledge workers. The knowledge worker in today's world owns the means of doing work. This ownership of knowledge, innovation, and technology by individuals changes the locus of control with regard to the means and resources essential to organizational success. Human capital is now equal to financial and material capital in ensuring the viability and sustainability of any economic or institutional enterprise. This creates a challenging situation for the manager.

First, the manager can no longer unilaterally direct work that is dependent on the knowledge of those who do it. Second, the knowledge worker has as much investment in the exercise of his or her knowledge and the unfolding of the related work as the manager has investment in the system. In fact, the investments of both the knowledge worker and a manager (representing ownership) in the system is equated. There now must be a convergence between the two roles so that the appropriate integration and desired outcomes are achieved.

The problems arise as a result of the shift between the industrial model and the new quantum framework needed to support the contribution of the knowledge worker. The old expectations regarding workers and work are now in conflict with the new reality related to the role of the knowledge worker. Because of the tradition of "parenting" (verticalism and hierarchy) by management over decades, even centuries, workers have become essentially dependent in mindset and behavior.

Because managers have a history of directing and controlling and the workers have a history of doing as told, contradictions now emerge between the behavior of the players and the expectations of the workplace. It is these contradictions that create the foundations for significant change processing and for shifting both role and structure in the organization to support a different understanding of relationships in the emerging sociotechnical (quantum) age.

As mentioned in Chapter 5, the patient care council and the service framework are designed specifically to ensure that 90 percent of the decisions that depend on the knowledge worker at the point of service are made there (and that generally decisions are made where they belong). Although in the past most decisions were made in the management structure, in knowledge-driven approaches managers must now be precluded from making decisions that do not belong to them. In fact, in accountability-based organizations structured for knowledge/technology work, ownership of decisions is a critical organizational construct. In such systems, managers must focus on contextual accountabilities while the professional knowledge/technical worker focuses on accountability related to the content of the work.

This creates a huge challenge for the organization. One new expectation is that managers will focus on different areas of accountability than they did before. The role of manager is directly limited to the management of the system (context). Therefore, the manager represents the system and all of the efforts that the system undertakes to fulfill its mission, manage its resources, and ensure that those at the point of service are supported in a way that is consistent with the organization's purposes.

DISTINCTION OF ACCOUNTABILITY

One of the chief characteristics of shared governance is the clear distinction that is necessary between areas of accountability and between associated roles. Indeed, as indicated in Chapter 2, clarity of accountability is an important foundation of shared governance. This is certainly true for the role of manager, which must be a clearly defined range of accountability that does not overlap the accountability that belongs to others (knowledge workers, professionals) or diminish their accountability. Accountability cannot be delegated or supervised. It is applied and evaluated within the context of the role of those who possess it, although all who depend upon the accountability are involved in its evaluation.

Everybody whom the accountability affects has a right to address its appropriateness. Therefore, hierarchical notions of supervision and unilateral control and delegation have relevance. Indeed, in knowledge-dependent organizations, the relationships in the organization must become increasingly horizontal, equitable, and communication driven.

Horizontal relationships require adult-to-adult interchanges, collateral communication, equality in the roles around the point of service, and mutuality of accountability. It is the obligation of each player to be aware of the impact of the activities done to meet his or her accountability and also to be aware of the impact of others' accountability-related activities.

MANAGEMENT ACCOUNTABILITY

The need to limit the role of manager to its proper range of accountability requires an investigation into what the proper range of accountability might be. Further, it is important to understand the difference between the accountability around *context* and accountability that represents the *content* of work.

There should be as few levels of management as possible in the organization. The greater the number of managers, the less efficient the system becomes. There is an inverse relationship between the number of managers and the effectiveness of a system.

The providers (knowledge workers) at the point of service have the predominant accountability for the content of work and for achieving meaningful outcomes. That accountability can be characterized as content accountability. On the other hand, the manager, who is not accountable for undertaking the activities associated with producing clinical outcomes at the point of service, is accountable for ensuring that the support given to the providers is appropriate and effective. In other words, the role of management is basically to create a supporting context for the performance of work. Contextual accountability relates specifically to the stewardship of the organizational resources directed toward supporting those who do knowledge work. It is fundamentally reflective of the organization's linkage and support functions—the functions that allow those at the point of service to undertake the clinical work which depends on the exercise of their own knowledge competence.

Contextual accountability is essentially resources driven. All the functional roles of the manager are resource based, and the fundamental accountability of the manager usually relates to the delineation, distribution, and utilization of resources in support of the mission and objectives of the organization and its point-of-service activities.

Using Mintzberg's framework, we can identify the following areas of resource accountability: human, fiscal, material, support, and systems resources. Together these areas form the central core of the management role. Accountability for the right use of resources belongs both to individual managers and to management as a whole.

Each area of the resource accountability has specific functional requirements. Each is also defined in terms of outcomes so that the focus of managers is not so much on process as on achievement of goals (Exhibit 6-2). Obviously, there must be a mechanism or process for articulating what is expected of each manager.

THE TWO LEVELS OF MANAGEMENT

In the approach to management presented in this book, there are essentially only two types of managers—those who integrate the system and those who integrate the service. The nature of the accountability of the types is fundamentally the same, but the breadth of accountability and the obligations associated with the types differ.

For example, those who act as system integrators have an obligation to maintain a linkage with the external community (e.g., the board of trustees, other health agencies, health partners). On the other hand, each leader of a service pathway has an obligation to maintain linkages with other pathways as well as

Exhibit 6-2   Management Accountability

Human Resources
- A unit staffing plan takes into account staffing guidelines, productivity measures, and the hospital plan of care.
- A staffing system meets identified customer and service needs through the utilization of available resources.
- A mechanism exists for selecting personnel who meet the identified needs of the unit.
- A mechanism exists for removing personnel who do not meet the identified needs of the unit.
- There is compliance with all applicable policies, regulations, and laws.

Fiscal Resources
- A unit business plan based on products and services provided is in alignment with the overall goals of the organization.
- A system for effective management of the business plan is based on monitoring and modification of operations.
- A process is in place for communicating the business plan to all involved parties.

Material Resources
- There is an ongoing mechanism for assessing material and capital needs.
- An effective plan for meeting material and capital needs utilizing available resources is consistent with the goals of the organization.
- There is an ongoing system for effectively managing material and supplies usage on the unit.

Support Resources
- The work environment effectively achieves the goals of the organization.
- A process that empowers employees through the relocation of decision making is in place.
- A mechanism is in place to measure quality and to ensure that quality relates to goals.
- A system that facilitates staff development, including a performance appraisal process, is in place.
- The approach to problem solving utilizes facilitation skills and tools to achieve unit objectives.
- There is a plan that assesses and meets the ongoing developmental needs of the manager.

System Resources
- The approach to work systems is multifocal, multidisciplinary, and patient based.
- The approach to operational systems ensures effective interdepartmental linkages.
- The approach to technological systems ensures support for work and operational systems.
- A mechanism is in place for integrating and evaluating systems within and across units to support partnerships.

linkages between the various components of the service customers and their knowledge workers. Although each pathway is functionally complete (in the sense that it has its own accountability and focus), all the pathways are interdependent. For example, no system integrator (senior manager) could undertake the implementation of change in community health priorities without first consulting the service pathway leaders (unit managers) whose services would be affected by the change. Conversely, no service pathway leader would undertake a strategic change in the service content of the pathway without consulting system integrators about the possible effects on the organization's mission, objectives, integrity, and linkages. The range of accountability of each type of manager differs, but both types depend on each other in their attempts to support the integrity of the system and the functional efficiency of the service pathways.

Although the accountability of each of the roles can be clearly defined, this is not true for the interface between the roles—or the impact that a manager's actions can have on the organization and the individual players. One of the drawbacks of an accountability-based organization is the ability of any one player to make decisions independent of other people and to have a dramatic and possibly negative impact on the integrity and effectiveness of the organization. The fact that each leadership role is a locus of control entails that destructive conflicts will arise if there is no mechanism for ensuring that the decisions made are consistent with the organization's strategy, tactics, and direction. The operations council is created to address this problem.

THE FOUNDATION OF THE OPERATIONS COUNCIL

In the operations council, the management team meets to create a broad-based framework for ensuring the integrity of the system and the effectiveness of resource decisions made throughout the system. The same objectives pursued by the patient care council—integration, seamlessness, effectiveness, broad-based accountability—give direction to the activities of the operations council. The main difference is that the operations council acts as an organ of the system and focuses on the delineation and integration of resources from the perspective of the whole. Although its structure is similar to the nursing structure, it has a much broader set of obligations (see Table 6-1).

In fact, its obligations will broaden as departmental structures diminish and the organization begins to configure itself around services, components, and pathways. The organization now is built on its functional services and the methods and mechanisms through which those services are provided. The linkages in shared governance are predominantly horizontal (see Figure 6-1), and thus the council's focus is on addressing linkage, integration, and intersection

Table 6-1   Comparison of Nursing Management Council and Operations Council

Nursing Management Council	Operations Council
Limited to nursing	Multidisciplinary (includes support areas)
Single facility	Corporate accountability across individual facilities
Narrow scope	Broad, whole-system scope

of decision making in a way that enhances the effectiveness of the system. Because of the pathway format, we must emphasize the role of the councils in ensuring appropriate linkage and facilitation of decisions likely to affect the system as a whole or alter any component of the system.

Figure 6-1   Process Elements of the Service Organization

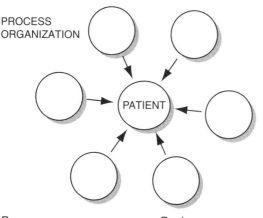

PROCESS ORGANIZATION

PATIENT

- No more departments
- Only patient service teams and supporters of the caregivers!

Purpose
Customer satisfaction
Individualized service
All those served become
   our friends

Design
Customer driven
Worker partnerships
Roles
Accountability

Human Resources
Team based
Process proficiency
Team competencies
Service competencies

Performance Evaluation
Outcomes
Team accomplishments
Individual competencies
Customer satisfaction

Rewards
Proficiencies and team competencies
Team-based outcomes
Career-based benefits
Capacity, not expertise, valued

Support for the Management Role

Before we can clearly delineate the role of the operations council, other changes in the management structure must be enumerated. Because the point-of-service leaders assume the critical leadership role in the system, other roles in the system once thought of as line roles (with specific summary responsibility for the functions and decisions at the point of service) now change in both character and content. Some senior management roles even disappear.

In the old approach, there were often senior-level administrators for finance, human resources, planning, marketing, and development as well as various other operational vice presidents, and all of the organization's functions, activities, departments, and structures were essentially distributed among the various vice-presidential roles. In the shared governance approach, the distribution occurs within a service pathways framework. First, there are the services provided directly to patients, and these are configured within a specific service pathway; second, there are services oriented toward the whole system or intended to support the individuals in direct contact with the patients (Table 6-2).

As for the old administrative senior-level positions, the majority no longer remain line positions in shared governance. Instead, they become administrative/consulting positions whose purpose is to translate strategy, assist implementation, and provide service to the system and the service pathway leaders and others in the system. Because summary line responsibility cannot unilaterally act as a frame of reference for the organization's design in shared governance, the identification of certain individuals as senior managers ceases to have value.

Real value in the organization now depends on the relationship of all roles and functions in the system to the service pathway and the point of service. In keeping with Deming's challenge, shared governance requires that each person either be providing a service or serving someone who is. One consequence is that senior management plays a stronger support role in the system.

Purpose of the Operations Council

The operations council is the gathering place for the management leaders accountable for the resources of the organization. Both levels of management (system and service) are represented on the operations council. In this council the leaders meet to delineate issues affecting the system and the services. Also present are the systems administrative/consulting partners (formerly senior administrators), whose role is to provide information and support to the council during deliberations and decision making. The primary focus of the council's

Table 6-2   Comparison of Service Integrator and Service Coordinator Roles

Service Leader	Service Coordinator
Management-level position	Staff-level position
Accountable for resource management	Accountable for coordinating daily activity in a functional area
Accountable for budget development	Accountable for operating within budgeted guidelines
Overview perspective of operations	Involved at the point of service with daily operations
Organized around pathways	Organized around points of service

work comprises linkage, integration, effectiveness, and the tactics intended to achieve the objectives set by the governance council.

The operations council also deals with capital planning, operational budget, and strategic initiative issues that mainly concern one pathway but may affect the integrity of the system. The council is in fact the place where the managers of the organization make decisions that affect the integrity and efficacy of the organization as a whole.

The council deliberates issues related to its fundamental accountability for the management of resources throughout the system. Elements of the council's accountability might include the following:

- Delineation and distribution of resources, including budgetary, operational, capital, and contingent financial resources
- Delineation of issues associated with the provision of the material resources necessary to meet the service needs of the system and the individual service pathways
- Delineation and provision of support and clerical services
- Delineation and evaluation of the resource distribution system (service/value chain) to ensure equitable, appropriate, service-based distribution
- Design and implementation of an appropriate management and resource information network to ensure that the appropriate informational components are available to monitor the effectiveness of resource distribution and use
- Delineation of human resource requirements and a legal framework to meet applicable federal, state, and organizational standards regarding the management of human resources

- Provision of an operational and leadership connection between the various service pathways as a means of problem identification and solution seeking in an effort to reduce policy, priority, service, and mission conflicts
- Integration of the decisions and activities of the various service pathways to ensure congruence in decision making and service provision
- Identification of organizational and service pathway problems and conflicts and establishment of a mechanism for deliberation about and resolution of these problems and conflicts
- Establishment and maintenance of communication routes between councils, between pathways, and between councils and pathways to facilitate the delineation and sharing of information
- Creation of a mechanism for developing the management leadership of the organization both individually and in groups to ensure that leaders can meet the different role expectations associated with shared governance
- Appropriate operations council representation on other councils and on task forces, workgroups, and other functional groups needing the insight of operations council members and their integration and leadership skills
- Deliberation and decisions resolving conflicts of accountability between system and service leadership.

These tasks are indicative of the accountability of the operations council, but each individual organization will add other obligations. The main point to keep in mind is that the organization's environment, framework, and support structures and the information foundations necessary to support the work at the point of service and to link it with mission and objectives of the organization lie at the center of the operations council's role.

As with the patient care and governance councils, any group, committee, task force, or functional group focusing on any specific task or requirement of the operations council must be appointed by the operations council. In addition, all of these appointed groups are accountable to the operations council. The council is the appropriate locus of control for the work that relates to its accountability. It also has the right to delineate how that work is to be done. If the work is assigned, accountability for its completion remains with the council and cannot be delegated away.

The incapacity to delegate accountability away from its legitimate locus of control is a critical element of shared governance. In the vertical/hierarchical organizational system, accountability was erroneously believed to be delegated from management to staff. Because by definition, professional accountability is inherent or embedded in a role (comes with it), it is not possible to delegate it away from the role that owns it. This illegitimate locus of control related to accountability is problematic insofar as the wrong people presumed or assumed control over accountability and in doing so have been unable to achieve outcomes that can be obtained only through the expression of the ownership of accountability.

Because locating professional accountability requires ownership by practitioners at the point of service, it creates "noise" in the system when autonomy, authority, and competence are seen dead in practitioners deciding and acting within their councils. Therefore, caution must be exhibited in the formation of committees so as not to remove the locus of control from the councils that are the location for the accountability of the work of the committees they might appoint. The formation of committees and other kinds of workgroups can tend to fractionalize the organization and diminish its effectiveness. The councils must maintain control over the work of the organization in a disciplined way and make certain that accountability for its outcomes never shifts from the councils and that any functional activities associated with this accountability are carefully managed by the councils.

The Role of the Operations Council

The role of the operations council is to bring managers and their patient pathway perspectives (including units/departmental point-of-service driven) together to facilitate the decision making related to resource management. In the old hierarchical structure, a project or proposed system change may have been initiated by a manager, and its success was directly related to the manager's ability to persuade or cajole necessary top-level stakeholders into supporting the initiative and providing the necessary staff. Staff at the point of service may not have been involved at all in developing the plan or have any ownership of the project. Indeed, they may not even be aware a change in their functional area was being developed.

The move toward shared governance always causes some leaders to complain that it represents "decision making by committee" and that group decision making is inefficient and expensive. Such complaints are based on a misunderstanding of system constructs and how to design decision work. In the past, in a number of workgroups, the decision-making process was undisciplined, group techniques were almost never used, and process skills were almost never present. It is rarely true that engaging stakeholders in decisions that will have an impact on their lives is a poor strategy. However, it is true that, unless a well-structured decision-making process and a disciplined deliberation methodology are in place, both time and money can be lost in the engagement of others in decision making.

Furthermore, when such processes are not consistently undertaken and efficiently designed and implemented, the decisions made tend to be incremental and short term. Also, because the decisions require continual repetition, the staff becomes more passive and dependent on leaders for making the decisions. It is not that groups are incapable of good decision making but that they need appropriate accountability and the necessary tools and skills. Decisions made by the right people, in the right place, at the right time, for the right purpose will always trump unilateral decisions made by people solely by virtue of their position and role assignment in a system. It is only because accountability is the cornerstone of effective shared governance decisions that the system is more effective than traditional hierarchical or any other vertically oriented decisional model in all but critical or crisis-oriented decisions.

Decisions do not move from their locus of control. If the decision needs to be informed or approved, move the decision maker(s) to the decision. Decisions should never travel!

The Operations Council Membership

The membership of the operations council should reflect the resource leadership configuration of the organization (see Table 6-3). It is critical that the operations council be composed of decision makers and representatives from all service pathways so that all perspectives have a hearing. The consequences of not having the complete representation include the making of decisions that neglect the needs of a stakeholder group or that have little credibility in the rest of the organization.

In many settings, the council membership is determined initially by the shared governance steering group (SGSG) during management restructuring deliberations. Often, the SGSG organizes the council membership around the newly developed pathway structure by including representatives from all pathways on the council. And not only are clinical service areas from all over the organization included, but support areas are often included, which brings a valuable support perspective to decision making. In this approach, such areas as information systems and finance are actually involved in making clinically related decisions and the implementation issues surrounding them. Having a full range of perspectives results in everyone having a better understanding of each other's perspectives and in better overall decision-making and implementation processes.

The operations council provides a forum for resource-based decisions around which all the stakeholders are configured.

Table 6-3   Operations Council Membership

Member	Expectations
Service integrator	• To bring a systems overview perspective to the council's deliberations • To help ensure that the focus of the council is appropriate
Service leader	• To bring the individual pathway perspective to the council's deliberations • To participate in deliberations as an objective steward of corporate resources
Physicians	• To bring the physicians' clinical perspective to the council's deliberations • To act as a communication link to other members of the medical staff
Chief financial officer	• To bring financial expertise to the work of the council • To assist council members in developing their financial understanding and analytical ability

Individuals who represent significant stakeholder groups should be considered for membership. These include the chief financial officer (CFO), an administrative/consulting partner, someone from medical affairs, several service integrators (one, two, or three senior administrators), and a member of the board of directors (trustees). As the medical staff structure becomes more fully incorporated into the shared governance structure, the president/chief of the medical staff is also added to the operations council membership.

These individuals bring specialized and invaluable experience and viewpoints to the process. The CFO can help raise the council members' level of understanding of the financial workings of the organization. The consulting partner, the medical affairs member, and the president (or other officer) of the medical staff bring a physician perspective to decision making. The service integrators are in a position to provide a broad systems overview and needed context. The board member brings knowledge of the workings of the board as well as a community perspective.

All members of the operations council face a steep learning curve. Not only must they understand the strategic priorities and management structure of the organization, but they must also have a thorough understanding of shared governance principles. Most members will find themselves gaining a new perspective on the financial operations of the corporation and will need education on basic business tasks, such as strategic visioning, budget development, capital planning, and financial statement review, as well as basic accounting practices. They will also need education on the current stage of certain business processes, such as predictive and adaptive strategic visioning and site planning. It is critical that the council identify as many educational needs early in the development process so that adequate resources can be found to educate members fully. At the end of their term on the council, members will have gained a level of understanding of the business of health care comparable to what used to be attained by a chief operating officer or divisional vice president.

> **The operations council requires that each member maintains a view of the whole system, not simply a view of the part he or she represents.**

Initially (and sometimes thereafter) the chair of the operations council, like the chairs of the service and governance councils, is selected from the SGSG. This ensures continuity with the original work performed in laying out the new structure and defining the new roles of managers. The council's first order of business, besides determining its accountability, is to decide on the functional aspects of its operation, including the selection process for members, term limits, meeting times and locations, and other details. The role of the chair is to lead the meetings in a manner that focuses the participants on the core issues, disciplines the dialogue on the issues, and facilitates decision making by consensus. The chair is also empowered to make critical decisions on behalf of the council (as is the case for all council chairs), including the commitment of corporate resources when time does not allow for a council meeting. When a critical decision is made by the chair, he or she has an obligation to report the decision back to the council at the earliest opportunity.

> **The chair has power to act delegated by the council. It is characteristic of the governance notion as applied to a system.**

The role of the manager in shared governance shifts in content and expression. It now involves supporting, mentoring, and coaching staff at the point of service so that they will better understand the truly empowered nature of their positions. With the move to a flatter organization and the relocation of decision making comes the need for a decision-making body to deal with operational and resource issues that cross the boundaries between areas of the organization. It is this need that the corporate operations council is intended to meet.

The tearing down of the old hierarchical power base and the move to a council structure based on evidence, data, and outcomes are a paradigm shift for everyone involved. A great deal of education and development of council members is required if the council is to achieve full functionality. Former managers and administrators who now find themselves without a hierarchical power base will need to adapt to the new structure and to the new management role.

Making the Operations Council Work

In the operations council, projects related to the organization's priorities are scrutinized by a management panel and by the organization's financial experts. Because the council includes representatives from all pathways, all perspectives are shared at the table during the process. The council focuses on data "fit" within the context of a strategic plan or priority list, so politicking for a particular project or idea is excluded from the decision-making process. The council also serves as a focal point for systems, processes, and projects that span multiple pathways. Although it is primarily a decision-making body, the council is accountable for ensuring that certain tasks are completed and certain outcomes achieved. Thus, it is required to delegate responsibilities to facilitate the completion of tasks.

> **The role of manager must be broadened in a way that makes it impossible for the manager to continue to do the work that has always been expected.**

One of the major challenges facing a newly formed operations council is to find the right context for decisions. In the old hierarchical structure, the context may have been as simple as one administrator's feeling that a particular idea was a good one and should be acted upon. At other times, administrators or managers might have translated the application of a strategic or tactical imperative in a way they thought was best for the organization. In both these cases, decisions became the subset of role and choice of the manager rather than the more desirable decision and action of those most accountable for translating, defining, and performing within the context of a particular strategic or tactical trajectory with which professional staff have some measure of ownership. As decision making becomes more of a council-driven, data-based process, an overriding context must be found that facilitates the comparison of projects, priority setting, and the arrival at satisfactory decisions.

The Operations Council Process

> In the operations council approach, it is not possible for an individual to control decisions or project a personal agenda.

A good example of a major operations council issue would be the capital purchase of a new treatment technology. In the old structure, a physician (or department manager) might research a new technology and decide unilaterally that it would make life easier or achieve better outcomes within the organization's scope of care and service. The physician would then try to "sell" an administrator on the need for the technology by pointing to a currently important issue (e.g., cost containment, poor patient satisfaction). The administrator might then try to sell the idea to senior management stakeholders depending on the size of the purchase, and ultimately the CFO would have to buy into the idea. This process is typically very time consuming because an individual meeting has to be held with each stakeholder. Different questions might be asked at each meeting, requiring additional research and investigation. Each person might have unique issues in mind as he or she evaluates the purchase, and the feelings and viewpoints of the stakeholders may not be congruent with the overall goals of the organization. At the end of the process, the involved parties, strategic committees, strategy task forces, or the capital planning committee become tired of being hounded by the champions of the new technology and may cave in and agree with the purchase or even may reject it. By this time, supplier discounts may have been missed because of the length of time required to get approval, or the scope of the project may have grown or shrunk and might be completely different from the original proposal (see Table 6-4).

> There are no other approval mechanisms outside the council structure. There is a single locus of control for all decisions.

CLARITY OF ISSUES

The operations council provides an opportunity to expedite the planning and decision process and keep the discussion focused on the key issues. For example, a capital purchase may be identified by a service coordinator or a provider team and communicated to the service manager/integrator associated with the pathway. The service manager/integrator is accountable for ensuring that all the necessary homework is completed for a purchase, including a detailed

Table 6-4   Old and New Decision Processes

Old Process	Operations Council
No shared understanding of standard	Projects are evaluated based on an understanding of fit
No context for consistency	Operations council approves all major processes and items
Narrow point of review and approval	Projects are evaluated by a diverse group of stakeholders
Ability to project a personal agenda	Decisions are made by consensus
Ability to force a request or demand through the system	All decisions reflect the organization's priorities and goals

financial analysis for presentation to the operations council. At the council meeting, members hear the presentation (see Exhibit 6-3) and discuss the fit of the purchase with organizational strategies and capital resources. Because the discussion takes place with all the stakeholders in the room, a decision can be made immediately. Politicking and hidden agendas become nonissues because the justification for the purchase is based on data and the purchase's fit with the priorities of the system. Once the decision is made, no further approval process is required. A service leader presents his or her proposal only once.

The challenge for the council is to clarify the context for decision making. There is generally no shortage of good ideas coming forward for approval. Trying to understand what resources are available or clarifying strategies to a point where they are helpful in the decision process can be the biggest challenge for the council. In the old hierarchy, vague strategies or a fuzzy logic and/or indicators of available capital could be used to move personal agendas forward. In data-driven discussions, the source of information must be clear and to the point. This may require a review of existing strategic plans including implementation details and generation of new financial reports that give a good picture of capital availability to the organization. Furthermore, engaging the right stakeholders with the breadth of responsibilities that relates to the challenges of choice and use of technology or application of strategic imperatives ensures a higher level of mutuality and collateral ownership. Both degree of risk and required impact on individual departments when contrasted with the general benefit to the system engage stakeholders and force them to confront the practical realities and vagaries associated with making the best decision versus the decision that may be compartmentally and unilaterally advantageous.

Exhibit 6-3   Presentation Guidelines

1. Project steps
   - Problem statement
   - "As is" statement
   - Brainstorming
   - Option design and selection
   - Implementation plan
   - Follow-up and benefits statement

2. Checklist
   - Does project meet strategic requirements?
   - Is project budgeted?
   - Does project exceed budgeted dollars?
   - Is project consistent with capital plan?
   - Is this a subproject of previously approved project?
   - Are stakeholders identified and included in project process?
   - Did physicians have input and express agreement?

3. Option selection
   - List of benefits
   - Cost analysis
   - Type of decision requested
   - Nonbudgeted projects (add justification or reasoning)

CLARIFYING OPERATIONS COUNCIL ACCOUNTABILITY

One of the critical first steps to undertake in developing any council is to firmly establish in writing the accountability of the council (see Exhibit 6-4). This provides a focus for council members and serves as a tool for communicating the purpose of the council to stakeholders. It also establishes the foundations for what will ultimately become the bylaws of reorganization. This work requires creativity and perseverance until all members feel comfortable with the wording of the accountability statement and fully understand its meaning. It is important that each organization take the time to develop its own accountability statement to take into account its unique characteristics. The accountability statement, which should clearly define the charge of the council in a theoretical fashion, must delineate the council's specific areas of control, authority, and decision making. Noted should be the absence of control of or accountability for work, quality, competence, and the outcomes of the relationships between team members at the point of service.

Exhibit 6-4   Operations Council Accountability Statement

Material Resources

To provide the linkage, communication, and action between service and governance as it relates to material resources within the corporation and the community as evidenced by the following:

- Capital priorities that are consistent with the corporate mission and strategies
- A corporate capital plan based on products and services provided that is in alignment with the health goals and mission of the organization
- Establishment of parameters for monitoring and evaluating material resources
- A process for communicating the capital plan, material resources parameters, and other actions of the council

Human Resources

- Corporate policies and strategies regarding recruitment, retention, and utilization of human resources reflect the philosophy, mission, and values of the organization and are consistent with applicable laws.
- A communication and action linkage exists between the service and governance councils regarding human resources.

Support Resources

There is a framework in place that accomplishes the following:

- Facilitates the transition to shared governance
- Provides educational resources for the development of staff and management
- Supports the relocation of decision making and redefining of management accountability
- Facilitates the removal of organizational obstacles to point-of-service decision making at all places they exist in the organization

Fiscal Resources

There is collaboration between leaders and representatives from the appropriate disciplines and services to develop an annual operating budget and a long-term capital plan, including a strategy to monitor the implementation of the plan. The budget review process includes consideration of the appropriateness of the organization's plan for providing care to meet patient needs.

A communication and action linkage exists between service and governance regarding fiscal resources within the organization and the community, as evidenced by the following:

- Program evaluation consistent with the organizational mission
- Consistent linkage and integration of strategies, service pathways, and prioritized budgetary resources

(continues)

Exhibit 6-4   Operations Council Accountability Statement (continued)

- Facilitation of the fiscal activities of the service pathways, including the following:
  - The monitoring of appropriate budget indicators
  - The monitoring of appropriate business plans
  - The sharing of resources across service pathways
  - The removal of obstacles to fiscal integrity
  - A corporate business plan based on products and services provided that is in alignment with the health goals and mission of the organization
  - A process for communicating the business plan and other actions of the council

Systems Resources

There is evidence that each service pathway, discipline, or service group has established and individualized its functional accountability within the context of a whole-systems shared governance framework.

Integrated information systems serve as a foundation for the linkage of all services across the continuum, as evidenced by the following:

- An approach to work systems that is multifocal, multidisciplinary, and patient based
- A method of determining and interpreting systems models, policies, and strategies to create a shared governance systems framework
- An approach to new technological systems that ensures support for work and operations, with attention to work flow and how work flow will change
- A mechanism for integrating and evaluating systems within and across work areas to support partnerships
- A mechanism to deal with systems problems at the level where they occur

Appropriate application of systems resources will be evidenced by the following:

- The linking of systems within the work area and across the service pathways and the defining of their purpose
- The utilization of a project management or continuous quality improvement (CQI) process for systems development, maintenance, and improvement
- The assurance of work area system alignment with the organizational mission, goals, and values
- The implementation of systems in the work area within the context of a whole-systems shared governance framework
- The implementation of a clinical information system to meet the needs of patient-focused care

As the operations council, we define the following terms as follows:

- Linkage as the flow of communication between related points

Exhibit 6-4   Operations Council Accountability Statement (continued)

- Multifocal as the viewing of an issue or a system from more than one perspective
- Partnership as the organizational relationship between stakeholders who have shared accountability
- Systems as tasks, activities, and information flows that are interconnected (every change in a system has potential repercussions in every other system)
- Whole-systems shared governance as the organizational system that supports the work of the organization through the application of the principles of partnership, equity, accountability, and ownership

Stewardship is a key role of the leader. Control of the resources facilitates growth when done well and ensures decline when done poorly.

THE OPERATING BUDGET PROCESS

As previously mentioned, many activities formerly performed in different areas of the old hierarchy become included in the accountability of the operations council in a shared governance structure. For example, development of capital and operating budgets is overseen by the operations council rather than only by the CFO or finance department. The council monitors the budget process at certain checkpoints to ensure that financial targets are being met and budget assumptions and implementation plans are coordinated across pathways. Much of the coordination of the process remains with the technical experts, who facilitate the completion of large fiscal projects. However, the locus of control rests with the operations council.

Once the budget is developed, the operations council monitors the financial performance of the organization and makes the decisions necessary to ensure that targets are met. Individual department or service leaders monitor and manage their own budgets including their variance reporting. Variance reporting is aggregated in a way that can be shared and evaluated by the operations council as a part of its responsibility to ensure appropriate distribution, application, and use of resources. Variance reports generated by the finance office are reviewed monthly by the council. Action plans submitted by service leaders are reviewed to ensure the correction of any performance shortfalls.

The accountability for financial performance provides discipline when targets are not met. The operations council serves as a support for service leaders, reviews all variance reports with a systems perspective, and looks for trends or patterns across pathways. Using tools generated by the finance department in conjunction with their monitoring activities, the council can direct resources to be rerouted from one pathway to another or can balance budget shortfalls with budget overages in other areas. Note that the role of the council is not to control or manipulate point-of-service leaders but to support them in meeting their particular accountability for financial performance. Thus, council members must have a clear understanding of the personal accountability of individual service leaders. If a service leader continually demonstrates a pattern of nonperformance, the operations council recommends actions to be taken by the appropriate council or organizational leader. Individual leadership discipline is not undertaken by the operations council. The role of the operations council is to note patterns of variance and recommend appropriate corrective action or follow-up. If management or leadership behavior is at issue with regard to repeated variance or compliance with operation council expectations and standards, the leadership reporting structure is the vehicle used for specific corrective action or disciplinary processes.

THE CAPITAL BUDGET PROCESS

All workers are stakeholders in the sharing of the resources of an organization. Each must play a part if the resources are to be equitably distributed.

As previously mentioned, the operations council spends a good portion of time reviewing capital purchases. Although routine capital budgeted items fall within the high signature limits of individual point-of-service leaders, items that are unbudgeted or that require expenditures over the relevant signature levels must be reviewed by the council prior to purchase. The purpose of this review, which represents another clear departure from the way a hierarchical organization functions, is to determine the priority of the item being requested. The council members must therefore be aware of the amount of capital resources available and the strategic priorities of the organization. In many cases, the discussion centers on the consequences of trading one capital expenditure for another.

This type of capital analysis may require new reports to be generated by the finance consultants. Monthly reports of capital purchases need to be reviewed to understand how much of the available capital has been spent to date, how much was budgeted initially, how much capacity remains in the system, and what major expenses loom on the horizon that may change the financial picture.

Capital Project Presentations

Another aspect of the council review process involves development of all leaders, clinical and management, in the art of project presentation. Guidelines need to be developed by the council that indicate what kinds of questions may be asked during a presentation and thus provide a framework for the presentation. Leaders with previous management experience in a hierarchical organization may have been conditioned to "sell" capital items. A selling type of presentation has no place in the operations council. Discussion of the merits of a project should be based on organizational priorities, data, and financial analysis rather than intangible benefits that cannot be measured.

> **In all proposals for consideration by the operations council, the goal is not to convince others of the value of the proposal. Instead, proposals simply validate through data analysis the central viability and outcome they are supposed to address.**

Prior to each project presentation, the chair must carefully preview the presentation to ensure that the necessary facts are included, its relationship to the strategic and tactical priorities established for the organization or department, and all questions are anticipated by the presenter, with adequate answers at the ready. As experience is gained, the discussion of projects in the council becomes more and more disciplined. Use of evidence-based management, the strategic process, operational priorities, and continuous quality improvement (CQI) techniques, such as process flowcharts and a formal project management process, help further regulate the dialogue so that frustration is minimized for both the council and the presenter.

The Primacy of Financial Accountability

Although the accountability of the council covers all five categories of resource management, the majority of council time will likely be taken up dealing with the financial matters. Development of the operating and capital budgets, variance monitoring, and capital purchase review are basic functions that dominate the work of the council. These are common business functions, but performing these tasks in a shared governance structure means the routine steps may require modification. The challenge for the council is to understand where accountability lies for completion of tasks, set expectations for performance, and take appropriate action when targets are not met.

Setting Targets

If you do not know where you are going, anything will get you there.

Important components of operations leadership include understanding the importance of target setting and placing the accountability for outcomes in its proper place. It is common knowledge that in the current healthcare environment, most healthcare organizations are experiencing decreasing revenues and increasing challenges to their revenues and growing costs. As a consequence, an organization's financial picture influences nearly every decision made. It is not possible to focus on any patient care issue without considering the financial implications, nor is it possible to focus on financial performance without considering its impact on quality. The balance of cost and quality defines value. If this balance is used as the overall template for the organization—setting financial targets to achieve maximum value—the result will be a good fit between cost and quality. In other words, all financial activities should be disciplined by the mission and purposes (and evidenced by relevant strategy) of the organization and ultimately generate real value for the organization and the people it serves.

OPERATIONS COUNCIL COMMITMENT

Membership on the operations council demands a significant commitment of time and energy. There is generally enough business in a large organization to require biweekly meetings of the council. In the early stages of council formation and development, a great deal of time is spent discussing the accountability of the council and other details of its implementation and operation. As the council begins to take on the real business of the organization, every presentation or process becomes a learning experience for the council members.

Discovering which questions are important in getting to the bottom of an issue takes time and experience (and can be facilitated by problem solving and a wide variety of quality improvement techniques). Likewise, presenters must

Exhibit 6-5   Rules for Building a Consensus

A consensus requires that everyone involved in the decision must agree on the individual points discussed before the points become part of the decision. Not every point will meet with everyone's complete approval. Unanimity is not the goal, although it may be reached unintentionally. It is not necessary that everyone be satisfied, but everyone's ideas should be thoroughly reviewed. The goal is for individuals to understand the relevant data and, if need be, accept the logic of differing points of view.

The following rules are helpful in reaching a consensus:

- Avoid arguing over individual ranking or position. Present a position as lucidly as possible, but seriously consider what the other group members are presenting.
- Avoid win–lose stalemates. Discard the notion that someone must win and thus someone else must lose. When an impasse occurs, look for the next most acceptable alternative for both parties.
- Avoid trying to change minds only to avoid conflict and achieve harmony. Withstand the pressure to yield to views that have no basis in logic or the supporting data.
- Avoid majority voting, averaging, bargaining, or coin flipping. These techniques do not lead to a consensus. Treat differences of opinion as indicative of an incomplete sharing of information, so keep probing.
- Keep the attitude that the holding of different views by group members is both natural and healthy. Diversity is a normal state; continuous agreement is not.
- View initial agreement as suspect. Explore the reasons underlying apparent agreement on a decision and make sure that all members understand the implications of the decision and willingly support it.

learn how to formulate presentations based on strategic priorities, evidence, and data—a process that may take time for those who have had years of experience playing political games rather than responding to fact-based arguments. The council must constantly remind itself that its role is to provide support for managers and act as the steward of the resources of the system, not function as a high court handing down summary judgments (see Exhibit 6-5).

CONSENSUS-BASED DECISION MAKING

Council members need a thorough understanding of the consensus-based decision making. Most of us have experience with groups that make decisions using a voting process. Although this process results in majority support for decisions, it is not the best process for an accountability-based model.

> Consensus is not simply agreement. Instead, it involves the group's acknowledging what is right, and then doing it.

In reaching a decision by consensus, every participant in the decision process must understand and agree on the points that make up the decision. This does not mean that every point will meet with everyone's complete approval. The end result of a consensus process is a decision that everyone understands as the right one that can be supported because all the relevant data have been analyzed. Some participants may not be totally satisfied, but all can support the decision based on logic, data, and fit. It is potentially the most right decision at the time it is made.

There is no voting in consensus decision making; instead, there is a determination of where the group is with its understanding of the pertinent issues. Included is a strategy to broaden understanding and knowledge and to provide sufficient data to form a solid foundation for whatever decision is reached. Seeking a consensus in this way prevents members from holding on to a minority view and sabotaging the decision. It also prevents issues from being constantly revisited. In explaining his or her attitude toward a consensus decision, a participant might state, "I do not fully agree with the outcome of the decision-making process, but I understand the reasons why this decision was chosen and I can support it."

When an organization moves toward a shared governance council model in which participants are truly empowered, managers are forced to cope with their perceived loss of power. The loss of power is difficult for anyone but can be especially traumatic for individuals positioned at higher levels. Directors, administrators, vice presidents, and even presidents must all come to terms with the fact that either their role no longer serves the same purpose in the new organization or has changed into a stronger support role. The shared governance organization does not place any value on the symbolism or trappings of hierarchy. Large offices, individual secretaries, and special privileges are all looked at carefully during the transition. Although they certainly do not necessarily all disappear, they may be distributed differently to reflect a new emphasis on the point of service and the more clearly defined and dispersed point-of-service-driven accountability for achievement of goals.

This attitude toward the trappings of power is inconsistent with the rewards managers (including senior-level managers) have grown to associate with power and authority and "climbing the ladder." Many who have spent their work lives climbing to the top of the organization may feel like the rug has been pulled out from under them. A sense of concern and confusion may also permeate the staff as the power base of individuals they have worked for is considerably reconfigured. During this transition, the chief executive officer (CEO) plays an essential role in holding things together while pushing the parameters of the organizational hierarchy toward a more effective point-of-service decision-making framework. With feelings of loss experienced by everyone on the leadership team, the CEO's ability to motivate leaders in the change of their roles during this shift to shared governance is critical.

> **There is nothing that causes more fear and pain than a shift in the power base of a leader. All the work done to obtain power and keep it is lost in the "noise" resulting from a change in the locus of control.**

SHARED VISION

One common consequence of the move toward shared governance is the discovery that the organizational vision is not broadly shared. In a hierarchical structure, senior management may have a common understanding of the organization's mission and major strategies, but their penetration to the lower levels of management may be suspect. When a project or tactic is discussed in a council meeting, it must be debated within the context of the mission, vision, and strategic plan of the organization by the real stakeholders in the implementation of vision and strategy. All council members must have a common understanding of these before a well-founded conclusion can be reached. In most healthcare organizations, a great deal of time is spent in efforts aimed at adding clarity and specificity to the strategic plan, by providing supporting documents and relevant information, for example, in the attempt to build a solid foundation for determining tactics.

The operations council must be given substantial authority, and decisions should require no further approval than that obtained at the council. In an empowered shared governance organization, the chair of the operations council (always a point-of-service manager) has the same signature limit as the CEO (see Exhibit 6-6). Decisions of the operations council are final unless they involve a capital expenditure above a dollar amount that requires board of directors approval. The transition to this type of approval process requires an education process not only for the council chair but for all stakeholders who have resource stewardship or fiscal accountability. Everyone who is affected must be educated, including the board and the accounts payable and materials management staff because they may be involved in the purchase process.

Exhibit 6-6   Council Chair Duties and Powers

- Calling meetings
- Controlling the agenda
- Moving the council to a consensus on decisions
- Removing nonparticipating members
- Making group assignments
- Making critical decisions on behalf of the council as needed
- Calling emergency meetings if needed
- Acting as mentor of the chair-elect
- Executing signature authority for the council

There cannot be two places where a decision is made. Preference is always given to decisions made closest to the point of service.

In a shared governance organization, the operations council assumes areas of accountability that formerly belonged to the chief operations officer or the CFO. Rather than simply being a new place to perform old tasks, however, the operations council plays an important role in supporting the entire shared governance structure. Besides reviewing capital purchases and projects, the operations council is accountable for all resources at the corporate level. When the administrative process does not give way to the council's role, the council's involvement simply evaporates in the face of the administrative control where the "real" power to decide resides. This "escape option" must be eliminated if true accountability is to exist and be expressed by the council.

Whereas service leaders are accountable for managing human, fiscal, material, system, and support resources within their service pathways, issues that involve multiple pathways or have a substantial impact on the organization are handled by the operations council. For example, although daily staffing is managed at the point of service by service coordinators, service leaders are accountable for acquiring an adequate staff with the necessary qualifications to meet the needs of the pathway for which they are responsible. The operations council, with its systems perspective, is accountable for the compensation system used to pay all staff members within the organization. This illustrates the difference in focus at different levels of accountability. The operations council is mainly accountable for translating the strategies of the system into actions and outcomes consistent with the mission, purposes, and objectives (including strategic imperatives) of the system (see Figure 6-2).

Figure 6-2   Operations Council Accountability

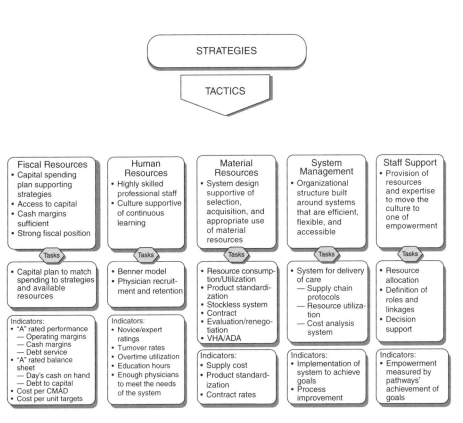

SYSTEMS ACCOUNTABILITY AND SUPPORT ACCOUNTABILITY

All work, all relationships, must be seen from the perspective of the whole, not of each part. A system is not simply the sum of its parts.

Although human, fiscal, and material resource accountability is fairly self-explanatory, systems accountability and support accountability require further elaboration. While the term *systems* may suggest that the focus is on the organization's computer system and information system, the operations council's definition encompasses all systems that form the organization. In fact, there is a connection between its understanding of the concept and "systems thinking" (see Chapter 4). As noted already, the interrelationships between all business processes must be understood in addition to the subsystems and the individual tasks.

This concept is often difficult for many in the organization to embrace. It is one primary reason that the learning organization approach plays a central role in the development of all personnel. It should be expected that everyone who is part of the organization will have role transitions to confront and they will need the insight gained from engaging in an effort to understand and work within an interdisciplinary shared governance framework. The operations council has an obligation to ensure that everyone has the opportunity to learn and adapt. If the council does not facilitate the achievement of a higher level of systems understanding, the organization will fail to undergo essential change.

Its accountability for support requires that the council must provide a framework for supporting behaviors that resonate with shared governance throughout the organization. The leadership must commit to removing obstacles to full implementation of the values that will undergird the restructured organization. The operations council is the locus of the debate about how the new structure should work, how roles may need to change, and what systems may need to be altered. Therefore, its members must exhibit a high degree of creativity and develop a thorough understanding of the basic principles of shared governance.

LINKAGE TO THE OTHER COUNCILS

Linkage between the councils is critical to the integrity of a shared governance system. As should be clear to the reader, communication and interaction in the building of collateral relationships are requisites of shared governance. Consequently, considerable attention must be paid to the linkage and communication processes that support accountability and effectiveness within the councils.

Council representation is one important means of linking councils to each other. Just as the operations council leadership should be represented on the patient care council, so should the patient care council leadership be represented on the operations council (and both should be represented on the governance council). This type of cross-representation helps ensure that decisions made in any one part of the organization do not impede the decisions made in another part. It also begins to address the issues of equity and integrity in a horizontal or equity-based organizational system. Shared governance demands that no one part of the system either make decisions that belong in another part or jeopardize the integrity of decisions made elsewhere. The only way to guarantee that this does not happen is to create linkages throughout the system.

Each of the council leaders represented on the operations council has the full right of participation in the decisions of that council. Indeed, it is expected that the patient care council's chair will articulate the impact of budgetary consid-erations and tactical planning on the decisions made in the patient care/service council. Further, the patient care /service council's chair communicates the framework for decisions generated in the operations council in conjunction with the operations council leadership representatives on the patient care/service council. The same strategy is used in the operations council—the chair and the patient care/service council leadership representatives communicate decisions made in the patient care council.

CAUTIONS ABOUT CONTROL

One of the most challenging shifts in the locus of control in a shared gover-nance organization relates to the authority of the manager and the framework for decision making. In the old model, ego rewards, personal fulfillment, and role expectations centered around the authority of managers to make summary decisions regarding the services that they led, and those old expectations and behaviors are hard to extinguish. Yet they need to be eliminated if the new man-agement role expectations are to be met.

One major focus of the operations council is to develop new leadership skills and to establish a behavioral framework for the new management role. Coaching, development, education, mentoring, and other tactics for changing behavior become essential. The operations council should look carefully at the new role, the shift in expectations, the shift in evaluation of performance, and the new behavioral models of leadership as part of its accountability for supporting the transition to shared governance.

It should be understood that not every manager will be able to make the move to a new kind of leadership. Managers who obtained personal rewards and satisfaction in the exercise of the old role may find the new role to be unful-filling. The operations council should recognize this reality and make it possible for individuals to move out of unsatisfying roles and into roles that fit their needs and likes. Although the transition to shared governance can be a challenging and traumatic time for the organization, it is also a time when the organization can configure its support structure so as to provide a solid foundation for the cre-ation of effective and meaningful roles.

SUPPORT FROM THE CEO

The position of CEO remains a critical leadership position in interdisciplinary shared governance. While operational concerns are transferred to the operations council and the lean point-of-service management structure, the CEO remains a visible figure focused on the community interface and serves as a focal point in guiding the organization into the new paradigm. During the transition, while the staff are learning their new empowered roles, they may continue to look for leadership from their traditional leaders, who are themselves learning new roles—or even changing them. The CEO is in a position to send a powerful message to the staff and provide strong support for the new values. For this reason, it is critical that the CEO be brought along during the entire process. Without the support of the CEO, the predicted chaos of the transition may be amplified.

The CEO, although a leadership figure in a visible position, is also vulnerable to attack from all sides during the transition. Physicians, board members, and staff will all turn to the CEO at some point for support and reassurance. For this reason, the CEO must have a firm grasp of the theory and application of interdisciplinary shared governance, fully understand who is accountable for problem solving, and be willing to take great criticism from nearly everyone while providing an anchor for the organization. The CEO must demonstrate a sensitivity to the traumatic changes the organization is going through and be willing to direct people to the right place in the new structure to get problems and concerns dealt with. Even the slightest wavering in the CEO's commitment will be amplified and used as evidence that the new structure is not working.

OTHER ADMINISTRATOR CHANGES

Whereas the role of the CEO remains basically intact in the new structure, the roles of other senior managers become more developmental and consultative in nature. The need for many senior management roles alters considerably in the new structure as staff members assume accountability for decision making, and the remaining senior managers are required to provide special expertise throughout the organization and develop a teaching–learning relationship with the point-of-service managers (see also Chapter 8). These consulting managers/administrators (called consulting partners in this text) also play a very important role at the council level.

> In shared governance, the old vice president or senior management roles disappear. Instead, the role of systems consultant emerges, available to all who need support for decision making.

Because the operations council assumes accountability for many of the critical financial decisions, the expertise of the former CFO is essential for operations council deliberations, and thus this particular administrative/consulting partner is in regular attendance at the council meetings. As the need arises for different types of expertise, other administrator/consulting partners can be accessed by the council. Indeed, the administrative/consulting partners are expected to be present at the operations council meetings so that the council can obtain any information it needs to make good decisions. Also, the other councils and unit or point-of-service groups and teams have the right to access these administrators/consultants for deliberations and problem solving whenever it becomes apparent they need expert assistance.

OTHER MANAGER TRANSITIONS

For some members of the senior management group, the loss of perceived power resulting from surrendering ownership of "their" employees and budget cost centers presents substantial difficulties. The ones who adapt more easily will be those who come to understand they are being offered an opportunity to become more deeply involved with interesting projects and to have a broader impact on the organization by improving the skill level of new managers. It is here where the learning character of the new organization becomes critical to the role change of the leadership. Strong support and a learning framework provide the bridge between old and new role behaviors and performance expectations.

CONCLUSION

Even with a fully empowered work staff and flat management structure, not all decisions can be made at the point of service. For very large projects that cross multiple clinical services and pathways and exceed the scope of the point-of-service leader, a forum must be established to review the projects and act as a steward for the major categories of resources.

The operations council brings together managerial stakeholders with a variety of perspectives and acts as a decision-making body for far-reaching systems issues. Decisions are made faster and are of higher quality because the issues are examined in the open by leaders with a wide range of perspectives and expertise. By fulfilling its role, the operations council contributes substantially to the implementation of shared governance and ensures the long-term viability of the organization.

SUGGESTED READING

Bodaken, B., & Fritz, R. (2006). *The managerial moment of truth.* New York: Free Press.

Charan, R. (2005). *Boards that deliver: Advancing corporate governance from compliance to competitive advantage* (1st ed.). San Francisco: Jossey-Bass.

Coakes, E. (2003). *Knowledge management: Current issues and challenges.* Hershey, PA: IRM Press.

Hosmer, L. T. (2006). *The ethics of management* (5th ed.). Boston: McGraw-Hill/Irwin.

Kaplan, R., & Norton, D. (2008). Mastering the management system. *Harvard Business Review, 86*(1), 26–44.

Kim, C., & Mauborgne, R. (2005). *Blue ocean strategy* (Vol. 86). Boston: Harvard Business School Press.

Riggio, R. E., & Orr, S. S. (2004). *Improving leadership in nonprofit organizations* (1st ed.). San Francisco: Jossey-Bass.

Ulrich, D., & Smallwood, W. N. (2003). *Why the bottom line isn't!: How to build value through people and organization.* Hoboken: John Wiley.

Weisbord, M. R. (2004). *Productive workplaces revisited: Dignity, meaning, and community in the 21st century* (2nd ed.). San Francisco: Jossey-Bass.

CHAPTER 7

Transforming Governance: Linking Strategy with Practice

Tim Porter-O'Grady and Kathryn J. McDonagh

*With input from stakeholders inside and outside the organization,
leaders are expected to shape agendas, not impose priorities;
to allocate attention, not dictate results; and to define problems,
not mandate solutions. These expectations we now have for leaders
closely resemble conventional notions of governing.*

—RICHARD P. CHAIT, WILLIAM P. RYAN, AND BARBARA E. TAYLOR,
GOVERNANCE AS LEADERSHIP

LINKING THE SYSTEM

So far, this book has covered the service and operational components of the clinical health system as it reconfigures itself for an integrated continuum of care approach to health services. Now is the time to address the governance and linkage components of the organization.

> The system focuses on the entire community. The point of service focuses on the community one member at a time.

Shared governance is fundamentally a point-of-service framework that tends to link the greater community with specific patients and the internal community (Porter-O'Grady, 1992). The assumption is that, although the organization serves the community as a part of its mission, each provider can serve only one patient at a time. Consequently, providing excellent service to an individual patient is a way of serving the community as a whole.

Linking the external and internal communities previously has been a function of the board of trustees (Brown, 1994), whose main goal, of course, is to help achieve the mission and objectives of the organization within the context of the community. However, in the emerging integrated environment, linking activities can no longer be looked at in the same way, and neither is the traditional view of governance appropriate for an integrated health system (Block, 1993).

NEW NOTIONS OF LEADERSHIP

In the new paradigm, a new set of rules applies to all the functions of the organization, including those related to governance. The clear distinctions between the roles of one level of an organization and another (vertical design) are no longer sufficient to delineate new kinds of relationships. In the movement from vertically integrated structures to horizontally integrated systems, a large-scale change occurs in the relationship between the functional elements of each part of the organization (Beneveniste, 1994). The clear distinction between such elements no longer has meaning and value, for the following reasons:

- Ownership is no longer a model for control in horizontal systems. Shared risks now become the foundation for relationships.
- Functional integrity at the point of service requires a clear understanding of the system's mission and objectives.
- The fit between decisions that relate to the system as a whole and those that affect work at the point of service must be clearly understood. It can no longer be assumed that a governance decision need not have the same content or context as a point-of-service decision.
- To ensure the continuing engagement of empowered individuals, some reference to and linkage with governance in functional decisions must be maintained as an ongoing part of the organization's work.
- Effective decisions are made as close as possible to the place where they will be carried out. Therefore, anything that impedes the ability of those at the point of service to understand the implications of governance decisions can no longer be tolerated. Decisions that affect a group of individuals should not be made without somehow including those individuals in the decision-making process.

This integrated approach to decision making and governance is a novel concept for many healthcare organizations that have been steeped in a hierarchical model rooted in such a model's military and religious histories. Many clinicians lack awareness of the functions of the governing board and view it as a "mysterious" body. This lack of understanding of governing boards may be a result of the historically more dominant role of the medical staff and professional management that traditionally superseded the authority and contribution of hospital governing boards (Pointer & Ewell, 1995). Therefore, it is imperative for organizations to undertake an educational process to transition to more contemporary notions of leadership and governance.

GOVERNING BOARDS IN TRANSITION

Just as notions of leadership have evolved, so too are the concepts and practices of governing boards changing. Rapidly evolving business environments and tumultuous dynamics in health care call for more effective boards and the need to strengthen performance of governance (McDonagh, 2005).

Assuming governance decisions can be made without including those they will affect is no longer tenable in the new systems paradigm.

Charan (2005) describes the evolutionary stages of governing boards. The first phase included ceremonial boards that performed their duties in a perfunctory manner. This was often seen in hospital and healthcare system boards when local leaders were chosen for the board more as a position of status than as a service to the community. The second evolutionary phase was a more chief executive officer–dominated board that resulted in many public governance scandals. The prime example of this type of board in health care was the Alleghany Health, Education and Research Foundation (AHERF) in Pittsburgh, Pennsylvania. The AHERF case study is replete with examples of weak governance structures, conflicts of interest, and an excessive domination by the chief executive in the face of poor decision making. The liberated board is the third phase, where board members assume a more active role in governance. An emerging phase is the progressive board, which moves from individual contributions to a cohesive approach that adds value to the corporation. This board enjoys lively debate, focuses on the important issues, and learns from each other. A progressive board leads to better governance through a focus on group dynamics, appropriate information architecture, and substantive issues. The governance council structure within a whole-systems shared governance organization is a most appropriate prototype for this effective governance model (Charan, 2005; McDonagh, 2005, pp. 13–14).

Once the locus of control for a decision is determined, the major task is determining how to engage those whom the decision will affect directly.

Governance experts Chait, Ryan, and Taylor (2005) framed a theory described as *governance as leadership* that includes the concept of generative governance. Generative governance is a collaborative process between board and management and from a shared governance perspective; this engagement includes clinicians as well. The process includes shared, creative thinking that makes sense of data and deliberates issues through robust and meaningful dialogue. Generative boards are more engaging and reflective and provide a vital sense of purpose for leaders (Chait, Ryan, & Taylor, 2005).

As governance theory and practices evolve to a more collaborative and inclusive approach, the movement toward whole-systems shared governance will strengthen. The trends toward more clinical involvement in decision making and the recruitment of more enlightened board members support a transformation in board culture that will then cascade throughout the organization.

LINKING GOVERNANCE AND FUNCTION

In an accountability-based framework, the linking of all components of the organization is essential for the judicious exercise of accountability (see Figure 7-1). Decisions regarding the organization's mission and objectives (decisions typically made by the board) are usually carried out by those at the point of service. In an empowered organization, those at the point of service are expected to play some role in making such decisions and in determining how they will be implemented (Graham & Lebaron, 1994).

> **In shared governance, the status of one's position is no longer a viable determinant of value. It is instead the consonance between the decision and the accountability for its implementation that defines role value.**

Linkage of decisions between one component of the organization and another depends on understanding the implications of the decisions throughout the system, especially the places they will be implemented. Decisions made at some point always affect decisions made elsewhere. Consequently it is appropriate to delineate decisions in an accountability-driven system based on their appropriate locus of control, and then to intersect the decisions in a way that engages the individuals who will carry them out. Also, work related to decisions depends on the decisions having legitimacy where they are made (Maurer, 1995). For example, making a decision about a way in which care will be delivered should be made in the places where accountability for providing the care exists.

Figure 7-1   Whole-Systems Shared Governance: Integrating the System

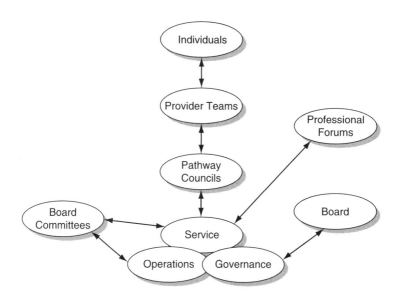

The delivery model and clinical framework should not be the province of the administrative leadership—and in shared governance they are not (McDonagh, 1991). Therefore, empowering an administrative group or board group to choose the model for the delivery of care is inappropriate. It is equivalent to precluding certain decisions from being made in certain parts of the organization regardless of who might be there and what perceptions of their authority might exist.

In shared governance organizations, it is critical to view decision making as a partnership activity. Each partner in a partnership has a specified role to play—a role that contributes to achieving the goals of the partnership (Coeling & Wilcox, 1994). What is essential is for each partner to be clear about the functions and extent of decision making that falls within the ambit of his or her role (see Figure 7-2).

> If outcomes are to be sustained, those at the point of service must exhibit as strong a sense of ownership and investment in the system as those at the "point of governance."

Figure 7-2   Whole-Systems Shared Governance: Structural Interface

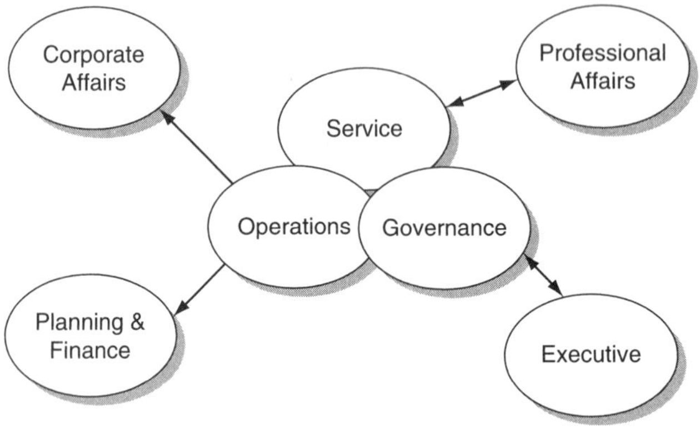

In an organizational system, such as a healthcare organization, the partnership framework works in the same way. When a partnership has been forged between the various components, it becomes imperative to delineate what roles and functions are appropriate for which partners. The concept of partnership is inconsistent with the concept of hierarchy, but decision making among partners still requires the delineation of decision-making obligations. The *Report of the Blue Ribbon Panel on Health Care Governance* (Center for Healthcare Governance, 2007) recommends the use of a policy and diagram for decision-making authority. This written decision authority matrix, which outlines the shared governance structure and accountabilities, can help avoid confusion and conflict about how decisions are made.

> The board is obligated to ensure an appropriate interface exists between the system and the community it serves. It is primarily a steward of relationships rather than resources.

This is also true at the council level. A partnership between the councils is created to ensure that specific decisions are made, work is accomplished, and desired outcomes are achieved (Jenkins, 1991). Each role and function, range of accountability, and outcome expectation is delineated by the stakeholders. Because there is a recognition of stakeholder obligations, stakeholders can negotiate to clarify their obligations. Once the obligations have been clarified, it is expected that they will be met. The checks and balances in the system are designed to ensure that accountability is exercised and desired outcomes are achieved.

> **In shared governance, the board is as accountable to its internal community as it is to its external community.**

TRANSLATING BOARD ACCOUNTABILITY

One of the biggest challenges presented by point-of-service models is to ensure that the goals envisioned by the board are translated into functions and activities at the point of service and implemented in some sustainable format (Lorsch, 1995). It is clear that, in a point-of-service model, sustainable outcomes can be achieved only by those who have a strong sense of ownership and have fully participated in the activities related to their functions and work. Consequently, decisions must not limit the ability of those at the point of service to own and influence the processes and outcomes of their work. This principle is critical for understanding the shared governance process and point-of-service models.

Increasingly it is apparent that whole-systems ownership and the investment of all of the stakeholders in the work of the system and the achievement of outcomes are necessary to make that achievement sustainable and gain everyone's commitment to continuous improvement (Nirenberg, 1993). Performance improvement is a critical and highly visible issue in healthcare today. Accountability for sustained performance improvement requires clear roles and responsibilities, accurate data and reporting, and a systematic approach to understanding, measuring, and improving performance (McDonagh, Chenoweth, Totten, & Orlikoff, 2008). Whole-systems shared governance provides the structural model to achieve these important outcomes.

> **In shared governance, there is a linkage between the decisions of any of the operating bodies of the system, no matter whether vertically or horizontally related.**

There must also be a clear understanding of the accountability and expectations that relate to the functions of the various components of the organization and the people who work there. The board, for example, is expected to act as a liaison between the organization and the community that it serves. In that capacity, the board defines the relationship of the organization to the community (Johnson, 1994). One priority of the board is to identify functions and activities that support that relationship (as well as the organization's viability).

Unfortunately, the fulfillment of its stewardship responsibilities at the community level does not necessarily mean that the board's wishes and desires are translated into daily work. Indeed, there is often a disconnect between the perceptions of those who are doing the daily work and those who are prescribing the overall direction and goals of the organization—a disconnect that tends to create "systems noise." It is often only through the authority and energy of the administrative leadership that any portion of the board's vision ever gets translated into functions and activities at the point of service, and this is one reason hospitals and healthcare systems can wind up looking extremely faddish, frequently shifting between a whole range of initiatives and innovations that rarely are substantiated by any long-term process or by sustainable outcomes (Kochan & Osterman, 1994). The high turnover of healthcare chief executive officers also contributes to this disruption and lack of continuity.

> **In shared governance, the governance council replaces all executive-level groups as the core point of integration in the system.**

Generative boards can prevent this lack of coordination by working at two boundaries: the internal boundary between the board and the organization, and the external boundary between the board and the wider environment such as the community it serves. Because it ultimately enables group decision making, trustees should do boundary work in groups (Chait et al., 2005, pp. 111–118). The shared governance structure that includes the perspectives of trustees, administration, clinicians, and staff promotes shared experiences and meaning related to the mission of the organization.

TRANSLATING DIRECTION

To provide a meaningful linkage between the components of a shared governance organization, some process must occur that motivates the stakeholders to invest, either directly or indirectly, in the organization's operating system. Part of this process involves creating an interface between the stakeholders that engages them and facilitates their investment in the work and the outcomes envisioned by the board. Therefore, the board should be linked directly at key decision points in the shared governance system (see Exhibit 7-1).

In a shared governance framework, it is essential that there be linkages between all types of decision making along the vertical and horizontal continuum and that the players be enlisted in a meaningful and direct way in estab-

Exhibit 7-1   Governance Council Accountability

The governance council does the following activities:

* Translates the board's mission and objectives into strategies
* Sets policy and priorities
* Ties corporate goals to the organizational strategy
* Ensures system integration
* Resolves conflicts between councils

lishing direction, setting up objectives, and unfolding work. It is also essential that there be full participation by responsible individuals in decisions that affect their accountability. Through the representative process, the stakeholders at every level of the organization must be invested in a way that ensures both their understanding of the mission and objectives of the organization and their implementation of decisions that are made. The following principles apply:

* The mission and objectives mean nothing if the language of shared governance is all that is generated throughout the organization.
* The mission and objectives must be translated into functions and activities.
* The daily activities and insights of those at the point of service must be consistent with the purpose and structure of the organization.
* The organization's mission must be translated into strategies, which must be further refined into tactics and processes. Consequently, the mechanism for decision making must get designated stakeholders to invest in each type of decision making—strategic, tactical, and functional.
* Equity demands that players throughout the organization be equally involved in establishing the strategies and tactics chosen to fulfill the organization's mission.

Further, there must be a place within the organization where all of the activities, from direction setting to care provision, converge—indeed, where linkage occurs. Principles that should guide this include the following:

* Strategy formation must occur in one place, yet involve all the necessary stakeholders. A joint strategic planning process should be formalized for the organization to ensure this participative plan.
* The fit between the strategies of the organization and their direction must be defined as clearly as possible.
* The strategies and their relationship to the tactics must be identified in a clear, succinct way.

- Individual and team performance must reflect the tactics chosen to carry out each strategy.
- Performance measurement and outcomes determination must be linked to expectations in every type of decision making, including the direction setting, strategy development, formation of tactics, and development of the personal objectives of individual workers. A common performance scorecard or dashboard should be shared with all constituents throughout the organization so that success is measured and rewarded with consistency. This range of activities is central to the work of the governance council.

In shared governance, structures are locations for the convergence of decision making. Linkages between the various components of the system require an identifiable structural format. It is critical to the integrity of the system that there be a place where the leaders representing the stakeholders come together. In a whole-systems shared governance structure, that place of convergence is the governance council.

The governance council replaces all executive-level groups, presidents, councils, cabinets, or other groups that reflected the hierarchical relationships that existed previously. Much of the value of those roles is diminished or eliminated with the change to shared governance. Consequently, having a body at the executive level whose role is to make direction-setting decisions no longer makes sense. In a shared governance framework, the governance council assumes the accountability for tying the components and configurations of the organization together as well as the strategies and tactics that the organization undertakes to fulfill its mission (Evans et al., 1995). Like all councils, the governance council is a decision-making body. Its decisions, however, are specifically related to the following issues:

- Translating the direction, mission, and objectives set by the board of trustees into specified strategies that give form to the work of the organization
- Linking decision-making loci to ensure that each component of the organization is meeting its obligation to achieve its assigned goals
- Dealing with linkage, intersection, and integration issues to ensure the fluid and effective functioning of all of the components of the organization
- Addressing problems with linkage and integration as well as the implementation of tactics related to the strategies for which it is accountable
- Evaluating the extent to which the strategies and tactics identified, agreed upon, and implemented by the councils and pathways are contributing to the achievement of the organization's objectives and the fulfillment of its mission

- Reviewing the interface between capital initiatives and strategic plans to ensure that resources are directed to the priorities it has established for the organization

The governance council is a place where the key designated leaders meet to focus on issues of direction and integration. It serves as a forum for delineating and assessing both the integrity and the effectiveness of the organization's work.

Governance Council Membership

The leadership of the governance council represents the leadership of all the major components of the system, not just the administrators and the board.

The governance council includes as members the key decision makers and stakeholders in the organization. Because it is responsible for integrating the organization and ensuring that the work being done is fulfilling the mission and objectives set by the board of trustees, leaders who are accountable for achieving objectives properly belong on the council. Therefore, at a minimum the members of the governance council include the following:

- The chair of the board of trustees (or a designee)
- The chair of the service (patient care) council
- The chair of the operations council
- The chief of the medical staff
- The CEO (and designated senior leaders)
- All senior leaders and consultants (ex officio)

This list covers the primary members (see also Figure 7-3). It is important to note that senior leaders and consultants are present as ex officio members because of their involvement in whole-systems applications across components. The leaders are mainly responsible for making critical decisions regarding the integration of the organization and the fulfillment of its mission, and the consultants provide information and support to the leaders.

THE ROLE OF THE CEO

The CEO is the agent of the organization and an officer of the system. As the designated link to the board, the CEO must ensure that the work of the governance

Figure 7-3   Governance Council Membership

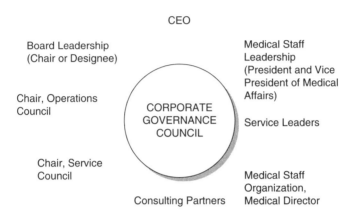

council fits the mission and objectives set by the board. As noted, the governance council is primarily responsible for translating the mission and objectives into the work activities performed in all parts of the organization. It is thus secondarily responsible for developing and promulgating strategies to fulfill the mission. To meet its responsibilities, it uses its links with the patient care council, the operations council, and the service pathway leadership.

A further obligation of the governance council is to ensure that all leaders pursue the strategic priorities in a disciplined manner. Because the governance council constructs the priorities, it has an interest in seeing to it that everyone is focused on them and that no one gets sidetracked into spending undue energy on unimportant projects.

ROLE OF THE CONSULTING PARTNERS

The greatest barrier to innovation is conventional wisdom.

As the old leadership team disappears from the organization, a new set of relationships emerges. In the hierarchical approach to senior-level structuring, a specific range of authority and accountability was associated with each role. The chief financial officer had accountability for all financial issues. The human resources senior officer dealt with all human resource issues. Authority and accountability for anything involving those issues fell under the auspices of the senior officers (presidents, vice presidents, administrators, etc.).

In a point-of-service system, as much authority and accountability for issues of control and revenue generation, for example, lie at the point of service as with the financial leadership. Utilization and regulation of human resources are also largely a point-of-service responsibility. The role of senior leaders is primarily to provide support to the point of service and the decision makers located there. Indeed, in some models the leaders who were designated vice president delineations are now called consulting partners. For example, the chief financial officer may now be the consulting partner for finance. This consulting partner's role is to ensure that the various responsible decision-making groups and individuals at the point of service have the information, tools, resources, and guidance they need to make good finance-related decisions.

> **Hierarchy has no inherent validity. It is merely the accommodation to our failing to do the real work of relationship building in organizational and work systems.**

This same role shift occurs for human resources, information, marketing, planning, and other officers. The consulting partners have an obligation to be accessible to anyone making decisions about the utilization of resources or other key matters.

Consulting partners operate like any consultants. They seek to market their services to those who need them (at the pathway level and in the councils) and validate their performance effectiveness by their degree of availability, their impact on decision making, and the number of consulting relationships they establish in a given period of time. Consequently, they accomplish the following activities:

- Are available at all levels of the organization upon demand for their services from the internal customers or point-of-service decision makers
- Are prepared to provide educational and support services to advance the skill base of the point-of-service decision makers
- Accept task assignments for research and planning related to major strategic initiatives
- Provide advice and assistance to pathway leaders for decision making related to the management of their particular service pathways
- Continue to refine the systems, services, and structures required for supporting point-of-service decision makers in all the places where decisions must be made

> The old vice presidents now become consulting partners, providing resources and support to decision makers closer to the point of service.

Needless to say, the shift to consulting partner for the system requires tremendous changes in behavior and function. Not all senior leaders can make this transition. A sense of loss and diminishment is sometimes associated with the movement of authority to the point of service and the change from being key decision maker to being key decision maker consultant. The organization must be prepared to meet the challenges presented by the dramatic change in role. The chief human resources officer plays a critical role in this transformation by developing new position descriptions, advising and supporting leaders in their new roles, and ensuring the recruitment process for new leaders is adapted to this new model of governance.

Much of the importance of the role of consulting partner derives from the value of the advice the consultants give key decision makers at the council or pathway level. Because councils and pathways in interdisciplinary shared governance are the only two loci of resource-related decisions, providing the information and advice is critical to the quality of the decisions made there. Indeed, the pathway leaders and council members require the same level of insight and knowledge as was once required of senior-level administrators. Moving decisions closer to the point of service does not reduce the need for good insights and comprehensive information. In fact, it is becoming apparent that high-quality decision making needs to occur more frequently at the point of service than at any other point in the organization (Russell & Evans, 1992).

> A shift from senior officer in the system to consulting partner requires a major shift in role and behavior. Not all people can make this shift successfully.

The consulting partners also have an obligation to the governance council. Because the governance council's role is to ensure the integration of the whole system, the governance council leadership needs the insights and the skills of the consulting partners to recognize the implications of strategic decisions and the linkages required to make the strategic initiatives successful.

The consulting partners usually have defined roles delegated to them by the governance council leadership to facilitate the translation of strategies into tactics at the pathway and point-of-service levels. The governance council does not develop tactics. It simply develops strategies. It does, however, have the expectation that tactics will be developed in the operations and service councils as well as in the service pathways. The main duty of the consulting partners is to help translate the strategies into tactics.

The consulting partner role is becoming increasingly important to the organizational integrity. Indeed, it can be argued that this role has broader implications than did the old vice-presidential roles that were defined compartmentally or by divisional allocations in the hospital structure. In the new approach, the consulting partners have a broad impact on the integrity of the organization, the effectiveness of decision making, and the delineation of expectations.

> **There is no value or future in believing something cannot be done. The future is always in making things happen.**

GOVERNANCE COUNCIL ACCOUNTABILITY

Like all other councils, the governance council has defined areas of accountability that determine its parameters and give it direction.

The areas of accountability of the governance council are necessarily broad because its role is to ensure the translation of the organization's mission and objectives into strategies, tactics, and ultimately functions and activities. In particular, the council is accountable for ensuring the existence of the following:

- A mechanism for reviewing evidence that the organization is achieving its goals, which typically takes the form of a scorecard or dashboard format so that all constituents are working toward the common direction
- A process for establishing priorities for the organizational strategies and initiatives
- A mechanism for ensuring that strategic initiatives support the achievement of the mission and objectives of the organization
- A framework for translating the organizational mission and objectives into strategies and tactics
- A mechanism for ensuring that all councils fulfill their obligations in a manner consistent with the mission and objectives of the organization
- A structure to ensure that all councils meet their accountability for making necessary decisions in a timely manner
- A system that provides necessary information to decision makers throughout the organization
- Evidence that all work performed by the councils and pathways is consistent with the strategies selected by the governance council

- A clear linkage between the organization and the external community so that the needs of the community are met by the services of the organization
- An information infrastructure to support decision making throughout the organization
- A mechanism to ensure that all decision processes support each other and that the decisions made at the point of service and the team, pathway, and council levels are integrated in a way that contributes to the fulfillment of the organization's mission
- A decision-making review process that regularly examines decisions made against their objectives for success factors and lessons learned

BREADTH OF ACCOUNTABILITY

The governance council has general accountability for the effectiveness of the system as a whole. Consequently, it is especially concerned with the linkages between internal structures as well as the organization's linkage to the greater community. It has an obligation to make certain that the perspectives of the community and the organization's mission are what drive its own deliberations.

> **The governance council ensures that there is a seamless linkage between all the points of decision making throughout the system and that they all work to fulfill the mission of the system.**

Ensuring seamless connections between the decision-making components of the organization is a critical goal of the governance council. Seamlessness is important to the integrity of decision making in point-of-service systems. Therefore, the governance council is always assessing the "fit" of the components with each other. The integrity of decision making at one place in the organization becomes a serious concern if it affects the viability of decision making in another place.

The whole-systems perspective of the governance council leadership is critical for the ability of the whole council to perform its role. The council uses various information strategies and the reports to determine whether the decisions made throughout the organization are consistent with the strategies it has selected.

> **The governance council leadership is concerned with the "fit" of the components of the system and their congruence with the system's mission.**

Evaluating individual performance is not nearly as important as evaluating the integration of components committed to fulfilling their obligation to provide patient care services. However, the provision of patient care services may have a positive or negative impact on other components of the organization. Each component must operate within concerted service parameters yet facilitate the work of the other components if the continuum of services is to be viable over the long term. One part of the system (e.g., one pathway) operating in a way that creates an impediment for another part vital to its integrity results in an unsustainable activity. If the pathways do not intersect appropriately or if the work of one pathway is in conflict with that of another, some mechanism must be used to find a solution. It is the duty of the governance council to ensure that there are mechanisms for the following tasks:

- Measuring the dissonance between the pathways
- Identifying the source and nature of the problem(s) causing the dissonance
- Linking each of the players involved so that a meaningful dialogue may occur
- Identifying and clarifying appropriate methods for problem resolution
- Selecting a method and measuring its impact
- Evaluating performance

The governance council also has an obligation to ensure that there are assessment mechanisms to measure the achievement of objectives. Note that rather than it being the identifier of problems, the governance council makes certain that there are strategies, mechanisms, and systems in place to assist those at the point of service in identifying incompatibility or performance interruptions and in resolving issues and concerns.

THE QUESTION OF SYSTEMS

Clearly, organizational effectiveness over the long term depends less on the ability of the governance council to resolve specific problems and more on its ability to identify imbedded processes that can be used to correct problems or address issues (Blendon & Brodie, 1994). The governance council has a predominant role in ensuring that such processes exist in the organization.

> **The governance council must be sure that the information infrastructure provides the range and depth of information necessary to clearly determine the seamless flow of data across the system supporting all outcome measurement.**

Key to the success of any systems approach is the quality of the information infrastructure. The internal information system (see Chapter 8) and the external information system (see Chapter 9) are critical tools for measuring the effectiveness of the organization. An information system is like a river that flows through the organizational system. Any player along the way should be able to "dip into the river" and obtain any information needed to guide decision making, correct deficiencies, and resolve problems. The insights, tools, and evaluative mechanisms necessary to determine effectiveness should be available at any given time to any player. It is the governance council's duty to see to it that the information system is in place, does operate, and meets the needs it was designed to meet. In the future, the information infrastructure of a healthcare organization will function as the framework for planning, implementing, and evaluating at every level. Because the governance council's focus is linkage and integration, the information system is a crucial vehicle for determining whether integration has occurred and how effectively goals are being achieved.

> **Attachment to the current structure always impedes the ability to conceive new structures. In general, conceptual capture by the passing age makes it difficult to see the emerging elements of the new age.**

THE GOVERNANCE COUNCIL AND THE CASCADE

Because there is no hierarchy in a shared governance system, the integration of decision making, the facilitation of partnership, and the interface between the components of the system are essential factors. In addition, a functioning system that assists the leadership in determining the proper direction for the organization and in moving the organization in that direction is critical to the organization's viability (Imparato & Harari, 1995).

> **The implementation of strategy is becoming increasingly dependent on the quality of the information infrastructure. Without it, data interface is virtually impossible in an integrated system.**

The success of a strategic approach is highly dependent on the quality, breadth, and integrity of the information system. Because control can no longer be achieved by ownership of all processes, a shared risk framework requires not only good information but a good informational structure supporting the activities of the organization and their linkage.

Figure 7-4   A Strategic Cascade

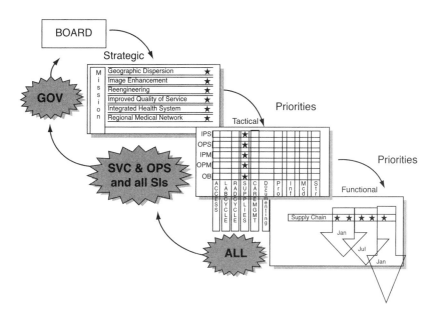

The board sets the direction for the system, the governance council translates that direction into specific strategies, and leadership of the system formulates tactics for their implementation.

A strategic cascade provides just such a structure. In this system, the board determines the organization's mission, objectives, and direction based on the demand and need for services within the community. As it links with the community, the organization defines its relationship to those it serves (see Figure 7-4). In fact, in a subscriber-based marketplace, the community is equivalent to the subscribers, both current and potential.

The governance council's role is to identify key strategies for fulfilling the mission established by the board. Although the strategies that define the organization's direction may be few, they are broadly encompassing and create the framework for subsequent activities by the councils, the pathways, and the service teams (see Figure 7-5).

Figure 7-5   Translating Mission into Strategy

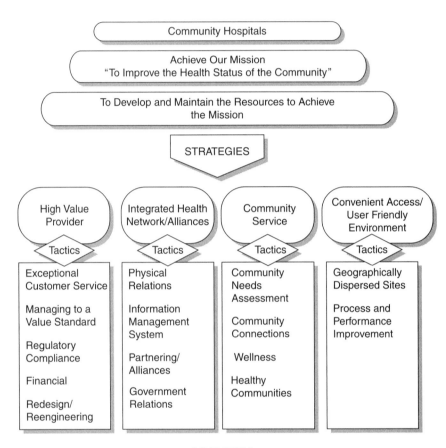

As noted already, the board's work is to set the direction. The governance council's role is to translate the direction into strategies, mandates, capital plans, and other functional elements, and the strategies determine the organizational priorities toward which the energies and work of the system are devoted (Wall & Shannon, 1995).

> **The strategic cascade provides the necessary tools to link strategy, tactics, and outcomes within a seamless connection between elements of the system and the mission to which the system is directed.**

Following the development of strategies, the governance council and the pathway leaders are required to develop specific tactics to carry out the strategies. These tactics identify sharply defined activities and functions that are intended ultimately to lead to the achievement of the objectives of the organization.

> **The governance council should bring a level of clarity to the intersection of the components of shared governance that will allow any person to enter it and easily know how it works and what people do within it.**

Because stakeholders are involved in every component of the system, staff at the team level, staff and management at the pathway level, staff representatives on the service council, management representatives on the operations council, and staff and management leaders as well as organizational leaders and consultants at the governance level all converge to provide a framework for the delineation and implementation of the tactics. Since the tactics are identified in an outcome format, the outcomes toward which the tactics are directed are identified in advance. Consequently, as the outcomes are defined, the organization simply backs into those behaviors, actions, or functions that will facilitate their achievement.

In the past, there was a heavy emphasis on process and action, but today the emphasis is on outcome. Recognition of the need to fit actions to outcomes is now part of the mindset of all leaders. Doing more work and using more resources are not equivalent to providing effective services, and much of the systems noise is caused by the conflict between the old functional expectations and the new focus on fit between resources and essential work.

The cascade from strategies to tactics to performance creates an organized and systematic mechanism to link all of the pieces of the organization together and create a seamless connection between process and outcome as well as a linkage to structure. It provides the governance council with a way to continually address the issues of integration and continuum and to identify those places where there are problems or issues or a break in the connection between components. Further, it also creates efficiencies in the system, narrows the place where decisions are made, clarifies accountability, and raises the level of performance expectations. Again, it does not increase the number of points of decision making. Only two points should exist in the organization: the point where decisions are made about service to patients and the point where decisions are made about service to providers. The structure, in other words, should support the providers in their work and the providers should support the patients in managing their lives and illness experiences along the continuum of service.

Hooking the cascade into the information infrastructure provides an ongoing interface between the daily activities, the clinical paths, the organizational goals and objectives, and the measurement of outcomes. Outcome measurement can occur all along the continuum so that at every place decisions are made, information that relates to the decisions or any associated decisions is available to whoever needs it. The governance council has the duty to push the organization to further refine information and the information structure to make it possible for more people to have more information about their performance and their relationship with other parts of the organization.

CHALLENGES TO EFFECTIVENESS

Many problems are associated with getting the governance council to work effectively. Many of them arise because of the major shift in the organizational structure that is occurring simultaneously.

> The most difficult challenge presented by the shift toward shared governance is changing parent–child behavioral dynamics into an adult-to-adult partnership at every level of the system.

Clearly, the total impact of the changes in roles, expectations, accountability, and functions creates a tremendous challenge for each player in the organization (Bennis & Mische, 1995). The move toward consulting rather than managing, for example, causes the leaders to experience extreme stress. Altering their behavior, changing their expectations, defining new roles, building new measures of evaluation, and determining new processes associated with the roles—all of this together can be overwhelming to those undergoing the switch.

No incremental system change can be sustained if it ultimately does not engage the whole system. No one can change one part of a system without ultimately affecting every part of the system.

The effectiveness of the governance council depends on the performance of the service and operations councils, the effectiveness of the pathways, the integration of the pathways, and the functioning of individuals at the point of service. Developments such as the increased involvement of the medical staff in point-of-service decision making and the closer linking of the medical staff organization and the entire system create substantial noise during the transformation process. For effectiveness to be maintained, those at the point of service need development as much as the erstwhile senior-level managers.

SHIFTING THE FOCUS OF WORK

The transfer of work formerly done by senior-level managers into the councils and the pathways is slow and traumatic. Assignments that once belonged to specific vice presidents now must move to the councils and to other players in the organization. The decision makers that are critical to the effectiveness of the pathways are now the pathway leaders (service leaders). As they develop and grow, they assume more of the responsibility appropriate to their roles. At the same time, responsibility is drawn away from the former vice presidents, who are now shifting into corporate consulting roles. They experience a sense of lost power and need special support. One good tactic is to maintain an ongoing dialogue so that everybody feels that they can have their say.

It cannot be expected that shifts in the context and content of work will be received by people with great joy and enthusiasm. The system must respond to loss as effectively as it deals with change.

Initially, this shift in the focus of the work can result in delays and unnecessarily long decision-making intervals. This is a natural stage of progression in a shared governance development process and can be mitigated by a focus on extensive communication and support between the consultants and pathway leaders. Eventually a rhythm will be developed and decision making can move at a pace appropriate to the outcomes needed.

Exhibit 7-2   The Governance Council–Physician Relationship

The governance council does the following activities:

- Translates the board's mission and objectives into strategy
- Interfaces with the physicians
- Ties its strategy regarding physicians to the organizational objectives
- Ensures physician integration
- Resolves conflicts with physicians

INTERFACE WITH THE MEDICAL STAFF

As the medical staff continue to refine their role as a partner in the process, their interface with the system becomes increasingly critical. It is important that the medical staff play roles at the governance, service, operations, and point-of-decision-making levels (see Exhibit 7-2). Unfortunately, the movement of physicians from customer to partner also creates much noise in the system.

Physicians play a more intimate role in the decisions of the system, but as partners, not customers. There is a greater focus on outcomes and relationships with other partners, requiring more integrating physician behavior.

Physicians have traditionally played a role on hospital governing boards for their clinical expertise, and now other clinicians, such as nurses, are important in that process as well. This clinical team collaborative approach is a change for many physicians from their traditional roles.

Physicians are accustomed to having summary authority and being the locus of control for clinical decision making. In a team-based format, responsibilities are more broadly defined, and a clear delineation of the accountability of each player is undertaken at the outset of each relationship.

In short, the physician's role undergoes a major change. The physicians must accept a loss of clinical control, develop a partnership orientation, and build relationships at the point of service with other providers. The challenges that these tasks present and the changes in the structure of the medical staff organization have an effect on the physicians' relationship to the shared governance structure.

ENHANCING EFFECTIVENESS IN SHARED GOVERNANCE

As the functional components of the organization move to higher levels of activity and achieve increasing success, the demand for the appropriate functioning of the governance council grows. Change is often slow. It becomes more evident every day during the shift to shared governance that the point-of-service functioning of the teams and pathways is an essential foundation of the viability of the evolving healthcare organization. As implementation of the whole-systems approach accelerates and begins to achieve desirable outcomes, the performance of the participants starts to stabilize.

> **Shared governance is a journey, not an event. It is not achieved overnight, and there is no conclusion—no point when it is fully in place. It only provides a foundation for further growth.**

The need for quality information, the development of a broad-based information infrastructure, the linkage of tactics to strategy, the need for increasing control over finances at the point of service, and the growing accountability of staff for effective utilization of resources all intensify the demand throughout the organization for support, for integration, and for clarity. It is to these ends that the governance council's work is directed.

CHECKS AND BALANCES

Because of the checks and balances that are inherent in an accountability-based approach, no one council can permanently or negatively affect the integrity of the organizational system. Clearly specified loci of control, point-of-service decision making, accountability-based expectations, a framework for clarifying the roles and functions of each council, and defined roles for managers—these are the types of checks and balances that ensure congruence, integrity, and effectiveness.

> **To create, to endure, and to create again—that is the requisite course of innovation. Creativity, like change, is a relentless taskmaster, always requiring more growth, more insight, more work.**

The governance council's focus on seamlessness of fit, the integrity of the relationship between the internal and external community, and the building of a supporting information infrastructure to help the system operate more effectively strengthens system-wide decision making. Of course, problems will still arise in clarifying roles and getting the players at the governance council level to agree to act within the context of their emerging roles and in concert with other leadership roles. The demand for role congruence increases in every part of the system and maintains the energy necessary to address issues that have not yet been resolved.

As the cascade becomes linked to the information infrastructure as well as the work process and as the accountability of the councils becomes clarified, effectiveness, measurability, and outcome determination become easier to achieve. The immediacy of decision making, the ability of those at the point of service to make high-level decisions, the timeliness of decision implementation, and the ability of the system to correct errors quickly all represent a level of effectiveness probably never before experienced by the organization. Because the governance council's primary role is to ensure the effectiveness of the system, it is rewarding to the leadership to see desired outcomes being achieved throughout the system at an unanticipated rate.

THE IMPORTANCE OF GOVERNANCE CULTURE

Although the structure and seamlessness of the shared governance system are vital, so too is the governance culture that is embedded in the organization. A governance culture includes the norms, values, and behaviors of the governing body—governance council—and how it works within that context as an effective team. For many years, there was a dearth of research in healthcare literature linking effective governance and organizational performance. Now there is a growing body of literature emerging, demonstrating that board culture has a significant impact on organizational outcomes (McDonagh et al., 2008). Thus, it is imperative for the governance council to develop a collaborative and cohesive team effort to ensure effective outcomes.

One study examined the effectiveness of governing boards and their respective hospital performance that supported the theory that governance effectiveness emanates from a sense of teamwork and cohesiveness of purpose. It supported a construct of governing boards as collaborative, community-oriented, socially dynamic networks of leaders dedicated to a unified purpose (McDonagh, 2005).

A part of the shared governance development process should include education about effective governance for all participants in the systems framework. This includes governing board members, governance council members, and all council and pathway leaders. This is imperative in developing the culture of cohesiveness and unified purpose that is so critical to the success of the organization's goals and the whole systems governance itself. All bodies in the governance structure (governing board, governance council, all councils) should also conduct annual self-evaluation surveys to measure the effectiveness of the governance process. Any issues that are raised can then be incorporated into an action plan to improve the performance of the governing bodies. This is truly leading by example because the entire organization is expected to continually improve its performance and the governing bodies should do the same by setting the standard for excellence.

CONCLUSION

The governance council's most critical role is to link the components of the system together to form a seamless whole. The goal of seamlessness demands that every component of the system serves the organization's objectives. As those objectives become more diverse, the various components must again focus on the outcomes identified at the point of service and evaluate them in light of the expectations of the board. Doing that as partners creates a definitive arena of accountability that ensures that the desired outcomes are achieved without violating the authority, autonomy, and control of any of the components. Every component, whether a council, pathway, or team, has clearly delineated accountability that at some level contributes to the fulfillment of the organization's mission in a very specific way.

Through integrating components, the governance council creates a mechanism for maintaining a focus on the organization's principles and mission. Further, all activities are tied to the direction of the organization as it responds to its obligation to serve the community.

At the governance council level, seamlessness becomes the driving force for effectiveness. The council's ability to support other components, its ability to act independently, its willingness to relate interdependently, and its respectfulness toward decisions made at the point of service create a framework for achieving the organization's objectives and sustaining the integrity of the shared governance process and the effectiveness of the organizational activities.

REFERENCES

Beneveniste, G. (1994). *The twenty-first century organization.* San Francisco: Jossey-Bass.

Bennis, W., & Mische, M. (1995). *The 21st century organization: Reinventing through reengineering.* San Diego, CA: Pfeiffer & Co.

Blendon, R., & Brodie, M. (1994). *Transforming the system: Building a new structure for a new century.* Vol. 4. Future of American Health Care series. New York: Faulkner & Grey.

Block, P. (1993). *Stewardship: Choosing service over self-interest.* San Francisco: Berrett-Koehler.

Brown, M. (1994). The purpose of hospital governance is purpose. *Health Care Management Review,* 19(2), 89–93.

Center for Healthcare Governance. (2007). *Building an exceptional board: Effective practices for health care governance, report of the Blue Ribbon Panel on Health Care Governance.* Chicago: Author.

Chait, R. P., Ryan, W. P., & Taylor, B. E. (2005). *Governance as leadership: Reframing the work of nonprofit boards.* Hoboken, NJ: John Wiley.

Charan, R. (2005). *Boards that deliver: Advancing corporate governance from compliance to competitive advantage.* San Francisco: Jossey-Bass.

Coeling, H., & Wilcox, J. (1994). Steps to collaboration. *Nursing Administration Quarterly, 18*(4), 44–55.

Evans, K., Takamoto, C., & Porter-O'Grady, T. (1995). Whole systems shared governance: A model for the integrated health system. *Journal of Nursing Administration, 25*(5), 18–27.

Graham, M., & Lebaron, M. (1994). *The horizontal revolution: Guiding the teaming takeover.* San Francisco: Jossey-Bass.

Imparato, N., & Harari, O. (1995). *Jumping the curve: Innovation and strategic choice in an age of transition.* San Francisco: Jossey-Bass.

Jenkins, J. (1991). Professional governance: The missing link. *Nursing Management, 22*(8), 26–30.

Johnson, R. (1994). The purpose of hospital governance. *Health Care Management Review, 19*(2), 81–88.

Kochan, T., & Osterman, P. (1994). *The mutual gains enterprise.* Boston: Harvard Business School Press.

Lorsch, J. (1995). Empowering the board. *Harvard Business Review, 72*(6), 107–118.

Maurer, G. (1995). True empowerment: From shared governance to self-managed work teams. *Journal of Shared Governance, 1*(1), 25–30.

McDonagh, K. (1991). *Nursing shared governance.* Atlanta, GA: KJ McDonagh Associates.

McDonagh, K. (2005). *Hospital governing boards: Study of the factors that measure governing board performance and the relationship to organizational performance in hospitals.* Doctoral dissertation, Tuoro University, Los Angeles, CA, Ann Arbor: UMI.

McDonagh, K., Chenoweth, J., Totten, M., & Orlikoff, J. (2008, April). Connecting governance culture and hospital performance improvement. *Trustee.* 11–14.

Nirenberg, J. (1993). *The living organization: Transforming teams into workplace communities.* Homewood, IL: Irwin Professional Publishing.

Pointer, D. D., & Ewell, C. M. (1995). Really governing: What type of work should boards be doing? *Hospital and Health Services Administration, 40*(3), 315.

Porter-O'Grady, T. (1992). *Implementing shared governance.* Baltimore, MD: Mosby.

Russell, P., & Evans, R. (1992). *The creative manager.* San Francisco: Jossey-Bass.

Wall, S., & Shannon, W. (1995). *The new strategists: Creating leaders at all levels.* New York: Free Press.

SUGGESTED READING

Hilb, M. (2005). *New corporate governance: Successful board management tools.* New York: Springer

Nadler, D., Behan, B., & Nadler, M. B. (2006). *Building better boards: A blueprint for effective governance.* (1st ed.). San Francisco: Jossey-Bass.

Oliver, R.W. (2004). *What is transparency?* New York: McGraw-Hill.

Wearing, R. (2005). *Cases in corporate governance.* Thousand Oaks, CA: Sage.

Integrating Physicians and Building Provider Partnerships: A Community Hospital System Approach

Phil Hinton, Marsha Parker, and Tim Porter-O'Grady

*The real voyage of discovery is not in
seeking new lands, but in having new eyes.*

—MARCEL PROUST

THE FORMAL MEDICAL STAFF

The medical staff in most hospital settings is an independent, self-governing organization that reports to the board of trustees, not the hospital administration. In most hospitals, a single medical staff organization serves the system, and the top-level physician committee is the medical executive committee, which has responsibility for quality of medical care within the hospital, medical staff credentialing, delineation of clinical privileges, and the disciplining of medical staff members. The medical executive committee usually consists of the president, the vice president (president-elect), the chairperson of each department (e.g., medicine, surgery, family practice, Ob-Gyn/peds, and clinical specialties), the chairperson of the credentials committee, the chairperson of the quality management committee, the chairperson of each medical staff council, and representatives from hospital management and the board (see Figure 8-1).

> Physicians are no longer customers in the health system. They are, instead, partners, creating a whole new set of relationships.

Although a number of simplifications have been made as a result of the evolution to a single integrated medical staff, the remnants of the individual medical staff councils at each of a system's acute facilities is a reminder that there is a long way to go. Those councils often no longer align with the rest of the structure and increasingly are an obstacle to decisions being made at the point

237

Figure 8-1   Sample Medical Staff Organizational Structure

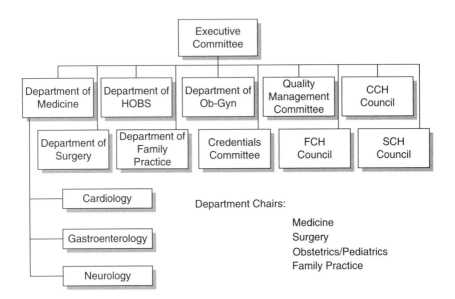

of service. They have less real authority, but everyone wants to include an informational step to the council before any final decisions are implemented. This often results in delays and turmoil that are not contributory to better decisions.

The current medical staff structure in most facilities is being redesigned to more closely align with the system's changing governance structure. Ideally, in a shared governance approach, medical directors are associated with each service line/pathway, and the aggregate group of service pathway directors constitutes the new medical executive committee. In this shared governance structure, then, the linkage between the medical staff committee work and the point of service is dramatically strengthened.

The redesign effort includes changing all medical director contracts to a performance-based format that accommodates medical director participation in the point-of-service multidisciplinary groups. This simplified, more aligned structure provides physicians more direct influence over practice in their most frequented areas. With the participation of physicians on the shared governance corporate councils, real collaboration can exist among the disciplines to govern and operate the whole system from the vantage of their own points of service. Unfortunately, there are some barriers to deal with along the way.

A PHYSICIAN'S VIEW OF BARRIERS TO SHARED GOVERNANCE

The bylaws of the medical staff at most health facilities are designed to protect the rights of the individual medical staff physicians rather than the rights of the patients (regardless of how they read). These bylaws are also intended to give the organized medical staff the maximum authority possible in how the hospital functions. The issue at the heart of the bylaws is control. Indeed, conflicts occasionally arise between the hospital and members of the medical staff, some of whom would like to believe that they should have veto power over changes in hospital staffing and organizational structure and decisions regarding hospital reorganizations or closures, mergers with other hospitals, and similar matters.

These same members threaten the hospital administration using time-honored tactics, including threatening to "vote with their feet" and move to other area hospitals if they are not afforded veto power over these decisions. Many members of the medical staff believe that their power rests in demands and threats—which may be true in the vertical, hierarchical power structures they are familiar with. Interdisciplinary shared governance approaches, however, hinge on team building, collaboration, partnership, interdependence, and accountability—a horizontal sharing of power (Coeling & Wilcox, 1994).

Informal Structures as Barriers

In addition to the formal medical staff structure, there exists another parallel system of informal physician political power related to personality strength, number of hospital admissions, abrasive behavior, racial alignment, religious affiliation, specialty association, heavy competition, referral relationships, and common economic benefits. Each physician feels that he or she is independent, is competent to make decisions of all kinds (regarding medical care, budgeting, planning, and personnel), and has a right to practice unilaterally and often without any constraint from the hospital or other physicians. Trying to organize physicians has often been likened to "herding cats."

In short, many physicians have felt that the hospital is simply their "workshop," a place that exists for their convenience and monetary gain. This historic cultural mindset is a major barrier to collaboration and partnership. Physicians have been acculturated to share power with no one, not even their own peers. In fact, the old medical staff structure is designed as an adversarial system, to protect individual physicians from the hospital and to protect individual physicians from the organized medical staff itself. As has been evidenced in a number of national cases, the rules as written often made it nearly impossible to discipline physicians for incompetence or intolerable behavior (Young, Rallison, & Eckman, 1995).

> The independent and unilateral practice of medicine in the United States is now dead. The physician of the future will exemplify a partner approach to practice in a much stronger team orientation.

In medical school and residency, deans and residency directors set clear boundaries to behavior. Breaking the rules of proper behavior at that level of training can result in suspension from the program, so trainees usually behave well. But when the physician is truly independent, having gained board certification and admission to the hospital medical staff, there are no such firm rules of behavior. The basic lessons learned in kindergarten, such as being nice, sharing, saying "please" and "thank you," are frequently forgotten, and physicians revert to adolescent behaviors when any conflict occurs, even a simple dispute over the requirement that a history and physical examination be in a patient's record before a surgical procedure is undertaken. It is hoped that recent behavioral requirements for hospitals from the Joint Commission will help facilitate the refinement of appropriate attitudinal and behavioral standards from this point forward.

Changes in Incentives

Before Medicare payments changed the landscape, physicians were paid on a fee-for-service basis, so their income went up as the number of hospital admissions and procedures performed went up. Similarly, the hospital was paid on a fee-for-service basis. Even with the advent of Medicare and hospital reimbursement by diagnosis-related group (DRG) and contemporary payment models and new outcomes, evidence, and performance-based approaches, the hospital has had an incentive to admit as many patients as possible and offer an intense level of care in the shortest possible time. This helped to decrease hospital costs and maximize income.

> There are no more resources. Anyone looking for more of anything in the current economic environment is engaged in a hopeless task.

Physicians' incentives have been somewhat different. Under the aegis of the new focus on quality of care, physicians gained maximum income by ordering multiple diagnostic tests and performing multiple procedures. Their physician colleagues historically benefited by multiple referrals during the hospital stay, and the longer the patient stayed in the hospital, the more money the physicians made.

With the implementation of managed care and subsequent performance-based payment models, both physicians and hospitals are paid by capitation, with a fixed fee for total care. This changed all the rules. With newer models of payment, the incentive for both the physicians and hospital is to manage care better. Most contracts provide for shared risks, value, and outcome so that excessive costs by either the hospital or the physicians come out of the pockets of both, and decreased costs by either the hospital or physicians advantages both (see Table 8-1).

> **When the price for service is negotiated in advance of service, everything changes in the health system.**

Table 8-1 Alignment of Incentives

	Hospital Admissions*	LOS†	Procedures‡	Patient Health§
Fee for Service				
Hospitals	+	+	+	−
Physicians	+	+	+	−
Medicare DRGs				
Hospitals	+	−	−	−
Physicians	+	+	+	−
Capitation				
Hospitals	−	−	−	+
Physicians	−	−	−	+

* Higher number of hospital admissions.
† Longer length of stay.
‡ Higher number of diagnostic and treatment procedures.
§ Better health for patients.

In this transformational time, with patients in many models of service management and cost control, many physicians do not fully like the fact that hospital admissions, stays, diagnostic tests, and procedures are costs to the system, not income generators. Many still dream of the old system. Some still envision the hospital as the enemy, trying to decrease physician income by encouraging best practices, good care management, early hospital discharge (decreasing length of stay [LOS]), and trying to maximize its own income by charging excessive amounts for services rendered and by cutting the number of caregivers to decrease salary expenses.

Physician Disconnection from a Systems Perspective

It should be clear that the medical staff functions in a way that keeps it disconnected from the core of the system. This disconnection, which results in delayed decision making and continuous conflict, weakens the care linkages to the point of service. One senior manager at a hospital created this personal breakthrough statement for working with the medical staff: "At this hospital the collaborative relationships among physician partners and hospital staff will be so smooth they will result in a complaint-free medical staff." The first reaction to that statement was uproarious laughter from hospital staff and physicians alike. Was the idea expressed really in the realm of the ridiculous? Apparently, it was thought to be.

> **The notion of integrating the medical staff is so unusual that many in the healthcare system see it as impossible, thus limiting the vision necessary to it ever happening.**

One of the learning outcomes from shared governance and whole-systems theory is that there should be no blame—every member of the system is accountable for the problems generated by the system. Yet in many hospital organizations, the historical relationship between physicians and administrators has been one of mutual blame. The physicians have often blamed the administrators for only caring about dollars, for making cost-cutting decisions that endanger the quality of care, for falling behind on spending for high-tech equipment, and so on. The administrators sometimes blamed physicians for not being enlightened about basic business necessities, for endangering the viability of the organization, for only wanting to further their own agenda to the detriment of their colleagues, and so on (see Figure 8-2).

Each side in this scenario expended a great deal of energy trying to find the pressure point that could gain it an advantage. At times, should either side get

Figure 8-2   Blame Cycle

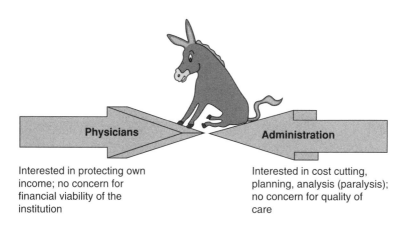

Physicians	Administration
Interested in protecting own income; no concern for financial viability of the institution	Interested in cost cutting, planning, analysis (paralysis); no concern for quality of care

too much control, something radical would be done to rebalance the scale. For example, the senior management team might be fired or the hospital system might set up physician organizations for the purpose of breaking old referral patterns and shifting power among the physicians. Neither of these solutions led to a healthy relationship between the hospital and the physicians.

> **In the past, physicians and hospitals bonded by offering more "goodies" to each other. Today there are precious few rewards that can be obtained without real partnership.**

Clearly, the hospital administrators and physicians have seen themselves as countervailing forces in a system, needing each other but lacking a mechanism for integrating the relationship. Each faction has operated as though their business affairs were completely independent of each other, as by law they have been. Each has tended to the belief that when push came to shove, new physician–hospital relationships could be set up—a belief that increased the risk of never developing committed and more sustainable relationships.

Physician bonding activities undertaken by hospitals are often based on the assumption that this kind of relationship is natural and attempt to create loyalty by offering more goodies to their physician customers. There is a great deal of effort spent on trying to understand the needs of physicians and appeasing them. There is often some short-term gain from such programs, but the reality of the provider–customer relationship between physicians and hospitals is that demands by one or the other continually become the focus of contention.

> **Each physician sees the world from his or her own perspective, not realizing that there is a broader frame of reference that is driving all change in the healthcare system.**

Adding to the dilemma are the difficulties that occur when a large organizational system interacts with small group systems or individual systems. Administrators agonize over the anecdotal complaints of physicians that seem so narrowly focused and so broadly communicated that they are frequently impossible to respond to. The example of the angry physician who, having had a frustrating day, storms into the administrative offices and accuses the administration of "lousy quality of care" because of staffing changes in a patient care unit is not an uncommon one. In a classic scenario, the physician loudly recounts a situation in which one staff member proved incompetent at observing symptoms and was bathing a patient when a crisis occurred. In another scenario, a physician demands the manager of the area be fired because "patients are being harmed." The appropriate response is to agree that there is a problem and to seek a resolution. However, it can happen that the manager, when researching the problem, finds that the problem occurred some time ago, has been corrected, and has nothing to do with why the physician is so angry. Yet the manager might well fail to provide feedback to the physician because there is no easy way to go back and tell the physician that there does not appear to be a replicability. Of course, the physician, receiving no satisfactory feedback, is reaffirmed in his or her belief that administration does not really want to work together on solving problems. It becomes a treadmill of failure, and the underlying causes remain unaddressed (see Figure 8-3).

Old structures and systems reinforce the problem of separateness. The medical staff structure is not only designed to be separate from the delivery structure, it is slow and cumbersome in its decision making so that any attempt at meaningful learning or collaboration is drained of energy. Old administrative structures can be rigid, and a morass of decision layers can effectively stymie any change efforts. The administration and the medical staff are each independent systems built on the assumption that they are distinct. This is a recipe for conflict. In this arrangement, there is little reason for the members of each of the structures to feel part of the larger whole and accountable for making the system work. When a medical staff committee votes to give itself approval powers over operational changes and when the administration assumes the right to control independent medical care decisions, conflict is engendered.

Figure 8-3   Paradigm Collision

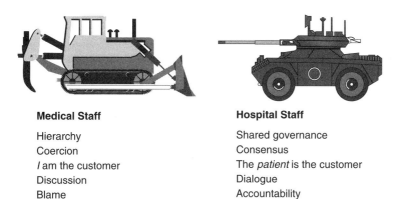

Medical Staff	Hospital Staff
Hierarchy	Shared governance
Coercion	Consensus
I am the customer	The *patient* is the customer
Discussion	Dialogue
Blame	Accountability

The dynamic at work here could be viewed from an entirely different perspective that offers up new solutions. If the relationship between the providers is assumed to be central and partner interaction is necessary to manage a patient population to a set of standards, the organization takes on a different character. When the living systems are seen by the people who make them up as so interrelated as to be inseparable, the anxiety, fear, and mistrust are offset by the mutual business of taking care of patients. Moving each patient to health becomes easier when the system is healthy.

A lack of understanding of what is to be gained by taking this perspective is the biggest obstacle to obtaining the benefits. The question then becomes, "How can we all begin to feel part of the system, an integral and necessary part of the whole?" This is the fundamental question of shared governance. The first step is to create some sort of vision or shared dream of what the end result could be.

> **Shared governance requires a vision of the interrelated aspects of all the elements of a system, not just the impact of any one component upon the whole.**

VISIONING WHOLE-SYSTEMS SHARED GOVERNANCE

The very first step in developing the vision is to try to get a grasp of what the system is all about. Too many old assumptions keep getting in the way. Demolishing the obstacles to understanding the relationships between living systems requires radical intervention. One good method is to engage in a "blank sheet exercise" in which groups sit down to a blank white board or flipchart and begin to discuss what it would take to manage a large, diverse patient population effectively and work toward an understanding of what would be needed beyond what currently exists. The first sessions foster the energy necessary to explore new solutions, and a shared view begins to emerge among the participants. These sessions can have shortcomings, however. If there are not enough physicians in the room when the exercise is done, the view is much too restrictive. In early discussions, the "whole system" is identified as the hospital system, the committed physician organization, and any contracted providers and suppliers. There is no consideration of the connections to other whole systems that significantly affect interrelatedness.

What will change the perspective is the possibility of merger or partnering with other facilities. Suddenly, the patient population numbers radically shift, and a new service mix is introduced. The obstacles to managing the patient population demand that the larger picture be considered. The overall impact serves to intensify the need for the key players to see themselves as part of the whole system rather than separate users of the system.

> The stakeholders in a system must be present at the making of decisions that affect what they do. In this case, you must be present to win.

The Vision

Once the view of the whole system and the shared governance framework emerge, the key players in the system begin to feel the need to restate the concept of their system in terms of a community integrated health network (IHN). This approach is not limited to a subset of the local patient population but is designed to take care of a large, diverse patient population along the entire continuum of care. Because the network model is based on whole-systems principles, the most important part of the system is the relationships between the elements of the network and the relationships with the other living systems that contribute to the functioning of the network (see Figure 8-4).

> The single greatest impediment to a new medical staff partnership is the old medical staff organization. One cannot hold onto yesterday while constructing tomorrow.

Figure 8-4   Systems Positions, Integrated Model

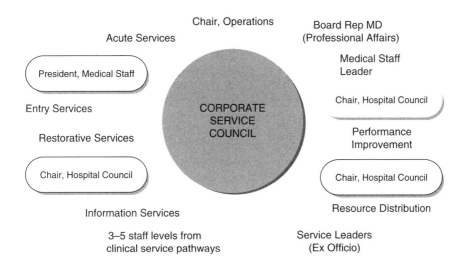

Interestingly, the physicians are going through significant turmoil in trying to get themselves organized at the same time. One of the major hurdles is their own political structure. Several groups exist in most health systems, such as practice groups, physician associations, an existing medical staff organization, and so forth. A number of players still have not yet committed to one of those groups and are watching the activity from a distance. Others have been deliberately excluded. Although many physicians realize the necessity of becoming organized to deal with the managed care pressures, they turn to political power and ownership control as a means of addressing the issues. As a consequence, the same dynamic that has kept physicians and administrators at odds for so long is also at work within the physicians' own ranks. Many fall back on old behaviors of mistrust and blame the hospital for their own leaders' inability to get the physicians organized.

Usually the physicians choose a "senior statesman" peer to help the various groups work through their issues and get organized into an interdependent physician association or a similar type of coalition made up of physicians committed to making the system succeed. When this strategy works and a significant breakthrough is achieved, the painful cost of the turmoil causes some physicians to leave the system. This radical change process reenergizes some of the hospital administrators to assist in integrating activities across the entire system, creating the IHN.

So, work on the vision results in some form of IHN identified as the services, systems, and relationships that support the provision of health services and the management of the health of a population up to a set of value standards. The value standard formula is:

Value standard = Quality (outcomes) / Cost (resources) × Time (service)

In managed care, the definition of the population served now encompasses not just the managed care members, but the whole community. It is the link with the community as a part of the network that helps illustrate how to better integrate the physician group.

Structuring to Support the Vision

Driving much of the new vision is the urgent need to move to a managed care type of organization and to stay strategically flexible in the rapidly changing environment. The strategy is to implement a continuum model of care.

The continuum can be identified here as a master pathway where users (people) are managed so that they reach best health status and different detour pathways are used when a user is having an acute episode. The goal of the health system is to manage care in a way that moves members (users) back to the master pathway as soon as possible. The master pathway is managed mostly by primary care physicians, and the detour pathways are managed mostly by specialists.

The detour pathways within an integrated care model are arranged into at least seven major pathways, three of which are continuum of care pathways (entry, acute, and restorative) and three support pathways (information management, performance improvement, and resource distribution). The seventh pathway is a standards pathway that might be called the "best practice institute," and it is there, in large part, that a link exists for connecting physicians, the community, and the rest of the delivery system. Using a structure of best practices, physicians can sit with other providers and community members to perform a truly interdisciplinary assessment of community and subset population health needs. They then can develop standards designed to meet those needs and measure outcomes.

Conceptually, members enter the master path after one of the following happens:

- They sign up for a plan served by the IHN.
- They go to any IHN system entry point.
- They apply for agency assistance as indigents.

The physician office and clinic are the most common entry points for most people. Interestingly, they offer the least information when the member arrives. In the new whole-systems vision, the physician-managed point of service (usually a physician's office) is the place with the most information related to management of the life of the individual member. The structuring of the information system around this vision and the whole-systems needs is one of the critical success factors in an interdisciplinary shared governance model.

Information system restructuring began with the evolution of the information systems departments into an information management pathway and the placement of all the old information-collecting, -processing, -analyzing, and -reporting jobs into process teams accountable for outcomes. Those outcomes relate back to the continuum tactics (the work of the patient care and operations councils). The next step is to integrate the information management efforts of the medical staff organization with the hospital system efforts to create an IHN.

During the struggles to find the right kind of organizational structure, an informal survey of key physicians can be useful. The single question is, "If you had a magic wand and could make anything at all happen, what questions about managed care would you have answered?" The following questions are commonly cited:

- Where do I learn how to manage care in a service-facilitating, cost-sensitive environment?
- How can I find out how I am performing compared with my peers?
- Where can I find the information and the method for managing a service budget so that I know whether I am making money doing this?
- How can I have input in setting the standards against which I am measured?

Answering these four questions provides a good foundation for the design of the organizational structure and the supporting systems. The design task is a huge undertaking and requires the board of directors to focus on the need for automated support for the whole integrated health network. The clinical information system, the network infrastructure, the shared governance decision support system, the office management systems, and electronic inpatient and outpatient medical record systems have to be selected and linked based on the answers to the preceding questions.

Physicians must be tied into the information system early to change their practice so that it is supportive of a systems approach.

In designing the information process, the physician member of the information management steering committee (the chair, if possible) must have the expertise to understand the greater system design needs and the importance of including physicians in the information system redesign process as early as possible. However, just because some physicians and hospital staff come up with a great vision does not mean it is an acceptable one. Aside from vision and structure, the following other elements of successful physician integration must be developed:

- Visible inclusionary activities
- Communication of the whole-systems view
- Results of best practice
- Finding and fixing underlying causes of conflict
- Participation in shared governance decision making

Seeing the Future

It is wise for hospital leadership to see the future clearly and make changes to prepare for managed care. This is easier for the hospital because it has an incentive, as it had with the old system, to manage costs for maximum benefit. Bringing the physicians along is more problematic. Even when presented with clear explanations of the changes, many physicians retain their fee-for-service mindset and sometimes refuse to let go of the idea that the hospital is their enemy (or at least their workshop, to do with as they like).

In the midst of this kind of turmoil, the hospital's leadership must look at the future anew. The CEO and the board must make a critical decision that in many ways will threaten the relationship between the physicians and the organization further—to proceed with a complete corporate reengineering, the institution of whole-systems shared governance, a radical flattening of corporate layers, and a redesign of processes to achieve breakthrough improvements in cost and quality. The hospital getting ready for the future must embrace change. Instituting shared governance entails a sweeping change of the corporate structure.

The Implementing Experience

Making a change of this nature requires both commitment and caution. The first steps taken to implement a different way of making decisions will create organizational noise and will be difficult for the physicians to accept.

The medical staff and the hospital experience a paradigm collision in implementing shared governance. Before shared governance, it is hierarchy versus hierarchy, raw political muscle versus backroom politics in a balance of power not unlike that brought about by a state of mutual assured destruction. With the new hospital structure, the medical staff bureaucracy can run headlong into shared governance councils. Coercion confronts decisions made by interdisciplinary caregivers (such as nurses and environmental workers). Physicians attempt to retain their customer orientation (I am the doctor, I am the customer). There is little evidence of a partnership mindset. There is still a desire to control (use of power to get what is wanted by avoiding facts that might be detrimental to a unilateral argument).

In the beginning, no dialogue is undertaken (no putting assumptions on the table, no inquiring whether other ideas might show assumptions to be incorrect), and much blame is present. There is little evidence of personal accountability (adult-to-adult interaction). Predictably, the medical staff's formal and informal structures are increasingly ineffective in communicating need or resolving problems in the emerging shared governance structure (see Figure 8-5). Indeed, without better characterizing the physician's relationship within the context of a partnership rather than the historic vertical relationship, it is difficult to build collaboration, engagement, ownership, and collateral relationships. The transition

Figure 8-5   Perceptual Conflict

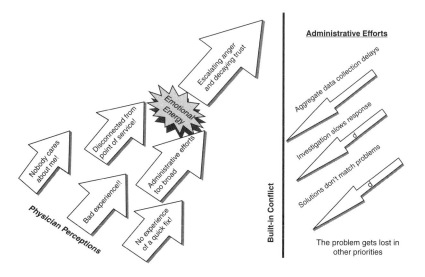

to these more horizontally oriented (adult-to-adult) patterns of behavior simply cannot be obtained or sustained without a clear delineation and expectation of partnership principles.

> **Polarization cannot survive in a partner-driven organization. No unilateral agenda processes can long thrive in such a system.**

Inviting the Medical Staff

The initial response of the hospital shared governance councils is to invite the formal medical staff organization into the "points of power," teach the staff to dialogue, allow their participation in decision making, and demand accountability. This is a major change from the usual structure, in which the physicians' responsibility is merely to identify problems, complain about them, and expect someone else to solve them. The best strategy is obvious: align incentives for the medical staff so that the success of the hospital is their success, and vice versa.

> **In health care, there is no us or them; there is only we.**

As the shared governance structure gets started (the experimental prototype for the whole system), the medical staff council soon realizes that decisions are being made by the governance councils rather than individual hospital administrators. Sometimes in the beginning, the organization, in driving the creation of shared governance, adds members to councils from nursing, the administration, and other hospital disciplines and gives them a defined role in council proceedings. Wise implementers of the governance council usually add physician members.

INTEGRATING PHYSICIANS INTO THE WHOLE SYSTEM

When interdisciplinary shared governance is structured within the health system redesign, the new single medical staff organization often deals with many of the same problems on a larger scale. Physician members of the medical staff should be invited to participate in the governance council, operations council, and patient care council. Meetings must be scheduled so that the physicians can attend without disrupting their office hours. Even if this is done, however, physician attendance at the outset is frequently poor. Reluctance to attend sometimes derives from the structure of the shared governance meetings.

Commitment to the decision-making process in shared governance is necessary to ensure the long-term efficacy of team activity.

When the physicians realize that decisions are made after extensive dialogue and the uncovering of assumptions, and that other caregivers have an equal voice, they are less interested in participating. Their idea of participation is that, if an issue is of interest to them, they will participate and have their solution adopted. Rarely have they been part of a diverse decision-making process in which they are not the only stakeholders who have an important role.

As an example of what can happen, consider this possible scenario. The entry pathway council is where decisions are made about the process of care in the emergency department. A key medical staff member, such as the physician in charge of quality in the ED, might be invited to participate in the new council's deliberations. He is well liked by the nurses, other caregivers, and the medical staff in general. He is viewed as fair, experienced, and open to change. But when his solutions to the ED problems are challenged, sometimes even by the least powerful people on the team (e.g., environmental workers, ward clerks, or administrative partners), his feelings become hurt and he might complain that his broader medical knowledge is not affording him the influence over the deci- sion-making process that he thought he deserved. He may characterize the shared decision-making process as "status collaboratis"—a condition similar to status epilepticus, where random chaotic flailing motions result in no forward motion. But suppose he is committed and persistent enough to stay in the process and does not quit the pathway council. As the council moves toward con- sensus on how to improve the processes in the ED, the physician might begin to understand the importance of looking at the process from the standpoint of the other stakeholders.

The final decisions that emerge from the team process are clearly superior to the physician's initial proposed solutions, and he eventually ceases to enu- merate at medical staff meetings the ways in which shared governance structure does not work. Indeed, he becomes a champion of the shared governance approach and defends the decisions of the council against the objections of his fellow physicians—and he might even seek their cooperation. He soon becomes accountable. Problems uncovered are owned and solved, not stated and com- plained about.

Physicians are members of the team. As members, they participate in the dialogue; they do not control it.

As the medical staff realize that their normal power base is eroding, their first reactionary move might be to demand veto power over all decisions of the shared governance councils. When this move is (predictably) rebuffed, their next request might be to be afforded input into administrative decisions that will affect physicians and their work. This is a step toward acting in concert with the councils because it fits with the shared governance principle that decisions should be made by those affected by the decision (stakeholders).

It is best to arrange a meeting between the medical staff leadership (members of the medical executive committee) and representatives of the shared governance and pathway councils at the beginning of the implementation effort. Each medical staff leadership position should be examined in light of its function and intended sphere of authority and responsibility and should be assigned a place in the shared governance structure. It should be recognized that a primary goal of shared governance is to bring 90 percent of all decision making to the point of service and that physicians retain power by being located at the provider team level, on the care units where the patients are served.

Physician Roles in the Corporate Shared Governance Councils

The membership of the patient care council, because this council deals with the way the work gets done, should include someone who represents the president of the medical staff. The decision to have broad-based medical staff representation is justified by the wide range of responsibilities of the medical staff members. The top leadership of the medical staff has primary accountability for the quality of medical care delivered by the medical staff members. Other medical staff leaders may have responsibility for site-specific issues (mainly quality issues) of interest to the medical staff, and they should also be members of the patient care council or present at its meetings.

Physicians must be present at critical decision making at the point of service where they have a major stake in its outcome.

In return for sitting on the councils, the medical staff members are expected to communicate the council's decisions to the rest of the medical staff and defend those decisions. They are expected to provide input regarding the needs of the medical staff, not to try to subvert the decision-making process for their own

Exhibit 8-1   Strategies to Win Over Physicians

- Role-model desired behaviors.
- Overeducate on concept.
- Keep overinformed.
- Ask advice frequently.
- Ask for help.
- Give credit freely.

ends. They are expected to respect the other members of the councils and treat them as equal representatives with viewpoints that must be considered before changes are made. Getting the medical staff to become invested in shared governance is a continuous, unending process that requires patience and persistence and an effective strategy (Exhibit 8-1).

The Medical Staff, Governance, and Operations

The operations council must also have a representative from the medical staff leadership. This is necessary because the medical staff share in the deliberations regarding capital requests and their priority. The consulting partner (VP) for medical affairs (see Chapter 5) is also a full participating member. The leadership of the operations council must realize that the hospital-based physicians are critical to decision making about infrastructure, such as the information system, facility construction, and clinical equipment.

Representation reflects ownership of decisions and influence over key outcomes that define the viability of the system.

The governance council, which devises strategies for the system and translates the board's direction into a practical plan for implementation, should have a key member of the medical staff as a member. It is preferable that the chief or president of the medical staff be that member because so much of the work of the organized medical staff must harmonize with the work of others in the system. Because setting policy, translating the mission into strategies, is the primary job of this council, this medical staff member is the most appropriate for the job.

Medical Staff Integration into the Pathways

The following are suggested assignments of the medical staff leaders to the decision groups developed within each pathway. The chair of the department of medicine sits on the medical pathway council, the chair of the department of surgery sits on the surgical pathway council, the chair of the Ob-Gyn/peds service sits on the maternal/child pathway council, and the chair of the department of family practice is assigned to primary care and sits on the home services pathway council.

The paid medical directors (e.g., the directors of cardiology, radiology, laboratory, rehab, and psych) are assigned to appropriate pathway councils and provider teams: The medical director of cardiology is assigned to the cardiopulmonary pathway (service line) council, the director of rehabilitation to the restorative pathway (service line) council, and so on. Many of the provider teams will want to participate in the orientation of the physician member to integrative and partner-based decision making.

The Medical Staff and Decision Making

A fundamental shared governance principle is that those who are affected by a decision should have a voice in making that decision. The major part of the medical staff input, therefore, is at the service level because the medical staff is primarily interested in how the work gets done, the quality of that work, the competency of the caregivers, and the education and health of patients. This means that the primary place to integrate physicians is in provider teams, pathway councils, and the patient care council. For issues related to resource use, such as capital requests and new services, the appropriate medical staff representative for the operations council is the medical staff officer usually assigned these duties. For policy and planning, especially strategic planning related to community needs assessment, governance council input from the president of the medical staff is important.

> **The key medical staff leaders are also key decision makers in the council format. All stakeholders are located in the same place.**

The object of integrating physicians and building provider relationships is to improve the care of the patient. The overall corporate mission is to improve the health of the entire community. Achieving improvement requires a whole-systems approach. Managing patients to a value standard is the method of choice for the enlightened health system. Managing patients to a value standard means using proven treatment methods routinely to achieve higher quality outcomes at lower cost.

The progressive medical staff, in partnership with all providers of service, select treatment methods based on best practices, evidence-based research (e.g., literature reviews), and expert decision methods (algorithms developed by experts in the field augmented by available research). Evidence-based and best practice models are those methods that achieve high-quality outcomes with low resource use. High-quality outcomes are defined as those including a low mortality rate compared with an expected rate adjusted for severity of illness and a low complication rate (a low morbidity rate compared with an expected rate). Low resource use means low rates of referral, low lab and X-ray usage, short hospital stays, low home health and medication costs, and so on. The highest possible health status and the lowest cost often go hand in hand, as in the case of surgical procedures. It is obvious (and easily documented) that surgical procedures performed smoothly cost far less than those plagued by untoward incidents, accidents, and complications. The shared governance process makes the obtaining of desired outcomes the work of all.

> **Managing to a value standard in shared governance becomes the work of every stakeholder. Outcomes are obtained through the efforts of the team, not just the work of any one member.**

To involve the physicians with the hospital in a partnership rather than a competition requires a change of tactics. Physicians are interested in quality care. Their entire training prepares them to engage in intense discussions on how to achieve better results. Even though their economic incentives are not always aligned with the hospital's, the clinical objectives are the same: excellent patient care and good clinical outcomes. Building on this shared vision, alignment of hospital and physicians is possible. If a method could be found to identify what type of care represents best practice, if the physicians could be convinced of the superiority of this type of care, and if the hospital systems could be modified to support it, the requirements for partnership would be met.

Physicians at the Point of Service

Locating the physician at the point of care is critical for successful physician investment in shared governance. If physician opinion is obtained at the provider team level about care, good decisions will result.

> **When outcomes require a different approach, it is the attachment to our rituals and routines that gets in the way of making any real change.**

An example of a successful process might be resolution of the chart location problem that exists in many hospitals. Because of the validating data in nursing research literature and a desire to simplify the charting process, nurses have often promoted the idea of moving the vital signs chart to the bedside. There is justification for this. If the person taking the vital signs records the data right away at the bedside, including intake and output (I&O) data, the accuracy of the data is enhanced and the chance for error is reduced. It is a simpler process, has fewer steps, and results in fewer delays. However, most hospitals are still on a paper chart system. If the decision to move to the electronic record is reevaluated, the physicians' and nurses' full adoption may still be years away.

Moving the vital signs record to the bedside affects more than the nursing caregivers. Frequently, after the decision to move the record is made, the physicians arrive on the unit to make rounds but cannot find the records because they are not where expected. It is then possible a physician might have to go into a room to see the patient and family without knowing the vital signs and fluid intake and output for the previous night and might have to struggle to obtain the information in the room in front of the patient and family. Even though the problem will ultimately be solved as the electronic medical record becomes the prevailing practice standard, in the interim dialogue and accommodation may need to be a part of the documentation management strategy.

Physicians and the Critical Path

The basic tool currently used for managing patients to a value standard is the evidence-driven clinical protocol, critical pathway, or care path. This protocol is a care plan for a particular diagnosis or problem, based on best practices, research, and algorithms. In the shared governance approach, it is developed at the point of service through engagement of the stakeholders on the individual provider teams. Each path includes multidisciplinary documentation that identifies expected outcomes on a shift-to-shift basis, an associated physician prescription set, a patient information brochure, and a pain control documentation sheet.

> **In systems approaches, problems do not belong to any one individual. If an issue affects the relationship between the partners and their work processes, it is everyone's problem.**

Good documentation sets forth the expected clinical activities, the proper treatments, the expected outcomes, the required labs, and the key decision points. Deviation from the plan requires reassessment of the patient, with changes in care and treatment aimed at getting the patient back on the path. Documentation menus are increasingly used, meaning that if the desired outcome is achieved, writing duplication is minimized. If a particular goal is not accomplished or a treatment not provided, documentation is required to identify the variance and to make plans for corrective action.

BECOMING INCLUSIVE

Just getting the hospital staff to begin including physicians in their decision making is usually more difficult than anticipated. Meeting times have to be changed so that physicians can attend (meetings before and after regular business hours and at noon are often more acceptable). Physicians are not prepared to function in groups that value and use dialogue and consensus processes. Many have difficulty in understanding and complying with the basic rules of engagement and often use old behaviors to attempt to control or influence outcomes. However, most are very valuable members of their groups and will attend more regularly when they realize there is no other means of influencing decisions in the shared governance approach. New partnership methods of linkage in decision making gradually eliminate the old methods (see Exhibit 8-2).

Once shared governance becomes the mode for decision making, the interest of physicians increases and their behavior becomes more consistent (their interest in attending meetings also improves). Collaboration among all the members of caregiving teams and physicians begins to develop, and the locus of control continues to shift toward the point of service.

> **In shared governance, the old method of deciding is ended. The new rules don't permit manipulation of the system in the interests of a single agenda.**

Exhibit 8-2   Operating Objectives for Physicians

- Continually improve quality of care and service
- Improve evidence-based continuity of care
- Create partnerships
- Increase resource and operations effectiveness
- Increase amount of teamwork and collaboration

COMMUNICATION: TRYING TO RECONNECT

One of the most visible inclusionary activities in shared governance is the assessment and implementation of new ways of working together. Because the new shared governance structure means that managers and staff council members become very mobile, the old office-based activities and meeting site gatherings become less effective. This is especially true in the emerging multiservice and multisite systems. The creation of the virtual office is going to change the way that people do business and make decisions in the future.

The way to connect to exchange information or to come to a decision is no longer just to call a meeting or invite someone to one's office. The establishment of an integrated information network infrastructure and the installation of Lotus Notes and comparable software allow everyone to communicate fluidly not only through e-mail but within whole projects because users can sit down in any workspace and access their work.

Perhaps the most interesting capability is the virtual meeting format that can be implemented by the point-of-service leadership. Any initiator of an idea or champion of an issue can hold a brainstorming session online. Options include participation by physicians in brainstorming, decision making, and project development—and all this is possible without the physicians having to leave their offices or attend meetings at inconvenient times.

Critical Communication

Communication in a shared governance system is usually less effective than it should be. Although every existing tool is used to communicate, there is often poor penetration. Suggested means of getting the messages out include these:

- *Newsletter.* A physician newsletter should be published every 2 weeks (if not more frequently).
- *Bulletin.* An online electronic bulletin should be published daily and posted on the units using the e-mail system. Most physicians should receive it electronically.

- *Memos and postings.* Cork boards in key places such as the physician lounge and the entrance to the cafeteria can be used to post information and use of online or e-mail-based means of communication.
- *Medical staff meetings.* Regular meetings are usually held monthly, and the minutes (electronic or online) are reviewed by many other groups as well. Staff members can routinely report changes.
- *Minutes.* Minutes from unit team meetings should be made available to anyone who has an interest in reading them.
- *The information network.* Information should be shared weekly through online computerized, personal digital assistant (PDA), portable, and virtual electronic means to reach those physicians not in attendance.

These usual means of communication do not always overcome the problem of penetration. Additional methods can be pursued:

- Shared points and the agenda from each shared governance meeting can be posted in the physician lounge and published in all the physicians' communication/electronic media.
- Cards (both manual and electronic) with contact person phone numbers by specialty can be created and distributed among the physicians.
- Storyboards showing changes being made, their targets, and their progress to date can be created. Eventually, most service areas should have permanent storyboard areas.
- Poster-size checkbook registers can be posted in all the care areas so that physicians can see how the care area money is being spent.
- Unit and special teams can meet with physicians individually and in groups to discuss specific changes. More than one meeting can be held on a specific change.
- Issues and changes and also how they fit into the whole system should be communicated. The context of an issue or change is as important as the issue or change itself.

Time must be allotted for the suggested "new way to work" systems to help increase penetration of information. In shared governance, it is affirmed that a new idea is never communicated enough, and it is worth a great deal of effort to repeat and repeat again the context for any communication.

Getting to the underlying causes of conflict is a painful process for all involved. A safe space must be available to confront the issues in a nonjudging but direct manner.

Results of the best practices process should be communicated only through an online/electronic protocol-tracking system. The results of the evidence-based practice protocol application process should show improvements in both cost and quality of care. In the development of protocols based on best practices, it takes at least a year of reporting, including physician reviews, before a critical mass of support and meaningful data are achieved. Protocol performance must be reported in all the medical staff committees as well as in the patient care and pathway councils. The ideal target for physicians is to manage at least 80 percent of the inpatient business according to value standards, creating a critical mass for faster implementation of value standard tools, evidence-based protocols, and information systems. Basing all practice standards on evidence-grounded best practices will energize more physicians, increasing their participation and improving outcomes.

RESOLVING CONFLICT

Finding and fixing underlying causes of conflict are especially challenging. The political uproar that accompanies reformatting the medical staff creates a terrible distraction and results in an environment bereft of trust for a period of time. Because only a few physicians fully grasp the concepts of shared governance, the discussions of conflict cannot start with causal loop illustrations. They must start at a more elementary point and build to the kind of trusting collaboration that gets into the more painful truths related to underlying causes. Using the work of the evidence-based best practice process as a vehicle to demonstrate, and not just propose, benefits is a method of validating whole-systems clinical processes and integrative decision making. Because evidence-based practice offers an opportunity for research and development and causes everyone to feel more open to new ideas, it provides fertile ground for real problem resolution for physicians and others.

GOVERNANCE FOR THE NEW VISION

The partnership between medical staff and system requires clear points of intersection where the interests of both can be negotiated and integrated.

Governance structures to support the pathways are always slow in being transformed into a truly integrated network model. The management service organization (medical staff organization [MSO]) usually has its own traditional structure, and this structure affects how the hospital system builds its shared governance structure. Throughout the process, teams of physicians and other partners must work on blending the functional areas of the two organizations based on clinical practice and their business interdependencies.

One team can be assigned the job of designing the way the whole service system should work over time. The process of physician–hospital partnership and integration is linked closely to the assessment of the community needs and to the ultimate structure of the IHN. This team can be a blend of physicians, nurses, hospital leaders, MSO leaders, and even community representatives. Discussions must at first center around the needs of the various elements of the network to have a say in decisions affecting the network. Because the recurring issue of control centers around ownership or partnership, the element of unilateral control is removed by creating a model showing the functional relationships of the network members supported through management service agreements that would link the MSO decision processes to that identified in the shared governance system, creating the foundation for real partnership (see Figure 8-6).

In the shared governance structure, a community development team can survey the community of users, prioritize their needs, and use the information for deliberations on how to achieve a truly integrated system. The group need not have line authority except that given it by all the members of the emerging network. It is empowered to review the community needs and the network needs

Figure 8-6   Medical Staff Linkage Diagram

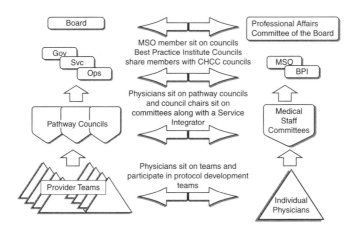

and propose changes to determine the organizing and relational priorities for the coming year (or years) for the new partners. Those priorities are then built into the management service agreements between the medical and health system partners. Everyone participates in the setting of service priorities, and each entity can feel comfortable that their particular needs and contributions have been considered.

Strategy Priorities

It is the job of the governance council and the MSO board to prioritize strategies for their organizations and to incorporate the recommendations of their workgroups (such as the community assessment group mentioned earlier) into those strategies. It is also their job to see to it that the objectives to be achieved by the strategies are clearly articulated and carried out as agreed to by their organizations. The communication responsibility of these two groups is twofold: They report the strategies to the operations and patient care groups in each of their organizations, and to the governance council and the governing board(s). The MSO board reports the strategies to the constituent organizations and physician members.

> **Many of the current separate functions of the medical staff will disappear as they become more integrated within the system.**

The MSO management leadership and the operations council focus on resource management in the five resource areas: fiscal, material, human, systems, and support (see Chapters 2 and 5). As the physicians become increasingly integrated, the two separate operations processes overlap more often. Having members from both systems (medical staff and provider partners) on all councils ensures that the work can be better organized and duplication avoided.

Through the evidence-based practice process, physicians can interact significantly with the patient care council (all providers). Both are accountable for how clinical work is done. The focus of these groups is the point-of-service connection between what the community needs and what is delivered. These are the groups that look at ways to continuously improve the quality of service delivery by using best practices principles in the development of practice standards (see Figure 8-7).

These network relationships exemplify the kind of functional relationships that hold the network together. There are many other tasks, such as contracting, community assessment, and claims management, that can be more efficiently

Figure 8-7   Integrated Health Network Shared Governance

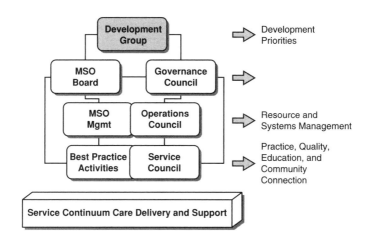

performed in a joint manner than done separately. Such tasks can be performed anywhere and are sometimes undertaken either by the health system or by the MSO. As long as there is agreement about the level of service to be provided and a group to determine priorities for development, the needs of the network should always be met.

Physician integration into the shared governance structure has already begun in many systems. The interfacing MSO should be designed to extend that integration. Each of the main shared governance corporate councils (governance, operations, and patient care) should have physician members, and the pathway and provider team groups at the point of service also should each have physician members. Early on, decisions shift closer to the point of service, and the corporate-level groups should be setting priorities, determining policies, and making any decisions that will have an impact across all service areas. The partnership between the medical staff organization and the system facilitates full continuum planning and decision making by paralleling the health system's work with the MSO and connecting physician-related structures through the application of shared governance concepts (see Figure 8-8).

> The real struggle for physicians is seeing themselves as partners in the health system rather than controllers of it.

Figure 8-8   Network Relationships Diagram

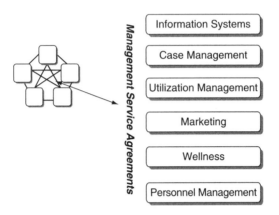

The goal of the medical staff and system leaders should be to ensure that all the medical staff committees eventually merge with pathway councils or corporate councils and that the joined yet parallel structures of the health system and MSO become completely merged. The whole system will thus become committed to addressing best practices for the community that they serve together. As this chapter indicates, there are clearly many barriers to overcome to realize this goal, but a careful and phased approach likely will be the most successful one.

Shared Governance and Value-Driven Care

As in many struggles, the real reasons for conflict are sometimes lost in the turmoil of raging emotions and feelings of the moment. The urge to strike out or retaliate for the painful parts of the change process often overcome the craving for an amicable settlement of the issue. In *Getting to Yes*, Fisher and Ury (1991) describe the dangers of position bargaining: "As more attention is paid to personal positions, less attention is devoted to meeting the underlying concerns of the parties. Agreement becomes less likely" (p. 36)

Talking about interests, options, and standards offers a basis for getting to an agreement. The principles of shared governance (equity, ownership, accountability, and partnership) reveal themselves through this same type of dialogue. But shared governance provides the option to go a step further than expressing these principles within the limits of a trained negotiating team. Instead, understanding the interests, options, and standards of another stakeholder group becomes the business of everyone in the system. This has extremely important implications for a physician in deciding whether or not to align with a particular system.

A scenario that exemplifies this dynamic is unfolding in one way or another in many health systems. It has to do with the security of livelihood and the quality of work life. It plays out daily through the point-of-service decisions that affect physician interests. When physicians are active collaborators in the processes associated with shared governance, whether it be in councils, provider teams, or at the point of service, the other members of the system begin to understand and appreciate their perspective and concerns.

Suppose, for example, an internist who serves on the patient care council is asked to address a provider team working on the new computer system. This physician has grown comfortable talking openly with multidisciplinary groups of providers with entirely different training and background from her own, and the team has also reached a comfort level and believes the physician to be reasonable and sensitive to her patients' needs. During the dialogue, the physician is asked to describe what her rounds are like. The entire team is shocked at the delays and barriers the physician states she must overcome every single time she makes rounds. Laying the information out on a flipchart, the team might find that the existing systems cause nearly 2 hours per day of wasted time—time spent waiting for, hunting down, or verifying information. Needless to say, this finding would have enormous implications for the design of a new information system.

How might the shared governance structure affect the physician's role and sense of security? By participating in the shared governance structure, the physician is more likely to know what is going on in the system as well as have an impact on decisions at the point of service. Indeed, substantial benefits—such as information about best practices for a particular diagnosis, a course on managing populations to a value standard, or case reviews and grand rounds—will be more readily available to this physician (and of course the system will gain from the physician's participation as well). When a new program is designed, for example, the physician is more likely to benefit from it if she was involved in the design process.

When an individual projects a unilateral agenda, there is no interest in what is best or right. Instead, there is an effort to achieve a singular goal without broad enough ownership to sustain it.

In the value-based market, a physician can lose huge chunks of his or her practice through the simple act of signing a contract. As long as the ebb and flow of the market tides continue to pull at physicians, there will be anxiety and concern. Investment in the emerging system offsets the dangers of wrong decisions and ties the physician's success to the success of the whole system.

> **Focusing on the same issues, partners can begin to really work on barriers to their relationship and the effectiveness of their work.**

In the process of implementing shared governance, physicians must keep in mind a few simple principles as they integrate with the health system. Shared governance is an accountability-based approach to structuring relationships. Therefore, personal and collective accountability are central to the success of decisions in the system. Physician members must apply the same rules of accountability as everyone if their role and participation in the system is to bear any real fruit. For example, they must do the following:

- Reach an understanding of commitment to a process and the accountability entailed by it before embarking
- Hold everyone accountable for his or her performance in and out of the meeting related to implementing the decision
- Never sway from the targets set by the group
- Be prepared for a large outlay of energy
- Never stop learning
- Respect all participants

A FEW QUESTIONS FOR THE PHYSICIAN'S SHARED GOVERNANCE JOURNEY

Implementing shared governance raises some unresolved questions for physicians as they confront the issues of health system integration:

- What benefits do physicians gain from being members of a system instead of independent practitioners?
- Market dynamics and healthcare economics are powerful and often negative forces that batter physician and healthcare system alike. Will membership in a system protect the physicians or make them more vulnerable? Can the system be protected without harming any individual physician?
- How can the long-term perceptual and cultural conflicts be removed to enhance the value of partnership and begin the long road to the trusting relationships characteristic of shared governance?

WHAT SEEMS TO BE WORKING SO FAR

The evidence for what works for physicians in a shared governance framework is growing. The consistent application of these rules, for example, seems to facilitate the achievement of sustainable outcomes:

- Locate physicians at power points for decision making, and then hold them accountable for decisions made there and for defending them to the rest of their medical staff partners.
- Move point-of-service decisions to the team of caregivers. Decisions are best made when the physician makes rounds with the care team.
- Convert waste time for physicians to productive time. Using communication tools set up in the units, surgical lounge, physician lounge, medical records completion areas, and offices allows physicians to focus on issues and their role in solution seeking. Tools for automated brainstorming, collecting input from physicians, information sharing for proposals, planning, and solution seeking must be provided.
- Dialogue, dialogue, dialogue—even when it is noisy and painful. Understanding the issues, interests, options, and standards that are important to work effectiveness and relationship building is the first step toward partnership.
- Take the broad view and try to grasp the whole system so that each piece can be kept in proper perspective.

THE FUTURE FOR PHYSICIAN PARTNERS IN SHARED GOVERNANCE

The term *evidence-based practice* has at least three meanings. It is used to define the philosophy of organizing all clinical functions to improve practices of any kind constantly. It is used to describe evidentiary practices that surpass all other practices commonly used in effectiveness and efficiency. Finally, it is used to refer to the process in which research and development of best practices anywhere in the organization are supported. No matter how evidence-based practice is defined, it can be used to help answer four questions that physicians feel are key:

1. Where do I learn how to manage care in a value-driven environment?
2. How can I find out how I am performing compared with my peers?
3. Where can I find the information and the method for managing a service budget so that I know whether I am making money providing services?
4. How can I have input into the creation of the standards against which I will be measured?

In committing resources to help the physicians answer these questions, the system is building partnership. When physicians create protocols designed around evidence-grounded best practices through their medical staff committee process, they are building a partnership. When physicians are fully invested in working with other providers at the point of service, that, too, is building partnership. When managing a member population to a value standard becomes the theme for the IHN and those efforts are supported by the evidence-based practice process, everyone is working as a partner—a fully engaged member of a health system that values his or her membership. The task of creating a structure that builds and sustains partnership lies at the heart of shared governance efforts.

CONCLUSION

It takes some real visible successes for everyone to feel the kind of trust in the system that will make it sustainable, but the foundations can be strongly laid and ready to support full physician integration into a shared decision-making framework. Such is the intent of the shared governance approach. Perhaps, through this approach the goal of a complaint-free and fully invested physician partnership is not so far-fetched after all.

REFERENCES

Coeling, H., & Wilcox, J. (1994). Steps to collaboration. *Nursing Administration Quarterly*, *18*(4), 44–55.

Fisher, R., & Ury, W. (1991). *Getting to yes: Negotiating agreement without giving in* (2nd ed.). New York: Penguin.

Young, M., Rallison, S., & Eckman, P. (1995). Patients, physicians, and professional knowledge. *Hospitals and Health Services Administration*, *40*(1), 40–49.

SUGGESTED READING

Moanojovich, M. (2005). Nurse-physician communication: An organizational accountability. *Journal of Nursing Scholarship*, *23*(2), 72–78.

Mullan, F. (2002). *Big doctoring: Primary care in America*. Berkeley: University of California Press.

Phillips, R., Harper, D., Wakefield, M., Green, L., & Fryer, G., Jr. (2002). Can nurse practitioners and physicians beat parochialism into plowshares. *Health Affairs*, *21*(5), 133–142.

Porter-O'Grady, T. (2001, January–February). 21st-century strategic thinking: Five insights for boards of trustees. *Health Progress*, 28–46.

Porter-O'Grady, T., & Afable, R. (2003). The technology of partnership. *Health Progress, 84*(3), 41–52.

Reinhardt, U. (2002). Dreaming the American dream: Once more around on physician workforce policy. *Health Affairs, 21*(5), 28–31.

Rosenstein, A. (2002). Nurse–physician relationships: Impact on nurse satisfaction and retention. *American Journal of Nursing, 102*(6), 26–34.

Smith, A. (2004). Partners at the bedside: The importance of nurse–physician relationships. *Nursing Economics, 22*(3), 161–164.

Thomson, S. (2007). Nurse–physician collaboration: A comparison of the attitudes of nurses and physicians. *Med-Surg Nursing, 16*(2), 87–93.

CHAPTER 9

Information Infrastructure for Interdisciplinary Decision Making

Marsha Parker, Lynn Neimeth, and Tim Porter-O'Grady

The Age of Technology will make neighbors of strangers,
and strangers of neighbors.

—MARSHALL McLUHAN

THE NEW INFORMATION INFRASTRUCTURE

Fostering the principles of shared governance (equity, accountability, partnership, and ownership) so that they are applied in daily decision making throughout an organization requires radical new approaches in organizational design (Porter-O'Grady & Krueger-Wilson, 1995). The most critical area needing redesign is the information management system. The components of information management in a shared governance organization are as follows:

- The structure, culture, training, information, and "systemness" embedded in the organization's activities
- The design of information flows between and among decision makers and councils
- Philosophical and conceptual modeling congruent with shared governance
- Data collection and delivery methodologies (procedural and design agreements that treat information as a dynamic)
- Hardware and software applications (putting the right pieces together to enable the flow of information)

THE IMPLICATIONS OF SHARED GOVERNANCE PRINCIPLES AND STRUCTURES FOR INFORMATION MANAGEMENT

Information is the new structure for society. It does not simply change what we do; it is defining what we will become.

The basic principles of shared governance all have a profound impact on the way information is conceptualized and the way systems for managing information are designed (Porter-O'Grady, 1992). The new design for information management must treat information as a dynamic rather than as a commodity. Or, as Margaret Wheatley has said, "The nut of the problem is that we've treated information as a 'thing,' as an inert entity to disseminate" (Wheatley, 1992). If the flow of information could be viewed as a river, currently only tiny tributaries flow from and to the point of service. Only the immediate information contained in the observations of the provider or the paper records of individual patients freely flows at the point of service. Even then, access is not unfettered.

The paper records are restricted resources that can be used by only one person at a time, and they never portray things as they are at the moment. Aggregated and trend data are the bulk of the river, and that river flows primarily toward management. Obstacles such as cataracts narrow the river and obstruct flow. These usually include the information experts, sometimes called analysts, who spend their time aggregating and trending information for others—again, usually managers. The more aggregated the data, the more senior the managers to which it is likely to be available, which means the flow is being further diverted away from the point of service.

Information is not a thing; it is a dynamic, a living process. It acts more like a river flowing than a machine producing.

One way to illustrate the problem is to view information from the perspective of a point-of-service decision maker. In this example, the point-of-service person, call her "Kelly Caregiver," is working in a shared governance organization. She is accountable not only for a daily caseload of patients but also for the outcomes of care for those patients' entire experience with the organization. Further, she is accountable, as part of a team council, for the improvement of the outcomes of her patients and many other patients like hers that make up the population served by her work team. Her job does not end there. She is accountable for the way the work is done, for the competence of the workers who provide the services, and for the appropriate use of the information that flows as a result of the work.

Kelly works in an environment that values her equally with every other provider of service in the organization, from the housekeeper to the radiologist to the CEO. Equity is built right into the structure and is enabled by such systems as the compensation management system and the communication system. The principle of partnership is that every individual is provided access to the capabilities and resources of every other individual in the organization. Ownership fosters a willingness to offer those capabilities to any other partner because it is the means of supporting the worker, the work, and its outcomes.

> **The information flow is continuous. It allows everyone to dip into it at any point along it when and where they need information in a format they can use.**

Information as a Resource

The most important thing Kelly needs to fulfill her accountability every day is information, but not information handled in the traditional way. Unfortunately, tradition still rules in the area of communication. Kelly comes to work at 7:00 a.m. and participates in clinical report, where she receives a flow of information lasting a few seconds or a few minutes about each of her assigned patients. That information contains some clinical indicators of the patients' status and problems. Major procedures pending are sometimes included and sometimes not. Kelly then goes to the many charts and lists used in her service area, checks the pending or open physician prescriptions for medical care, and creates her version of a worklist for the day. That worklist shows the tasks necessary for her to complete for her load of patients within her 12 hours. She measures her success by whether or not she is able to finish up the task list and handle the inevitable interruptions by the time her shift ends.

> **Information should help the provider make the decision that leads to the best outcome in the most timely fashion. It facilitates the provider's effort to do the right thing the first time, every time.**

The decisions Kelly makes throughout the day have to do with fitting together the tasks on the worklist with the immediate demands of her patients. She has an excellent education and knows the value of assessing and educating her patients. She is always driven by the need to do the right things and feels the pressure of her philosophical ideals, which frequently are at odds with the demands of the day. The kinds of things she must decide are, for example, "What is the most critical thing to do now? Ms. Smith must be ready for surgery in 15 minutes, and Dr. Jones is here demanding to know why his patient did not get the appropriate prep last night." Kelly has a "funny feeling" about Mr. Green but has not had time to get in the room to do an evaluation yet, and two members of her provider team do not understand their assignments.

The information required to support the decisions she must make is scattered: A paper chart she needs is in the possession of someone else at the moment; the nurse for Dr. Jones's patient is now at home asleep; the surgery schedule is posted on the wall behind the counter, where everyone is charting; the competency/skills checklists are in the manager's office; and the routine for prepping patients for surgery is on a form back in the unit clerk's area of the nurses' station. Gathering the data she needs is a formidable and time-consuming task. Furthermore, the difficulties she faces are not unusual, as every nurse can attest. Imagine the impact on the worklist if Mr. Green suddenly suffers an arrest and Kelly must manage a code. Will others help? Certainly, healthcare providers always rise to the occasion, regardless of what their workload is. But what happens when the providers Kelly hopes will ride to her rescue need rescuing themselves?

> Many times the real questions about information are who has the right to access it and how can it be controlled? In truth, however, information should be widely generated, not narrowly controlled.

Kelly has had some exposure to systems thinking and realizes, once she is home and rested, that several of the problems she typically must deal with have underlying causes. The team members should be better trained and more aware of their roles, two novices should not be scheduled together, there really should be a better way to handle the presurgical patients earlier than following report, and she has no idea whether cardiac arrest is common in the particular patient population that includes Mr. Green. Could Mr. Green's arrest have been avoided? Was her decision to quickly prepare Ms. Smith for surgery first an indirect cause of his arrest?

Where could she take all her concerns? Her supervisor? How many times has she complained without anything being done? Maybe she should air her concerns in the staff meeting. That is not for another week, and the meetings usually are not long enough or focused enough to deal with such issues. Maybe if she complained to Dr. Jones about her workload, he could get something done. Of course, she might then be viewed as a complainer. It is really not her job anyway, so maybe she should just keep quiet (Begun & White, 1995).

Shifting Control

In a shared governance model, the problems do not just go away, but there is a shift in the locus of decision making to the place where the problems occur and the means to uncover sustainable solutions exist (DeWoody & Price, 1994). One of the guiding ideas of shared governance is that the bulk of the decision making needs to occur at the place where the work is done (Chowaniec, 1994). How will Kelly be able to move decision making there? Although the answer is not complex, its implementation certainly will be. Kelly needs to bring about radical change in the following five elements before she will be effective in moving 90 percent of the decisions that most concern her to the point of service where she lives and works:

- Structure
- Culture
- Training
- Information
- Systemness

Structure

The shared governance model described in this book begins to put people with a point-of-service perspective into a structure that fosters seamless relationships throughout the system. People at the point of service begin to create the work practices, policies, and procedures that have real meaning—real impact (Evans et al., 1995). All the old stultifying administratively controlled three-ring binders are done away with, and only those few remaining rules that are fundamental to the integrity of the organization remain. The streamlined administrative framework makes those rules much easier to internalize and use in decision making than did the massive books that ostensibly governed behavior in the old system. Like boosting stations, the corporate councils become places to which information flows, is aggregated and made congruent with the needs and decision requirements of the organization, and then is distributed to those who may have need of it.

> **Information should always facilitate decision making. Information should support anyone attempting to make the right decision the first time and every time.**

When Kelly needs decisions made regarding issues in her service area, she has her own multidisciplinary provider team to assist her. If an issue affects more than just her service area or just her caseload of patients, Kelly can call on her pathway council to help. The object is to bring together the appropriate perspectives and disciplines to make the best possible decisions (Byrne, 1993).

Culture

The culture of the organization must support the empowerment of those providers who are struggling with the changes necessary to optimize their work (Albrecht, 2003, pp. xii, 260). Kelly, in our example, must feel confident that the values supporting her are uniformly held by all other members of the organization, including those in the management structure. All the usual checks, authorizations, and controls of the old system are replaced with enablers and empowerments, such as competency- and team-based compensation, evidence-based practice processes, peer review, and outcome-based evaluation.

The leaders of the organization, as information management role models, must exhibit openness and sharing. They must demonstrate the value of the learning organization. Kelly must be able to access the information that will help her find the right solutions quickly and easily, preferably wherever she happens to be when she needs it. Finally, resources must be put at her disposal to carry out the implementation of her decisions. For instance, if Kelly decides a patient would be much calmer if he knew his family had money for a meal and a motel room for the night, she could access organization funds set aside for such purposes with no need for any authorization (her service's "checkbook"). It should be that simple to facilitate the provision of good service!

> **In any system, it should be very simple for anyone at the point of service to satisfy a patient or family need.**

Training

Of course, Kelly does not instinctively know that aggregated and trended data for a patient population with Mr. Green's diagnosis might help her create a protocol of care based on best practices that would have reduced the chance of Mr. Green's having an arrest at that point in his course of illness. Neither would she automatically know that she could pull up flowcharts of the surgery preparation procedure and find that 6 of the 14 steps are no longer really necessary or that taking the old and new flowcharts to the councils would be an easy way to ensure that changes in procedure occur organization wide, thereby helping many surgical patients. But these are skills that are easily learned if training and education are made available.

Information

However, even if the structure, culture, and training were in place, there would still be little change in Kelly's daily life without information. It does her no good to know the techniques for reading and utilizing aggregated and trended data if they are exceptionally difficult to get or if she must know ahead of time the specifics or the sources of a report to even request it. There must be information—not just data, but usable information—available to Kelly when and where she needs it (Drucker, 1995) (see Figure 9-1). It is the food for thoughtful processing and decision crafting.

> **At the point of service, information should be both easy to get and easy to use. There is nothing worse than dealing with information that has no meaning or cannot be used.**

So, is the answer to anticipate what Kelly will need and create tidy routine reports by the cartload every month? That has been the method used in the past to send information to the vicinity of the decision maker. Unfortunately, it may not meet Kelly's need for availability and timeliness. Not many providers will take the time to wade through multiple reports to digest what is in each one, and then pull out items from each to put together in a meaningful final form. They will go with their intuitions instead and take the consequences. Something much different is needed.

Figure 9-1   Effect of Informed Decision Making on Patient Flow

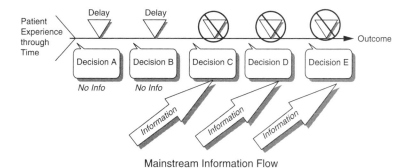

Technology is no longer the barrier. The only limit is the way information is conceptualized.

Systemness

Linkages and relationships create systemness (Wager, Wickham, & Glaser, 2005). The linkages that are supported in a shared governance environment not only must facilitate the daily work but must lead the organization as a whole to the next level of evolution (Porter-O'Grady, 1994). Shared governance supports point-of-service decision making and requires that the system be designed to ensure such decision making. User interface and ease are requisites for any data-based process that is intended to support decision making. They are also important for the relationship of the organization to its market and the community. It is not too much to expect every employee in an organization to "think globally and act locally" and to understand that every customer comes from and returns to a place that has contributed significantly to his or her being a customer in the first place.

> **In a shared governance system, all information is directed to supporting the point-of-service decision maker. It is there where the critical day-to-day issues are addressed and where most of the data support should be focused.**

So, how does information management systemness fit in a shared governance approach? The relationships and linkage of information flows make up the feedback mechanisms of communication, and communication feeds decision making. In a sense, systemness is equivalent to the essential data sharing that tells one part of the system how another is doing and how changes in one place cause changes in the other parts of the system—this systemness must be recognized and supported to sustain a shared governance approach.

If systemness could be visualized, it might look like a flow of work with decision loops all along it that relate to the patient experience through time. Whether the decisions support a smooth, unobstructed experience for the patient or become sources of delay and frustration depends on the stream of information that drives the decision process (see Figure 9-1).

INFORMATION FLOW AMONG SHARED GOVERNANCE ENTITIES

The shared governance structure comprises the corporate councils, the pathway (unit or service) councils, all the provider and service teams, and all the partners throughout the system, including suppliers, patients, individual staff partners, and physicians. In the old hierarchy, the lower down the person, the more dilute the information. Point-of-service personnel and customers got only what they could gather for themselves and what was immediately available in the provider–customer interaction (e.g., the medical record). The higher up the person, the more condensed the information. In the past, only senior management got aggregated, trended information that reflected the status of the entire organization. The result of this style of information flow was that each employee had no idea how his or her individual efforts affected the overall organizational outcomes—a form of isolation from the tactics and strategies upon which the decisions of the organization should be based.

> **In the past, only senior management got aggregated data. The point-of-service person never saw how his or her work affected the whole system or how others affected his or her work.**

In the shared governance system, strategic and tactical levels of information are routinely dealt with in all councils and provider team settings. The context for decisions is constantly being created jointly by the point of service and all levels of the structure. Because both formal and informal information exchange is vital, the informal "grapevine" is channeled by making the workings of the councils open to anyone.

Because there are no secrets, the informal networks should carry much more real information than they used to. Not that those incredibly imaginative and inventive individuals that exist in every organization will cease to feed the rumor mill; it is just easier to verify or discredit unsubstantiated stories. The formal information flow is supported by having the membership of each of the corporate councils assigned specific pathways (or unit and/or service councils) that they are responsible for keeping informed. It is also supported with all the typical tools, such as minutes, newsletters, share points, and bulletins, and everyone in the organization has access to the e-mail system and can have a personal e-mail address.

> The purpose of all information that flows through the shared governance system is to get the right data in the right form to the right person at the right time.

The purpose of all information flow in the shared governance decision-making groups is to get the right information to the right point of service at the right time. The corporate councils must ensure that the processes are designed, implemented, and maintained with that goal in mind.

Self-Directed Workgroups and Information Management

When planning how to use self-directed (point-of-service-driven) workgroups in the implementation of a major new clinical information system, several values, assumptions, and guiding ideas should be placed on the table. The backdrop for consideration is formed by the principles of shared governance: equity, ownership, accountability, and partnership. Secondary guiding values include openness, localness, and merit. And the main assumption should be that "any person, given the right information and the knowledge of how to use it, will make a sound decision" (Drucker, 1977).

> The most difficult challenge for team development is learning how to manage confrontation and conflict.

All these elements must be incorporated into the information management philosophy of the organization, and it makes sense to include them in the theme that will form the foundation for those designing any new organization-wide information system.

The self-directed teams should be put together using a mix of staff (some clinical practitioners and some technical experts) to keep the perspective as broad and whole-systems as possible. Each team should go through a rigorous training and on-the-job work experience program before the actual system development tasks begin. During development, the team members should familiarize themselves with shared governance principles and structure, shared leadership skills, and the many redesign and reengineering efforts going on throughout the organization.

Training encompasses the topics of project management, systems thinking (complex adaptive systems), systems assessment and design, shared governance principles, collaborative decision making, confrontation, presentation, continuous quality improvement, and basic problem solving. Each team member can then be given projects requiring the utilization of all the skills taught and be coached by other team members as well as by a service leader. The most difficult skills to master are those required for handling confrontation and conflict.

Self-directed information teams, like all teams, must learn their rules of engagement with each other in relation to the work they do. Outcomes of work cannot be obtained if there isn't a framework to facilitate and sustain them.

The evolution of the team during the first year involves intense learning, and some of the original members may exit as the team grows. Inevitably, problems bubble to the surface and demand changes in behavior. To the extent that the members can be flexible and adapt to the more sophisticated expectations, they will succeed. If a member cannot adapt, the rest of the team must address the problem and, if necessary, remove the member. This is the toughest side of accountability. It is not okay to accommodate an ineffective or inflexible member. Everyone must be capable of fulfilling his or her accountability. For the team to come to this understanding and then take the necessary action is a sign that it is becoming truly self-directed (Gottlieb, 2003).

To build a team context for their actions, the members usually spend a great deal of time in the early months developing the parameters within which they intend to work. Their activities include writing out the philosophy they will use to do their work, their goals and objectives as individuals and as a team, the rules they will use to deal with one another, and the behaviors they expect from one another. They can choose to coordinate their activities by rotating members into and out of a coordinator role. The coordinator is responsible for calling meetings and making sure the timelines are displayed so that any red flags can be picked up right away. The coordinator also has the primary duty of bringing together any team members in conflict and seeing to it that a resolution is reached.

Team-based evaluations can begin with a tool used by service leaders that everyone uses to evaluate everyone else—a 360° approach to performance review. The results can be aggregated and shared with the team members. The service leader can then follow up with any coaching or counseling indicated by the results. As the team matures (i.e., as the members become more comfortable with their own skills and with each other), the evaluation process involves more open dialogue within the team itself.

INFORMATION PROJECT TEAM

A good project team includes both clinical staff and technical staff. The team has a direct relationship to an information management steering committee (or some similar group). Each team member is accountable for the management of a piece of the project; and, of equal importance, each is accountable for his or her work and responsible to the other members. There is a role for a team leader or chair of the group, whose primary responsibilities are to run team meetings and to facilitate the activities. The team can decide that this role be rotated on a variable timeline basis so that all members have their turn. Project team assignments can be completely handled by the team, with input from its advisors, which should include the information systems service integrator, the consulting partner for information, the service leader, and the clinical information system vendor representatives.

> **Information development teams focus on the format for information generation. How it is used and applied at the point of service is determined in conjunction with the user.**

The team should apply standard project management techniques, such as the development of problem statements, the identification of agreed outcomes, and the measurement of progress toward these outcomes. One of the primary benefits of this approach is that a uniform, well-understood process for solving problems evolves. Each project manager is responsible for the development and maintenance of a Gantt chart for identifying barriers to achieving the desired outcomes or other issues that need resolution (Meyer, 1994).

> **Sustainable outcomes depend on the ownership of the work designed to produce them. The higher the level of ownership of the work, the more sustainable the outcomes. Although this is a simple truth, it is counter to the design of most organizations.**

THE TROUBLE WITH VENDOR PARTNERS

The self-directed work team concept is not generally well understood by software vendors, and shared governance or team leaders will have to take the time to explain the basic philosophy. The initial reaction will likely be skepticism based on a strong conviction that a major implementation effort must be supported by a hierarchical structure with "someone in control." Doubts about the concept usually emerge in the first 6 months, before the perseverance of the project team is able to change the vendors' perceptions of what works.

> **There is much talk of self-directed work teams. There is precious little evidence of belief in them in health care or in their real value to the organization.**

As the project approaches the completion of system tailoring and the beginning of integration testing, it often becomes apparent that not all of the objectives are being met. More important, it often becomes apparent that not all the objectives are clearly defined. When some objectives are not fully achieved, the leadership begins to assume more of the responsibility to ensure that the project schedule is not jeopardized rather than dealing head on with the noisy issue of individual accountability in a self-directed workgroup.

The chief information officer (CIO) can act as facilitator for the team in a series of sessions focused on assessing its strengths and weaknesses as a self-directed workgroup and determining its next steps. Three key outcomes should result from these sessions:

1. The team should remain a self-directed workgroup so that it can keep accountability for the work it does.
2. Continued emphasis should be placed on performance evaluation and continued attention paid to the kind and quality of the relationships between members.
3. The ability of team members to confront issues directly that belong to them and deal with each other honestly and frankly should continuously be developed.

The clinical information system project will not be successful if the system implementation stops at the creation of the self-directed work team. The ties between the developmental process and the operational units are key. The team, supplemented by pathway personnel, should engage in building a good information infrastructure. The time commitment of the pathway personnel varies by area, from minimal involvement (e.g., periodic meetings) up to a full slate of activities. The project managers also must work closely with the pathway councils and provider teams as they redesign the work flow to accommodate the new level of automation.

> In planning for effective information systems, it is important that the users be part of the team. Information should not be designed by the information senders without input from the end users.

To ensure appropriate linkage, a patient care task force should be involved in the project from the development of the request for proposal through implementation. The plan should be that this group, supplemented by representatives from other groups, will function as a user's group once the system is operational.

REAL-TIME INFORMATION ACCESS

One of the major challenges in ensuring appropriate information support is provided to individual users, councils, committees, decision makers, and user groups is real-time access to all current information available that may affect decision making. In open-systems decision making in a distributive decision-making environment, access to the universe of information is critical to effective decision consideration, processing, and rendering. Use of an organization-wide intranet containing the aggregate of all strategic, tactical, programmatic, initiative, council, committee, and administrative processes and decisions in real time is essential to effective well-informed point-of-service decision making.

Through use of laptop communication and wireless access, every decision maker and locus of control for decisions in the system using and accessing the same database should have available to them all the information sources and tools necessary for appropriate deliberation and consideration. Limiting the means of communication to the intranet as a single source of communication for the entire system creates a locus of control for information gathering and generating in a way that informs appropriate decision processes at every place in the organization. Using this real-time intranet-moderated communication and information infrastructure reduces duplication of non-cross-referenced decision making and uninformed decision processing, and limits decisions made not related to overall organizational priorities, strategic imperatives, and tactical objectives. Limiting the means of communication to the intranet-moderated communication information infrastructure and requiring that all decision makers use it create an effective operating information management dynamic that supports shared governance point-of-service decision-making approaches.

The Superusers

Another step necessary for moving an entire organization toward automation self-sufficiency is the development of *superusers*. These individuals' role is to help point-of-service staff identify problems, develop solutions, and answer questions. The superusers must fully understand the work flow in their areas and possess the information system skills necessary for superior first-line support.

The advantage of an interdisciplinary involvement process such as shared governance is that the major clinical information system is installed on time and on budget and there is a whole-systems perspective. Any member of the system can take the initiative to fix a problem when it arises to keep the project moving as it should. This approach provides the fast, fluid, and flexible teams of problem solvers and system designers. Whatever unpredictable shifts in the healthcare marketplace are thrown at the organization, it will have the resources to develop an effective response.

INFORMATION MANAGEMENT PHILOSOPHY

A view widely shared both inside and outside of the healthcare industry is that the industry comprises data-intensive, autonomous organizations. One common problem with the information transmitted, however, is that it is designed by the senders rather than the receivers. As a result, there is a mishmash of data processes and connections that are poorly integrated and not very effective (see Figure 9-2).

Over the course of the past few years, experts have recognized that an important part of the healthcare business is information management. Organizations that expect to survive as the healthcare environment undergoes major transitions must manage information as an asset and leverage it accordingly. In addition, health system leaders and vendors must continue to grow the concept that information systems are the organizational and architectural infrastructure of increasingly mobile and portable health systems and health services. Rather than seeing health information systems as strategic objectives and tactical goals, it is

Figure 9-2   Information Relationship Model: "As Is"

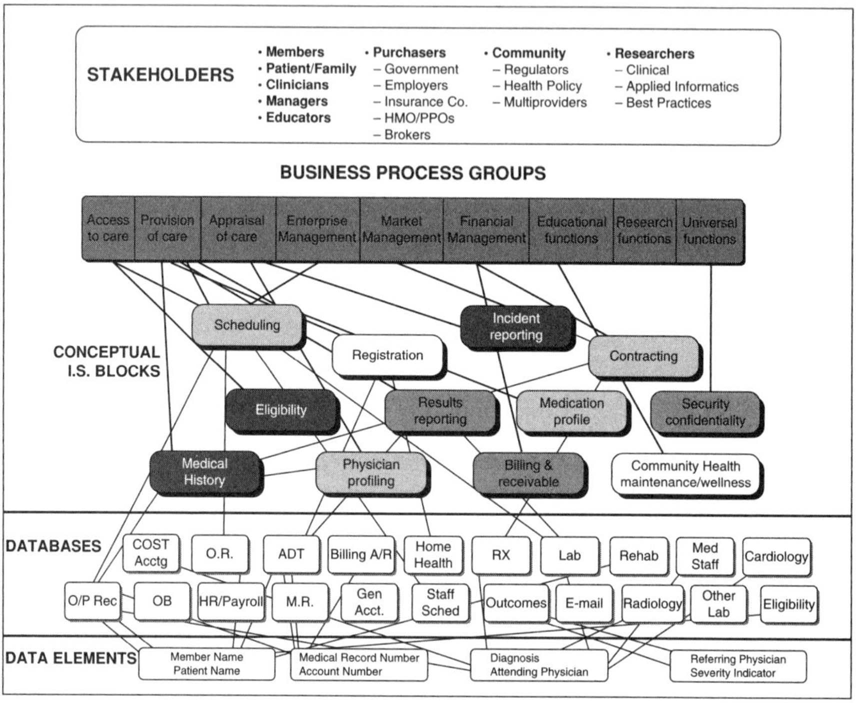

important for leaders to see the information infrastructure as the means, the vehicle, if you will, within which all service delivery processes operate and move.

The increasing portability of health service as a construct for service provision builds on the necessary foundations of real-time information and data management for the health service structure to operate at any level of effectiveness. Increasingly, all health service leaders, providers, professionals, and employees must see this continuous and dynamic information infrastructure as their means of doing business, recognizing now that it is impossible to do the work of health care at any level without the tight continuous interface between the information infrastructure and the service system.

Over the next decade, more than 50 percent of the capital outlays of the health system will be devoted to building a new information infrastructure for health care.

At most health systems, the largest capital investment by far is in the clinical information system. The largest investment of time and energy is in the people who will run and use the system. Information management requires a cultural change—a change in what happens in people's minds as they approach their work. Such a foundational change requires a whole new philosophy.

A well-developed philosophy of information management holds that the following points are true:

- Information is truly a shared resource for all members of the integrated health system.
- Access to information should be uniformly available to all authorized members of the integrated health system.
- Adequate education that allows the users to take advantage of the system's capabilities must be provided.
- Members of the integrated health network should be able to use information wherever their workplace is.

GOOD INFORMATION MANAGEMENT STRATEGIES

It is widely recognized that a health system's ability to compete and survive in a rapidly changing healthcare market is highly dependent upon the creation of information management strategies and the successful implementation of key information systems. Figure 9-3 shows that the information management strategies are in fact tactics with specific outcomes that tie directly back to one or more corporate strategies. The tactics in turn become drivers for specific information system projects that have specific goals as well. Perhaps the purpose of a single project (or multiple projects in various stages of implementation) is to support a given information management strategy. The following information management strategies can help enable operational improvements that in turn improve the value of the services:

- Provide for the integration of all network partners by providing the electronic communication linkages that support the collection and exchange of information.
- Provide a common set of information management tools so that individuals and teams can get the information they need to pursue their goals.
- Bring clinical and financial data to the point of service to support the timely, cost-effective, and high-quality decisions.
- Provide the information management support that enables the organizations within the integrated health network to evolve into knowledge-based learning organizations at the staff level.

Figure 9-3   The Information Management Cascade

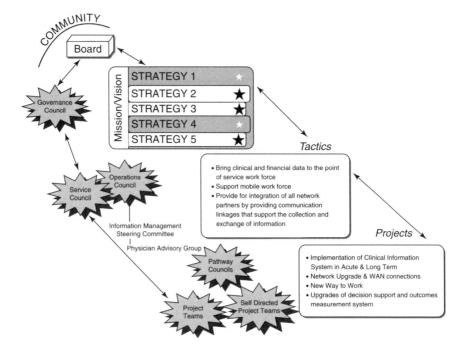

- Provide information management tools that support worker mobility and ensure access to needed information regardless of the workplace location.
- Make it feasible for all service providers to share applicable data about a customer.
- Ensure that the information system protects the customer and the user from the complexity of the system and safeguards confidentiality.
- Provide the information management tools that enable focused diagnosis, treatment, and business decisions to be made.
- Use aggregate data along with external databases and comparative data to pursue opportunities for improvement in practice.

TACTICAL IMPLEMENTATION: SOME SAMPLE PROJECTS

Several significant projects symbolize the drama of implementing information-based processes in a health system. One sample strategic and tactical cascade suggests some key information projects for the future of effective health systems:

- *Network upgrade.* This project encompasses a comprehensive data communication network plan that entails rewiring all existing facilities, includes installation of network management tools, and establishes high-speed wide area linkages between facilities. The data communication network provides the infrastructure foundation that enables all other information system endeavors to move forward. It ties directly to three information management strategies:
  - Provide for the integration of all network partners by providing the electronic communication linkages that support the collection and exchange of information.
  - Provide information management tools that allow mobility of the worker and ensure that the worker has access to the information he/she needs regardless of the workplace location.
  - Build the information infrastructure that will define the health system of the future and create the mobility necessary to bring health services to the subscriber rather than the subscriber to health services.

Virtual Office: New Ways to Work

The success of shared governance is highly dependent upon effective communication. The "new way to work" concept supports new ways of communicating. The concept also enables sharing of work information more quickly and allows widely disparate components to be brought together to form a whole. An integrated set of portability-based applications should be created for initial use by the service leadership team, the administrators, and some of the information service pathway self-directed work teams, and a plan should be devised for eventually deploying the tool set throughout the organization. The following applications might be included:

- Group scheduling (calendars)
- An improved portable electronic mail system
- Templates that provide for uniform problem solving
- Electronic opinion surveys with prioritization capabilities
- Work flow improvements supported by portability and electronic forms
- Electronic idea exchange brainstorming

The early users of these applications can be characterized as a mobile workforce. It is imperative that individuals have access to information they need to make decisions and perform their jobs from any location. Therefore, the term *virtual office* is appropriate. (What a virtual office approach entails is described in more detail later in the chapter.) Note that this approach is related to the following information management strategies:

- Provide for the integration of all network partners by providing electronic communication linkages that support the collection and exchange of information.
- Provide a common set of information management tools so that individuals and teams can get the information they need to pursue their goals.
- Provide the information management support that enables the organizations within the integrated health network to evolve into portability-enabled knowledge-based learning organizations at the staff level.
- Provide information management tools that support worker mobility and ensure access to needed information regardless of the workplace location.
- Provide information management tools that will enable portable focused diagnosis, treatment, and business decisions to be made.
- Enable decisions in the shared governance councils and pathways to be made quickly and effectively by providing the tools necessary for thorough deliberation and ready real-time access to relevant information.

Clinical Information System

The scope of this project is significant, and the implementation should be planned to last a minimum of 3 to 5 years. The first phase generally includes the replacement of the registration/admission, discharge and transfer, medical records coding and abstracting, chart deficiency tracking, radiology management, pharmacy, laboratory results reporting, and transcribed report viewing functions and the addition of new functionality for emergency department and automated worklists, order entry, and charge capture throughout the organization.

The implementation should occur at all facilities at the same time, including in physicians' offices that currently have access to the existing results reporting system. In subsequent phases, automated and portable documentation (charting and assessments), multidisciplinary care plans, enterprise scheduling, ancillary management, and patient accounting might be added. The clinical information system, which is further described later in the chapter, is related to these information management strategies:

- Provide for the integration of all network partners by providing the portable electronic communication linkages that support the collection and exchange of information.

- Provide a common set of information management tools so that individuals and teams can get the information they need to pursue their goals.
- Bring clinical and financial data to the point of service to support timely, cost-effective, and high-quality decisions.
- Provide the information management support that enables the organizations within the integrated health network to evolve into knowledge-based learning organizations at the staff level.
- Provide information management tools that support worker portability and mobility and ensure access to needed information regardless of the workplace location.
- Make it feasible for all service providers to share applicable data about a customer/patient.
- Ensure that the information system protects the customer and the user from the complexity of the system and safeguards confidentiality.
- Provide the information management tools that will enable focused diagnosis, treatment, and business decisions to be made.

All of the initiatives mentioned here should be a part of the organization's efforts to build true point-of-service information support. It is simply not possible to build a sustainable provider-driven system without offering the necessary assistance to providers where they live and practice. Furthermore, the empowerment approach simply will not work if it does not have the infrastructure it needs to sustain point-of-service control and foster good analysis and decision making. A commitment to creating an effective information systems infrastructure indicates the willingness of the organization to build structure to undergird the primary provider–patient relationship and the teams configured around it.

ROLES AND ACCOUNTABILITY

In recognition of the importance of devising information management strategies and implementing information systems that support the strategies (no minor undertaking), an information management steering committee should be established by the operations council. The role of this committee includes the following tasks:

- Develop information management strategies to facilitate managing care to a value standard.
- Engage in strategic information technology planning for voice, data, and image.
- Provide implementation oversight for key projects and initiatives.

- Review opportunities for utilizing information technology to improve value using the Malcolm Baldrige quality management framework or some other national standard.

> **All of the information system development means nothing if it does not enable those at the point of service to make better decisions and to evaluate their outcomes.**

The information management steering committee should be chaired by a nurse or physician, if possible, and should include a service integrator (service line, departmental, or unit manager), the service pathway leaders (preferably clinical leaders), at least two persons from the information services pathway, one person from the system leadership team, the CIO, the chief financial officer (CFO), a representative from the physician groups, and a project manager from the team responsible for implementing the clinical information system.

Establishing a clinical interdisciplinary advisory group is also wise. This can be chaired by the physician or nurse who chairs the information management committee. The role of the clinical advisory group is as follows:

- Standardize operational information flow for physician and clinical users
- Champion the use of the clinical information system by the nurses, physicians, and key clinical providers
- Participate in the ongoing design and development of the clinical information system (this entails participating in vendor–physician advisory group sessions)
- Evaluate recommendations for system modifications and enhancements
- Become superusers and advocates of the information management systems

Members of the information management steering committee provide a linkage to all three councils. The implications of information management strategy development and strategic information technology planning concern all three councils, whereas implementation oversight and information technology utilization review primarily concern the operations council.

THE CHANGING ROLE OF THE CHIEF INFORMATION OFFICER

> **In shared governance, the role of the chief information officer is primarily that of consultant to the system—the entire system, not just the information systems service.**

The terms *chief* and *officer* connote control and top-down management processes that do not have a place in a shared governance structure. The CIO's new role is to act as a senior advisor for information management and information services throughout the organization. The CIO helps to develop strategies and tactical plans that support a common vision of the ideal system, and the way of working requires that more time be devoted to educating and coaching everyone (not just a few leaders) and openly designing and facilitating information management initiatives (not creating mandates or dictating policies created with limited stakeholder involvement). The education process is not confined to information system staff but encompasses the board, the leadership team, physicians, and the provider teams.

> **Board support for the new information infrastructure services needs to be gained by involving the board members in the experience of the change through active learning rather than simple presentation.**

Power in the old model was held by controlling the purse strings for information system acquisitions and the information systems staff. In the shared governance structure, the service integrators have the accountability for the provision of resources, both staff and dollars. This relieves the CIO of having sole accountability for all operational decisions, which provides more time for focusing on strategy development. There are still opportunities to provide expert advice on operational matters, although the actual decision making is done by empowered individuals throughout the organization. The CIO should be invited to all shared governance council meetings and be highly encouraged to attend the operations council meetings, where tactics are formulated.

The specific responsibilities of the CIO might include these:

- Acting as advisor to the clinical information system project
- Assisting in the conceptual design of the integrated health network core system
- Facilitating whole-systems thinking and clinical information system template development
- Assisting in the design of the learning lab
- Facilitating problem-solving sessions
- Educating the leadership team, the information systems staff, and the board on information management matters
- Participating in redesign teams and system evaluation and selection processes
- Developing vendor partnerships and relationships
- Exploring telemedicine opportunities

Two of the preceding items deserve expansion. The first is integrated health network system design, which is covered in detail later in this chapter. The other is the board and the leadership team education.

Every presentation to the board should include the staff upon whom any change will have the greatest impact.

Board Support for the New Information Infrastructure

Specified board meetings should be devoted to understanding and supporting the construction of the information infrastructure. The CIO must act as a bridge between the board and the project team working on the CIS implementation, and between them and the information systems service integrator. Creating an interactive learning lab environment is the best method for indicating to the leadership team and the board what the future holds in store and for showing how the information infrastructure fits into an overall design of the integrated health network. The leadership team should format a dress rehearsal for the board meeting. In addition, an opportunity must exist to educate the leadership team on board dynamics.

The best way to approach educating the board is to develop a learning lab for them. Storyboards, workstation presentations, hands-on demonstrations, and video presentations are good learning tools. For getting across the nature of the clinical information system, areas should be set up to illustrate system use from the physician's and nurse's perspective, the caregiver's perspective, and the patient's perspective. In addition to CIS demonstrations, a workstation should be available that demonstrates the capability of the new system, a storyboard should provide a snapshot of where the project activities are relative to the schedule, and a description of the work team that is implementing the project should be available.

Another tool for giving the board a picture of the information systems is a demonstration of the capabilities of the "new way to work" project. A storyboard that describes the data communication network projects, including pictures of the wiring before and after, will allow the board to see the differences. A hands-on presentation built using computer-based training tools might be helpful. The presentation could describe, for example, the merits of the new information processes. Also, a video of the physician interface could be played for the members. Each learning area should be staffed with team members doing demonstrations or answering questions. The physician's perspective area should have tools that show the ease of use of the information system and its potential contribution toward physician inclusion in the organization, and it should offer a hands-on demonstration of a computer-based training module being developed specifically for physicians. The nurse's perspective could best be demonstrated by how the growing information infrastructure facilitates the nurse's role in facilitating, integrating, and coordinating all healthcare providers, clinical support, support departments, and the flow of activities necessary to move the patient along the continuum of care.

The impact of a learning lab in terms of increased support from the board can be formidable. In addition to letting the leadership and board learn about the information system efforts, it provides the individuals who are doing the actual system implementation an opportunity to respond to a broad spectrum of impressions and questions from board members. The effect on the entire organization can be very energizing.

In the old model, education of the board on information system matters usually involved a lecture delivered by the CIO and perhaps another senior vice president. The staff closest to the implementation projects would not have been engaged to participate, and it is unlikely that the entire leadership team would have had an opportunity to see the presentation and participate in refining it for the board. Bringing the stakeholders together creates further investment in and ownership of the challenging process of garnering board support.

INTEGRATED HEALTH NETWORK CORE SYSTEM DESIGN

The day is long past when a system can simply buy an information product and make it fit the needs of the system. The culture of a system drives all design.

It becomes clear early in the implementation of patient-based information systems and in the development of an electronic medical record that such a record will be of limited use unless key pieces of information are captured and documented in the physician's office (Tan, 1994). It should also become clear that an integrated health network needs a more global view of members or enrollees, many of whom are not ill but require health management services (e.g., well-baby checkups, screening exams). Therefore, the electronic health record must span the continuum of care, and the design of the information infrastructure must reflect this level of continuity (see Figure 9-4).

Even though the ideal is an electronic health record, it is not well understood exactly what an electronic health record should be. It is a myth, for example, that adequate health record software can currently be bought and installed. On the other hand, building an electronic health record in-house,

Figure 9-4   Information Relationship Model: "Ideal"

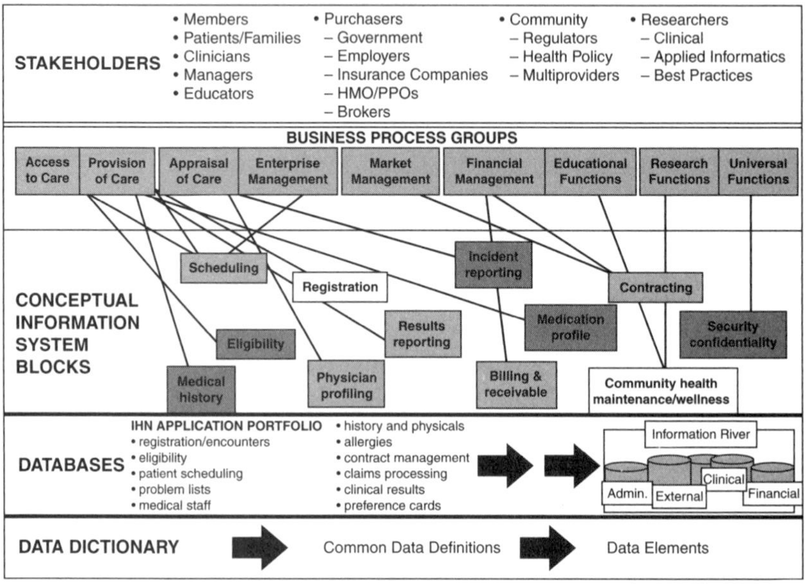

without support from vendors, is also problematic. Institutions that have taken this approach have typically spent millions of dollars and achieved only limited functionality. A significant portion of the development cycle is spent on designing the perfect system and never getting anything installed. Increasingly, however, the movement of large software vendors and online system utilities is increasing the potential for universality and portability of the patient's health record, making it increasingly possible to have patient-based mobile clinical records available across the breadth of the health system.

Any successful health system will need to go through a process of modifying and integrating its own application model of an integrated health record. After all, it is this record that will supply the data that will be fed into the dynamic river of information that will support decision making and enable improvements. The approach taken to developing the information system design should be guided by these rules:

- Develop an "as is" information relationship model (Figure 9-2) and an "ideal" information relationship model (Figure 9-4).
- Develop ideal flows from the perspective of each of these major stakeholders:

– Members (patients)
– Physicians and nurses
– Caregivers

* Develop a list of information management needs from an administrative perspective.
* Develop a system integration model (Figure 9-5) and continuum of care models for each layer (Figures 9-6 through 9-12).

A good integrated information model identifies the stakeholders, the primary business processes, the information system conceptual blocks, the databases that support the conceptual blocks, and, at the lowest level, the detailed data elements. The diagram seems fairly straightforward when the focus is on the relationship between a business process and the conceptual information system blocks that support the process. However, at the next level, the complexity of the existing environment is apparent. Multiple databases contain the same information. Some of the duplication is within network entities, and some is between entities (e.g., the medical staff organization, the physician's offices, and the payers or health plans). It is to be expected that the data element layer

Figure 9-5   System Integration Model

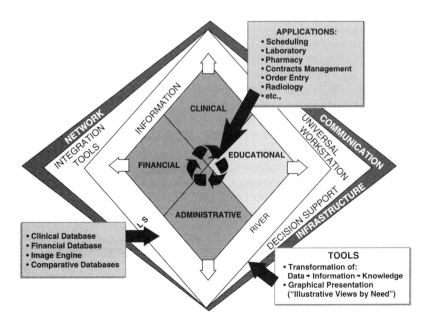

Figure 9-6   Core System Components: Clinical

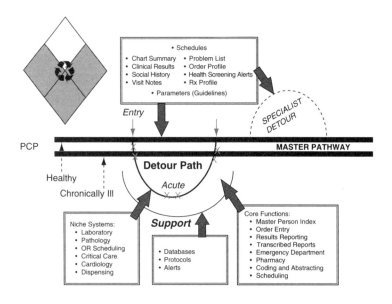

Figure 9-7   Core System Components: Financial

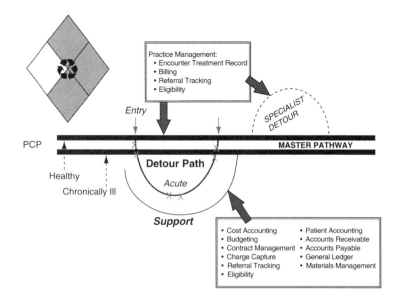

Figure 9-8   Core System Components: Educational

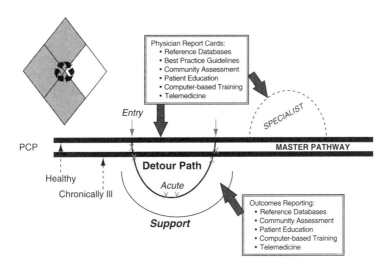

Figure 9-9   Core System Components: Administrative

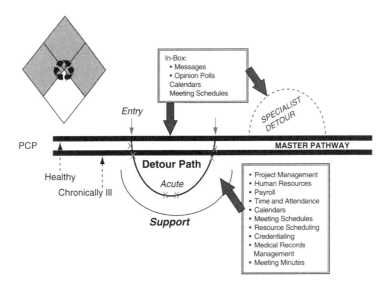

Figure 9-10   Core System Components: Software Components

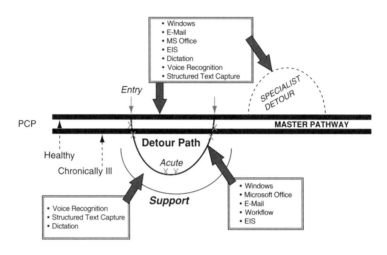

Figure 9-11   Core System Components: Reporting Process

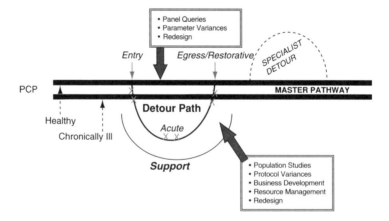

Figure 9-12   Core System Components: System Linkages

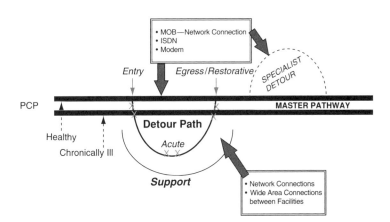

in an environment with multiple independent or loosely coupled databases would be as complex as a data system in which the data elements are in multiple places and have different definitions.

In an integrated system, the need for data duplication at any level is eliminated forever.

The ideal information relationship model (Figure 9-4) removes the duplicate databases from the picture completely. For example, there is no need for multiple laboratory systems in an integrated health network or operating room scheduling. The model also contains an "information river," which is a repository for data to flow throughout the system, and an organizational data dictionary, with common data definitions and mapping to the data sources. Without some model of the information relationships, the desired outcomes are unlikely to be achieved, and the complexity that prevailed in the past will grow to the point of causing the entire infrastructure to collapse.

As the ideal flow of information from a member's perspective is developed, it becomes clear that the following goals should be pursued—and that their achievement depends on the existence of a truly integrated information system that allows data to flow freely from the initial intake to wherever they are needed:

- Hassle-free care from the time of enrollment:
  - Coordinated appointment scheduling

– Data capture at the source (once and only once)
- System-wide identification of the patient and the patient's condition
- Orderly, caring, and sensitive service provision
- Desired outcomes ("feel better faster")
- Restricted access to sensitive data for those who do not have a need to know

Caregiver satisfaction will increase only if the information system achieves the following outcomes:

- Convenient access to all necessary information
- Access to reference data close to the point of care
- Faster turnaround of tests
- Accurate tracking of each patient's whereabouts
- Process improvements ("saves time")
- Desired outcomes
- Improved communication between healthcare team members
- Management of a patient population to a value standard

From an administrative perspective, the information system should achieve the following outcomes:

- Convenient access to information in support of decision making:
  – Financial indicators (e.g., volumes, revenues, contract performance)
  – Comparative information
  – Clinical outcomes
- High levels of member, physician, and staff satisfaction
- Increased market share

The system integration model diagram depicts the various layers of information technology that are necessary to provide various "views" of information for decision-making purposes:

- The outer layer is the communication layer—the network infrastructure that supports the rapid movement of data, voice, and image throughout the integrated health network.
- The next layer consists of the integration and decision support tools and the conceptual universal workstation.
- The information river provides for the combining of information to support the development of multifaceted views. It is commonly referred to as a *repository* or *information warehouse* in today's information technology terminology.
- The center depicts the four functional areas (clinical, financial, administrative, and educational) that are supported by applications that focus on the collection, manipulation, and reporting of data for a specific purpose.

The master path continuum of care model described in Chapter 4 should be used to further define the specific applications that are required to support each of the four functional areas along the continuum of care.

INFORMATION DEVELOPMENT AS EVOLUTION

Development of effective information systems unfolds over time, each piece relating to another. It cannot be constructed overnight.

The design and implementation of the integrated health record and the information management reporting system is an evolutionary process. The first step is to analyze data from external sources to begin to develop population studies. Initially, the reporting across the continuum of care will need to be derived from claims data and external sources.

The ideal information system allows for plug-and-play pieces that fit together seamlessly with little to no effort, similar to the systems that support banking and automated fund transfers. The reality is that health systems are still a long way away from achieving seamless integration. It is not financially feasible to replace all of the existing systems within any health system. The new systems must be truly open and support industry standards and open system protocols. Proprietary, closed systems simply do not work. Information islands are also not acceptable in an integrated health network. Members must be willing to contribute information if they wish to receive information.

Shared governance depends on the quality and effectiveness of data at the point of service and the ability of the provider and patient to use it.

Integrated health networks need to partner with vendors who are committed to their success and are willing to partner with other vendors to foster seamless integration. It is a common perception among information management executives and consultants that the majority of vendors today do not truly understand the nature of integrated delivery systems, and neither do they have a clue as to how to redesign the care delivery system. Off-the-shelf hospital information systems have an inherent structure that supports acute care processes (many of these systems are centered around charge capture, not true clinical care). Considering the ratio of physicians' office visits and ambulatory service visits to acute care hospitalizations, it does seem unlikely that systems with an acute care focus can be adapted for the outpatient setting. Likewise, systems that have been designed and developed for physicians' offices or ambulatory clinics probably do not have the capability to support acute care processes. This should not come as a surprise because relatively few acute care facilities have a single vendor that provides solutions for all of their information needs. Therefore, why expect there to be a single vendor offering a complete line of software for the emerging and rapidly changing integrated delivery systems? Nonetheless, it is important to maintain a whole-systems perspective and select the major components that will benefit the whole rather than a narrowly focused component.

CONCLUSION

Although it is apparent that there will be more integrated system solutions available in the next 2 to 5 years, healthcare organizations must begin to leverage information now to remain viable in today's market. This requires a significant investment to obtain the desired results. The service industries that are much further along than health care are now reaping the rewards of an effective information technology (see Figure 9-13). The information infrastructure is the future of health care.

Figure 9-13   Information Technology Expenditures as a Percentage of Annual Operating Expenses

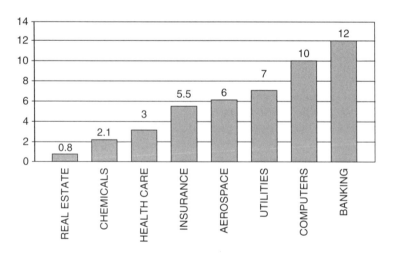

REFERENCES

Albrecht, K. (2003). The power of minds at work: Organizational intelligence in action. New York: AMACOM.

Begun, J., & White, K. (1995). Altering nursing's dominant logic: Guidelines from complex adaptive systems theory. *Complexity and Chaos in Nursing, 2*(1), 7–14.

Byrne, J. (1993, December 20). The horizontal corporation. *Business Week*, 76–81.

Chowaniec, C. (1994). Democracy and the living organization. *At Work, 3*(2), 17–19.

DeWoody, S., & Price, J. (1994). A systems approach to multidimensional critical paths. *Nursing Management, 25*(11), 47–51.

Drucker, P. (1977). *Management*. New York: Harper & Row.

Drucker, P. (1995). The information executives really need. *Harvard Business Review, 72*(6), 54–63.

Evans, K, Aubry, K., Hawkins, M., Curley, T. A., & Porter-O'Grady, T. (1995). Whole systems shared governance: A model for the integrated health system. *Journal of Nursing Administration, 25*(5), 18–27.

Gottlieb, M. (2003). *Managing group process*. Westport, CT: Praeger.

Meyer, C. (1994). How the right measures help teams excel. *Harvard Business Review, 72*(3), 95–103.

Porter-O'Grady, T. (1992). *Implementing shared governance*. Baltimore: Mosby.

Porter-O'Grady, T. (1994). Whole systems shared governance: Creating the seamless organization. *Nursing Economics, 12*, 187–195.

Porter-O'Grady, T., & Krueger-Wilson, C. (1995). *The leadership revolution in health care: Altering systems, changing behaviors*. (Gaithersburg, MD: Aspen Publishers.

Tan, J. (1994). Integrating health care with information technology. *Health Care Management Review, 19*(2), 72–80.

Wager, K., Wickham, F., & Glaser, J. (2005). Managing healthcare information systems: A practical approach for health executives. San Francisco: Jossey-Bass.

Wheatley, M. (1992). *Leadership and the new science*. San Francisco: Berrett-Koehler.

SUGGESTED READING

Goldstein, D., Groen, P., & Suniti, P. (2007). *Medical informatics 20/20: Quality and electronic health records through collaboration, open solutions, and innovation*. Sudbury, MA: Jones and Bartlett.

Maki, S., & Petterson, B. (2007). *Using the electronic health record in the health care provider practice*. Florence, KY: Delmar Learning.

Malloch, K., & Porter-O'Grady, T. (2006). *Introduction to evidence-based practice in nursing and healthcare*. Sudbury, MA: Jones and Bartlett.

Porter-O'Grady, T., & Malloch, K. (2007). *Quantum leadership: A resource for healthcare innovation*. Sudbury, MA: Jones and Bartlett.

Scott, T., Rundell, T., Vogt, T., & Hsu, J. (2007). *Implementing an electronic medical record system: Successes, failures, lessons*. Oxford, UK: Radcliffe.

Wager, K., Wickham, F., & Glaser, J. (2005). *Managing healthcare information systems: A practical approach for healthcare executives*. San Francisco: Jossey-Bass.

CHAPTER 10

Creating Sustainable Community in Health Care

Tim Porter-O'Grady and Marsha Parker

Loyalty to a petrified notion never broke a chain or freed a human soul.

—MARK TWAIN

HEALTH AND THE COMMUNITY

Implementing shared governance in a health system accomplishes nothing if the health of those served does not improve. The test of any renewal process is its impact on the purposes and work of the organization. Unfortunately, few measures exist yet to determine the relationship between restructuring health-care services and community health improvement. However, that does not diminish the need to uncover the relationship (Motes & Hess, 2007).

All the work undertaken at any integrated health network would have no long-term value if it did not address the issue of community health. Achieving the status of preferred health service provider depends on the fit between the populations served and the services offered. Further, patient satisfaction depends on the patients' obtaining health outcomes that can be directly related back to the services provided by the health network. All the shared decision making and seamless structure in the world are futile if enduring community health is not the main result (Porter-O'Grady, 2004).

The first step, of course, is to build a service community. That must be the central focus of the renewal and redesign work of shared governance and integration at any health system. The point-of-service design that has been created must support the system's purposes and work. The object is to engage the system at its center and force it to operate in a way that enhances provider–patient relationship. In our approach to shared governance in this book, service pathways now represent populations of patients, and the service constructs support their needs. All the providers are located in proximity to each other and are configured around the patients. Removed from the organization are most if not all of the barriers that impeded their relationships with each other and with the patients. Such are the structural shifts related to implementing interdisciplinary shared governance concepts (Batson, 2004) (see Figure 10-1).

309

**Figure 10-1   Integrating the System:
The Whole-Systems Shared Governance Model**

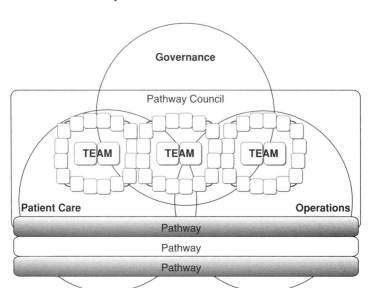

The critical issue then becomes, how does the organization, itself growing organizationally more healthy, move closer to the community to build the framework for creating a healthy community?

> **In the renewal process, there must ultimately be a fit between the changes undertaken within the system and the impact on those it serves.**

THE FIRST COMMUNITY: THE MEMBERSHIP COMMUNITY

Membership in the professions is not automatic. Each profession has its entrée obligations and requisites to obtain active practicing membership. In shared governance, it is important to perceive professions as membership communities. Failing to do so often creates an employee workgroup mental model subordinated to the institution rather than competency-based accountable membership in a profession that partners with the organization to which it has a specific relationship.

Licensed professions are enabled and empowered by society. They are not obligated to and neither are they controlled by the institutions with which they partner to undertake the work of the profession. It is the obligation of the profession in fulfilling its social mandate to ensure that its standards and practices advance the social interest, adhering to the highest ethical requisites. Membership in these professions is obtained through courses of study and rigorous vetting for both obtaining entrée and sustaining membership. The expectations and accountability for performance of members, therefore, must be as clear and precise as are the entry requirements.

In a professional frame of reference, clear expectations regarding the obligations of membership and the performance requisites that represent it are critical to the effectiveness and efficacy of the profession in undertaking its work as is clarity regarding the requirements of entry. It is here where the most significant issues of concern with regard to the activities and performance of professions are apparent. Lack of clarity with regard to membership expectations, performance, and accountability in the actual application of the work of the professions often creates critical dissonance between members within the profession and its relationship to other professions and the organizations within which they operate.

The individual professional community is the foundation upon which larger notions of community are constructed. The internal professional community must be as clearly representative of the obligations of community as the profession will make in its relationship with the larger community. The internal dynamics related to performance, peer behavior and relationships, accountability and contribution are the first critical indicators of the profession's own sense of community. Commitment to internal professional community and adherence between the members regarding common professional frames of reference, expectations, performance, values, relationships, and outcomes are the first phase necessary to initiating and sustaining the trajectory toward the larger reality of the healthy social community.

THE BASICS

Community health cannot be obtained without the community becoming involved in the effort. Allowing a dependent relationship between staff and community members to develop diminishes the members' accountability for their own health. However, for the community to become involved, positive relationships must already exist between providers all along the continuum of care. Therefore, the organization of the system must make possible broad-based relationships between the providers and must sustain those relationships through an effective communication and evaluation system (Mazur, 2003, pp. xvi, 187).

A health system cannot long sustain a real impact on the health of the community unless the system itself is healthy.

In newly integrating health systems, beginning parallel and horizontal relationships are being built between physicians and other providers. Linking the physicians together through the clinical network is critical for connecting the physicians to the system (see Chapter 8). Moving physicians to the center of the healthcare decision process is great, but that does not ensure that they will work collaboratively or effectively there. Making it impossible for them to be successful in any other way is an essential management strategy (Tourish & Hargie, 2004).

The need to pull the physicians permanently into a point-of-service partnership demands that every function and element of their practice of medicine be linked to the operating health system and support the partnership. To build a positive partnership between physicians and the health system, the support structure must tie the physicians tightly to the system. This is done, not to capture the physicians, but to give them no reason or need to operate outside of the system. In short, management, clinical, and information supports must work in concert to ensure that the physicians never have to go outside the system to get any practice issue addressed (Moanojovich, 2005).

This approach demands a continuous refinement of the partnership. Achieving a functional partnership does not happen overnight. In fact, it requires a long-term strategy. Such a strategy might well include the following tactics:

- Move the medical service organization the next step into a true committed clinical partnership between the physicians and the system. Make sure that physicians are located at every point where decisions that affect health service are made.
- Incorporate the medical staff problem-solving process into the partnership. This ensures that problems are identified and solved at the point of service. Remove any system or medical staff mechanism that would cause solution seeking to be moved away from the places where problems arise and have their impact.
- Ensure that the elected officers of the medical staff also serve on the organizational shared governance bodies so that physician practice and systems decision making are inexorably joined. This creates a seamless linkage between the organized medical staff and the system to which it is partnered.

• Connect the allied physician group to the information system at all levels, ensuring that all physician support and systems databases are integrated at every level of physician practice—from office management to patient clinical data—for every user in the system.

LINKAGE IS KEY

Although linking the physicians is a priority, it is only part of the work. This same kind of linkage must be forged for all the major providers. The nurses must be linked directly to all clinical partners in the system because they manage the patient-based relationships all along the clinical continuum. Pharmacists, therapists, social workers, and others must also be connected to each other along the continuum as a means of assuring the user that all the pieces of the service construct are in place and tracking the user at every level of interaction with the system (Carroll & Ameson, 2003).

The system must support, track, and follow the user through every level of need for the life of his or her relationship.

High-intensity connectedness ensures that the needs of the users are fully addressed, the costs associated with service provision are tracked, the outcomes are compared and contrasted within the system and between systems, and service value is continually evaluated. The effectiveness of the health system is determined by the intensity of connectedness at both the provider and the patient levels. The patient value stream is therefore emphasized as the core element that drives all others in the system. It is this framework that newly integrating health systems have yet to finalize but upon which they must build future viability.

THE INFORMATION INFRASTRUCTURE

The future of health care will be intricately intertwined with the development of information technology (Cassey, 2007). Likely half of all future capital resources of any healthcare organization will be devoted to building its information infrastructure. None of what is currently being constructed at health systems can be sustained without a well-linked information system that operates in a wide variety of areas affecting the community's health.

> **In the future, half of all the capital expenditures of a health system will go to find the information infrastructure of the system.**

The effectiveness of services and the linkage of service providers along the continuum depend for the most part on the quality of the information the providers have to manage the clinical relationship. Much of the service network depends on the information system for facilitating work and evaluating effectiveness. Because of the diversity of services and the various locations of the providers, a mechanism is needed to support them and to link them. It is not possible to sustain the decentralized and highly mobile workforce in a continuum-based organization without a good information infrastructure.

> **Information must flow smoothly across the continuum, and access to it must be fluid and friendly.**

The problem with most information systems, including those being constructed at integrating health systems, is that few people know what their structure should be and how best to design it to serve the needs of the potential users. The conflict between a vision and the technology needed to realize it is often considerable. Making a truly effective information system requires the joining together of a host of vendors in a cross-platform arrangement whose complexity and cost boggle the imagination. Further, integrating the various partners to the service arrangement creates all kinds of ownership, use, linkage, and confidentiality issues (Zuber, 2005).

> **The user must be able to know what to get from the information system. Having information is no good if it isn't used.**

Creating Useful Information Systems

Each of these issues must be confronted head on. The importance of good data for a highly decentralized operating and evidence-driven clinical system makes it necessary to ensure that the information system is well constructed and useful, and several considerations need to be taken into account when designing the system.

Future components of the information system must be compatible with existing hardware and software and easy to "plug into" the system. Adding some components of the system at later stages will be necessary because of cost considerations and the work related to building the continuum over time.

Information must be designed for the user. It needs to be in a language and a format that allows the user to interpret and apply it instantly. The user should not get information that is valuable to the sender but has no application to his or her work. Linking these systems with an interdisciplinary evidence-driven construct to meet obligations for demonstrating efficacy and clinical value will be essential to their applicability, viability, and sustainability.

It is no longer appropriate for financial information, operational information, and clinical information to be treated as distinct. Each is essential to determining what goes on at the point of service and what resources are needed for the work there. Tightening the relationships between the elements that influence effectiveness and demonstrate value becomes one of the major challenges in the design of an information system. Any separation of financial, operational, and service information tends to compartmentalize decision making and reduce its quality.

The data system should be designed by users, not by data management experts. Although the guidance and insight provided by the experts are essential to good design, investment in the information system must come from those who use it. If the barriers between information managers and clinical professionals are to ever be broken, both groups must join in the work of designing and evaluating the information system. Involving the user is a strong predictor of the utility, applicability, and adaptability of the information system at the point of service.

In the new paradigm, there is a central role for clinical data on the outcomes of treatment. These data allow sound judgments to be made as early as possible in the care cycle and can be used to adjust clinical processes that are not having the desired effect.

The hardware must be simple and convenient to use. If possible, it must be as portable as the provider is mobile. Portable hardware such as personal digital assistants (PDAs) need to interface as much as possible with the information system to ensure ready access to the user regardless of location. The more flexible it is, the more likely it will be used appropriately. Further, the more hardware pieces that can fit together or support other pieces, the greater the benefit to the providers. Cable and wireless linkages between computers and voice translation to hard data make the system more useful to a wider variety of people.

Supporting the Point of Service

Information is going to be as important to the point-of-service provider as it has been to the finance officer. The medical records function will change dramatically in the new age. Its responsibilities will include helping design the required formats and structures for information, and then generating the kind of information the clinical providers need to make their work simple and effective.

The main clinical use of the information technology will be to use and apply an evidence-based clinical protocol framework, document clinical events and processes, and access and record data in a way that facilitates patient care (Malloch & Porter-O'Grady, 2006). The information services need to make sure that providers have easy access to information on all users of the system.

It is no longer appropriate to view financial information as distinct from clinical information. Because the provider is increasingly the locus of control for service decision making, the financial implications of any decision must be available at the point of service. When price parameters are fixed in advance, as they increasingly are, it is important for providers to see how their decisions affect the expense framework for a particular patient and what options might be more cost effective and service efficient.

Clinical Support

Ongoing compilation of progress indicators regarding a patient's pathway and his or her position on it is also critical to provider decision making. The ability to lay out an evidence-validated critical path and the protocols becomes the foundation for evaluating response of the patient to treatment. Ultimately, of course, information on the outcome for a particular patient should be combined with information on the outcomes of like patients so that the most effective methods of practice can be discerned.

All users should have access wherever they serve patients. The physician in the office should be able to use the data set for his or her purposes with as much ease as the nurse in the field. The more fluid the information network, the more useful it is. The designers should see the network as the primary vehicle for hooking together all the key players along the continuum of care and providing them a platform for communicating with the system, the patients, and each other. All evidence-based activities should clearly reflect the integration of validated clinical approaches within each discipline. Those data should be aggregated to ensure that synthesis of discipline-specific clinical work as it affects the patient experience. Once a patient is within the service system, he or she should be easy to access and care should be easily managed from any place in the system. The quality of the community-system interface will depend almost entirely on the efficacy of the health systems information infrastructure.

Reduced Provider Competition

All providers are increasingly operating within the same frame of reference. There is less reason in the competitive marketplace for individual providers in the same system to be competing with each other. Physicians in an integrated practice system are actually supporting each other's practice (Porter-O'Grady & Afable, 2003). Increasingly, competition for patients and revenue will no longer characterize their relationship. Using the information system to make sure the physicians are connected to each other, to the nursing and other clinical staff, to clinical data, and to the patients is now the central work of the information services.

To get the physicians deeply invested in the system, it is important to fully connect them to the information structure. Everything linking their individual activities to the information system contributes to their partnership with the organization. For example, it would be ideal if the system allowed the physicians to do billing, patient scheduling, documentation, transcription, and record review from wherever they might be. In addition, providing a physician with the portable tools (such as PDAs) necessary to remain linked to the patient and to do business with the clinical staff and the organization creates an ongoing interdependence that advances the mutual relationship between clinical system and physician.

Information for Evaluation

Providers must also be able to use evidence-based strategies to evaluate groups of patients and their care over time. The team of providers who serve a defined patient population need to be able to determine what evidence-driven changes in activities or protocols are indicated by the aggregated data regarding that population. Data on care activities and their contribution to the clinical process and to total costs should be available to the team during evaluation. Adjustment of the team's activities, a shift in the team's standards and expectations, or a change in their relationship may entail a change in the database and a reconfiguration of the parameters of care. The system must facilitate this process and ensure that the adjustments can be incorporated when they do not violate other parameters of decision making (Hildreth & Kimble, 2004).

Linking the Internal and External Communities

One of the most important uses of information is to link the health system and the community it serves. After all, the ultimate goal of creating a user-driven clinical system is to ensure the ongoing health of the community of users while reducing the demand for illness-based, high-cost, high-intensity services. (The assumption is that cost control and service effectiveness are best obtained by decreasing the health system's dependence on such services.)

Simply designing effective evidence-based treatment protocols and establishing good clinical, operational, information, and financial systems will not accomplish this goal. These can be viewed as the foundation that must be laid to forge connections with the broader community and deal with issues of community health. It is in this context that community health service projects and community health information networks (CHINs) begin to have a defining role to play. It is ultimately the value of evidence-based practice to demonstrate the impact on health based on evidence of the specific activities that contribute to obtaining it. Creating the conditions for healthy individuals and a healthy community does not occur automatically or serendipitously. Instead, it is the result of well-validated protocols that, through evidence, establish a strong relationship between clinical process and health-giving clinical/community protocols and activities.

Community Health Information Networks

The use of information technology to construct a database focused on the health of a community and develop the connections to address it is just beginning, and the potential value of regional and community networks is just now being explored and refined. For information to be shared, it must exist, of course, but it also must be available in a useful form. Lack of utility is still an issue today. Ostensibly, regional and community networks would link health data from a wide range of sources—from public health services to statistical services to competing health systems (Thielst, 2007). The design of the information already existing at a number of these sources makes the linkage of the data feasible. This is especially important when one considers the need to build an aggregated clinical information repository where evidence of exemplary process and best practice can be stored and readily accessed as a way of ensuring that these evidence-based best practices will be quickly translated and applied in every relevant clinical setting.

> **Information underpins all service relationships. Outcomes cannot be assessed if information is not easily usable by the provider at the point of service.**

Most integrating health systems have been committed to building service-based information systems to link providers, patients, and operations together. It is expected that these networks will also help link the systems to their communities. However, other community connections must be initiated to build a strong community–health system relationship.

An information system must aid in dealing with the health needs and issues that emerge from the community–health system partnership. Keep the following several guidelines in mind when designing the information system:

- The information system must reflect some level of commitment to the health status of the community. It must be a place where the myriad categories of evidence-validated information can merge so that the community can gain an understanding of its needs.
- Data must be consolidated and reduced to a manageable level. Duplicate and nonessential information must be eliminated so that it does not reduce the usefulness of the data. This is especially important in the effort to delineate best practices to which all relevant stakeholders have access.
- Regardless of the purveyor of the system, the information it generates about the community's health and related best practices belongs to all the partners. The information must not be managed or manipulated in a way that obstructs the view of the stakeholders.
- The partners must be involved in designing and structuring the components of the information system so that it fits the needs of the users. For example, all users must have access to all the information generated by the system. Security and information protections should not be designed in a way that limits provider and user access to relevant and related information but, instead, protects that information from general visibility and inappropriate use by nonrelated parties. Ethical guidelines and use protocols must be incorporated into the developmental expectations of users so that the rules of engagement are clear and are consistently monitored and maintained.
- The information system must empower the partners to meet their obligations. For example, not only will data often reveal a need for action, but they can be crucial in determining what course of action is the best, which

is the foundation of an effective evidence-based infrastructure. The information system must provide the kinds of data that are essential for deliberation and decision making.

> **The information that is generated at the community level must prove itself to be of real value to the community.**

The development of community initiatives of any kind, including regional and community networks, requires a commitment to equity. As stated previously, equity is based on equality. No matter how large a partner's contribution to the community–health system partnership, it has the right to access whatever is necessary for facilitating its contribution.

Because care in a continuum-based health system is population based, the group of stakeholders reflects the makeup of the community. Indeed, the community leadership must be involved in decisions on how to respond to the issues brought to light by the health data generated by the regional and community networks.

Like most community-related activities, decision making regarding health care has political implications. For this reason, the data must be clear, frank, and available. Open data lines facilitate open dialogue. Although potential solutions to problems indicated by the data are subject to considerable dialogue and political processing, their effectiveness will be measurably enhanced by the directness and openness of the data generation.

Linking to the Political Structure

Linking the information system to local and regional political structure is a challenging yet essential task. It requires dialoguing with the political and bureaucratic leadership as early as possible and linking them to the regional and community network. The following guidelines should be kept in mind:

- The community expects its political leaders and structures to help it attain a state of improved health.
- The health systems must maintain direct communication linkages to individual political leaders at the local and regional levels.
- The political leadership should be included in institutional healthcare planning and policy formation.

- The linkage to the community should reflect the priorities of the political system in areas such as housing and education.
- The health system should become involved with the legislative process through offering testimony, constructing position papers, and engaging in policy development.
- The health system's database should be linked with public and government agency databases as a way of providing comprehensive information regarding the health needs of the community without violating the confidentiality of individual records and personal clinical information.

Integrated health systems have begun to make the initial linkages (through regional and community networks) necessary to establish a firm foundation for healthcare information database development. They undoubtedly will continue to recognize that at the center of any effective community–health system relationship will be a well-designed, clearly integrated regional/community health information network.

MAKING THE COMMUNITY CONNECTION

Many of the activities focused on community health depend on ongoing operational and functional linkages between the various health-related service industries (Farmer & Lawrenson, 2004). A number of principles pertain to developing these linkages. The following principles should guide the structural activities related to any work undertaken by any partner to the process.

Principle 1: The health system must play the lead role in providing the integration and linkage needed for the creation of healthy community initiatives. Because the focus of the health system is on generating health, it is reasonable to expect that the leadership for creating a healthy community network rests with the health system. The following expectations should flow out from the health system's commitment to creating a healthier community:

- The foundations of partnership are defined as part of the outreach of the health system.
- The responsibility for organizing and integrating healthy community initiative efforts belongs to the health system.
- Focusing on the education and development of the community partners and on the attainment of mutual understanding is essential.
- All the partners should be given an opportunity to be linked to the first activities related to building the community–health system relationship.
- The health system must provide the resources, location, time, and space necessary for the partners to gather.

Principle 2: All partners must be clear as to the vision, content, processes, and expectations of the healthy community initiatives. Without a clear understanding of the constructs and direction of the healthy community initiatives, the role of the partners becomes ambiguous and often skewed. Political and community fears, uncertainty, and lack of trust become accentuated when the contributions of the various partners are vague. Clarifying the significance of each partner's work and the expectations of each partner is an essential first step. Therefore, it is appropriate for these clarifying activities to be performed:

- A retreat for the partners should be utilized as a forum for developing a vision of a healthy community and setting the direction in which the partners should move.
- A facilitating process that includes the following elements should be undertaken:
  - A review of the factors that have led to the current need for an integrated approach to improving community health
  - An articulation of current circumstances and realities affecting community health
  - A delineation of stakeholder contributions to current and future efforts at improving health
  - Clarification and articulation of the factors that will likely affect the creation of sustainable healthy community initiatives
- A strategic process directed toward achieving the following should be designed and implemented:
  - An understanding of the priorities and essential components of any healthy community initiative
  - Clarification and articulation of the expectations of the partners regarding the improvement of community health
  - A delineation of the functional tasks and activities necessary to create sustainable healthy community initiatives
  - A definition of the strategic initiatives undertaken by the partners for the purpose of creating a model for building a healthy community
  - A commitment by all partners to the vision and direction defined by them during the leadership retreat and a clear delineation of the synthesis of the aggregated efforts the involved partner will produce and achieve in advancing the community's health

Principle 3: The accountability of and expectations for each of the partners committed to the implementation of a healthy community initiative must be clearly delineated. All the strategic planning in the world has no value if it cannot be translated into meaningful action. All of the partners to the undertaking should be clear about their role in performing the functions and activities necessary to achieve the desired outcome. A healthy community initiative will be successful only if the partners work to implement fully the components of the process for which they are uniquely accountable. To ensure that ownership of the components will result in the desired outcome, the following are necessary:

- A governing body whose role is to coordinate, integrate, and facilitate the work of the partners should be created.
- Resources necessary for the activities of the partnership must be provided.
- A method for ensuring that conflicts, uncertainty, lack of clarity, and compliance and performance problems are addressed as soon as they arise must be defined. The goal is to make sure that the partnership is not threatened by the complexity of implementing the initiative.
- The partners must commit to the linkage of the public and private information systems that will provide data to those responsible for implementing and evaluating the healthy community initiative.
- The partners must identify the efficiencies in current healthcare activities and processes so that they can be corrected.

Principle 4: A mechanism must exist for evaluating the implementation and ongoing operation of the healthy community initiative. Clearly, if there is no way of measuring the changes brought about by the initiative, its effectiveness will remain unknown—as will any modifications that might improve the initiative. Building evaluation activities into the process is a fundamental obligation of the partners, and the following elements should be considered to be requisite:

- A clear delineation of performance expectations and assignments for each of the partners
- Criteria for measuring individual contributions and the linkage between the partners including the measurement of the outcomes resulting from the synthesis of the aggregated effort of all partners.
- Regular points of reference when the partners regather to determine individual and collective progress
- A supporting data infrastructure that provides broad-based information on the progress of the partners in integrating activities
- A framework for collective action and a definition of the time parameters within which adjustments and performance changes are to be undertaken
- Generation of information regarding the healthy community initiative and communication of it to members of the community in a way that gets them invested in the processes related to their own health and the health of others

Principle 5: There is an ongoing process in place for maintaining a continuing dialogue with the community. Clearly, undertaking an initiative to improve the health of a community does nothing if the members of the community remain unengaged. The leadership should be expected to touch base with every level of the community and every cultural and social enclave (McAlearney, 2002). The following tools can help the leaders to reach out effectively:

- An ongoing reporting mechanism (including the use of online services) for reporting the developmental and initiating activities of the healthy community initiative
- Linkage with the press to ensure their investment in publicizing the healthy community initiative
- Periodic community or town hall meetings (these can be used as a forum for dialogue and education)
- Regular and ongoing generation of information about the health status of the community (using all available communication technology)

These principles should guide the implementation of healthy community activities and partnerships. However, there is plenty of room for individualization. The culture and character of the community and the economic and social conditions that exist will determine which particular approaches and methods should be chosen.

Healthy community initiatives require a commitment to partnership (Butterfoss, 2007). In fact, building equitable partnerships is the fundamental task of the leadership of a healthy community initiative. It is expected that the health system, which itself undergoes significant changes, will be the place where the integration of the implementation activities begins and is sustained.

> **Building healthy communities is not simple work. Most health systems know little about the health of the communities in which they reside.**

At most integrating health systems, building a foundation for a healthy community framework has already begun. Elements of the foundation include service pathways, population-based care design, a well-integrated and broad-based healthcare information system (including regional and community health information networks), a learning framework for internal community development, and linkages across the service region. Following are some of the activities that integrating health systems are undertaking to begin to extend their internal change process into the community and to provide initial linkages that will evolve into sustainable relationships.

COMMUNITY PARTNERSHIP ACTIVITIES

At many integrating health systems, the community–health system partnership began as an effort to coalesce fragmented pieces into a more focused system for determining whether the desired impact on community health status is being achieved. The steps that need to be undertaken by the health system leadership include these:

1. Inventory existing efforts within the system.
2. Inventory joint efforts with other agencies or delivery systems.
3. Inventory efforts going on anywhere to assess the health needs of the community (include new software capabilities for healthy community needs assessment).
4. Define *community* and develop population categories.
5. Inventory the resources currently available for the proposed initiative.
6. Inventory the interest of the board and senior management.
7. Inventory the interest of the system staff and medical staff.
8. Inventory the interest of the system partners.
9. Package the information.
10. Find a small group of committed individuals.
11. Plan a proposed system ("We have a dream!").
12. Take the show on the road.
13. Lock down baseline measures and put in place data collection mechanisms for ongoing measurement.
14. Implement the initiative internally and begin a dialogue on implementing it community wide.
15. Constantly give feedback to all stakeholders.

Getting Started

Most integrated health systems are currently in the "build the system" stage. The kinds of activities helping to focus staff on the community-centered work already ongoing might include the following:

- An executive roundtable to bring together community and hospital system leaders to discuss healthcare issues
- A healthy community task force made up of several local delivery systems to deal with needs and problems such as childhood immunization and teen pregnancy
- A community needs assessment effort

- Outreach programs, including prenatal education and diabetes education programs
- Roundtable discussions with specific stakeholder groups to uncover healthcare issues related to specific cultural beliefs and practices and to improve the cultural competence of the organization

Partnership for Children

Establishing a system of accessible services for children is often a good way to connect a broad cross-section of the community with the health system. Young teenagers are having children at an alarming rate in many communities. Most single teenage mothers are very likely to have a second or even third child while very young, are relatively uneducated, and live in deep poverty. In a health system's ZIP code area, a defined percentage of the children live below the poverty level. There may be no fluoride in the water supply, a constant fear of gang violence, and poor air quality. Here is a clear health challenge! These children are the healthcare consumers of today, and they will continue to be heavy users of health services unless some kind of intervention occurs before their environment causes them to need high-intensity care.

Along with the health system, often numerous community and church groups are working to improve the lives of the people in the community. Their work is inspiring and impressive. Partnership with them will be necessary to make sure children's needs are incorporated into the health system's community health plan.

A Community Dream

Imagine what it would be like if every healthcare delivery system and every employer in any market gave back a portion of its profits to improve the health of its community. If each hospital system in the area adopted one ZIP code or clearly defined a service support area and worked on improving the health status of the people in that area, the impact would be incredible. Imagine what could happen if all the agencies currently working in the community pooled their resources and worked toward the same health goals. The overwhelming difficulty of pulling such a diverse variety of political entities together is outweighed only by the outcome if nothing is done.

The healthcare system is a part of the community within which it resides. It has the same obligations of citizenship as anyone who is a member of the local community.

There is simply no reason why integrating health systems should not provide the leadership needed to structure their relationships with their users and others around the issues of community health. The goal should be to demonstrate a successful outcome with a defined and limited population, which will make the program more appealing to partner agencies and funding sources and allow the effort to become more horizontal.

Shared Governance and Community Health

As noted at the beginning of this book, shared governance is a structure, not a model. In fact, many models apply the principles and practices associated with the structure of shared governance. Whichever one fits the culture and purposes of the organization is the one that should be implemented. However, it is important to keep in mind that the principles of shared governance can be applied broadly—for example, to the integration of communities of any size. Indeed, shared governance is about building a construct, a structure that creates a frame for not only building but also sustaining community. If a community wants to improve the health of its members, various components need to be linked in a way that makes for effective joint action. The principles of shared governance are easily adaptable to a community frame of reference and can be used to develop the kind of partnerships between community organizations that will lead to improved health for the entire population.

Broader Notions of Health

Broader notions of health are essential to building toward healthier communities and to creating partnerships between health systems and the communities they serve.

What has been discussed in this chapter so far provides only a rudimentary foundation for a much broader concept of health and health service and for more intensive relationships along a longer continuum within a larger context. Clearly, for services provided in a community framework to be sustained, an organizational and systematic structure needs to be in place that gives form to the provision of services. The principles of shared governance can be used to support the enlarged set of organizational relationships entailed by such a structure.

No matter what a health system's size, the accountability of individual providers and the community of providers for the achievement of desired outcomes is essential for the system's effectiveness. In a community context, each health system must have accountability for the improvement of health for the members of the community. Furthermore, the demand for community integration and linkage of health systems throughout the community is no different from the demand for internal linkage within any particular system. Because shared governance is whole-systems thinking applied to organizational relationships, the breadth and depth of the requisite linkages do not change. Only the format of the linkages changes.

Shared governance principles require that systems address the whole range of health issues. Therefore, lack of linkage to the community is simply not an option.

Applying shared governance to a whole community health system (made up of individual health-related organizations) requires linkage at the governance, operations, and service levels. Institutions, services, structures, and resources must be connected in a way that provides a broad-based framework for decision making, service provision, evaluation, and governance. Among the activities associated with each component is the continuing assessment of the fluid boundaries of the shared governance structure and the impact of the social system on the character and the extent of those boundaries. As in all systems, boundaries between components or portions of a community health system need to change when the characteristics of the relationships call for a change.

The capacity to build toward health in the community is simply a broader view of the system. To do so creates more sustainable relationships.

Figure 10-2 Shared Governance Community Health System

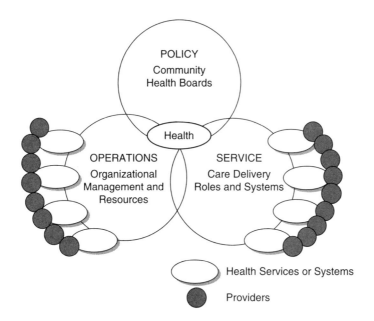

The application of shared governance to larger systems requires the application of the same principles. If these principles are applied, the integrity and effectiveness of the relationships between the components will undoubtedly be enhanced. The resulting seamless integration around purpose and service, the structural accountability of each of the components, and the linkage between governance, operations, and services will all contribute to the achievement of the ultimate goal—improved health for the members of the community (see Figure 10-2).

Organizing Around the Community

The leaders in integrated health systems should see no difference between organizing around a specific patient population and configuring around the entire community. The principles that govern the relationships between components remain essentially the same, although the structures and dynamics may be different. For example, a community health system governance council could do the following:

- Provide a place where leaders from all the partners in the community health system make decisions about the direction of the system
- Establish a mission and objectives for the community health system
- Identify priorities and service parameters
- Establish policies necessary for consistent behavior throughout the system
- Develop strategies and tactics
- Deal with integration issues, conflict, and barriers to seamlessness

The governance council could include representatives from all sectors of society, including the private sector, government, and the service agency sector. The governance process would focus on issues that might affect the long-term health of the community. It would truly link, especially at the local level, all of the elements needed to improve people's physical health as well as the social health of the community.

> **Shared governance at the community level has the same elements as at the point of service. Breadth does not alter principle.**

Guided by the community health system's governance council, the operations council (consisting of community service agency representatives) would deal with operations and resource issues. Its responsibilities would include the following:

- Budgeting and allocating resources
- Defining the functional accountability and obligations of various components of the system
- Defining the support and service structures necessary to integrate the continuum of care
- Refining and improving the community information and communication system
- Addressing the functional issues of relationship and partnership (those that facilitate or impede the ongoing activities necessary to maintain effective delivery of services within a community health framework)
- Building an evidence-based repository for community/regional clinical best practices.

Here again, the resource accountability of the operations council gets played out in the broad community context. Still, human, fiscal, material support, and systems resource distribution remain its core accountability.

At the service level of the community health system, integration around populations served is just as important as at the systems level. The main difference is that the populations are even more culturally and socially diverse.

The functional linkages and delivery structures still remain the essential core of the relationship between providers and consumers. However, linkage across the community continuum now becomes the framework for the activities of the community consumer services council. Here again, the issues that are deliberated at this level of decision making are those that directly and dramatically affect the achievement and maintenance of health within a community context by and with all those who comprise the community.

Community-Driven Service

At the community and consumer health services level, decisions that relate to the provision of service unfold within the broader context and include the following:

- Defining the delivery system, the models, and approaches to the delivery of care
- Outlining the linkages of the system along the continuum of care and all of the divisions of service provided within that context
- Outlining the delivery mechanisms and the team membership essential to building a multifocal multidisciplinary approach to providing health services
- Defining the interdisciplinary relationships, structures, processes, and evaluative activities to determine the successful intersection of disciplinary functions along a healthcare continuum
- Evaluating the effectiveness of the evidence-driven clinical infrastructure and services, identifying problems and concerns, moving to solution orientation, outlining responsive and change strategies for adjusting activities, and evaluating the quality of care within the context of preferable and defined outcomes
- Redefining and revising the models and approaches to care as the community demands for such changes are required

Here again, the framework remains focused on the point of service, the place where activities that support the outcomes of healthier communities unfold (Butterfoss, 2007). The intersection between consumers and providers is most intense where the community lives out its life and where the decisions made at the governance level are played out in the activities and functions of the point-of-service providers. Again, within the community context, the seamlessness of the linkages, the representative nature of the governance structure, the framework for decision making, and the point-of-service design work together to create the type of decision making and cooperation most likely to advance the health of the community.

CONCLUSION

The design and implementation of a shared governance approach provides a framework for achieving the broader agenda characteristic of the new health-care paradigm (Malloch & Porter-O'Grady, 2005). The new paradigm forms the impetus for changing structures and relationships in all health systems. As this book indicates, integrating health systems simply have to take the risk of redefining themselves within the context of the new paradigm—which entails redefining relationships between people, redefining systems, and redefining work.

> **Shared governance reflects the structural requisites of the new age: partnership, equity, accountability, and ownership.**

Certainly, the frameworks identified in this book are preliminary to a set of much broader based frameworks that will be needed. Society is in the midst of a fundamental change in social relationships driven by the impact of sociotechnology. Risk is inherent in creating new kinds of relationships—relationships, in this case, that reflect the interdependence of all people and systems (the quantum reality); the need for broad-based horizontal relationships between systems; the need for a strong, effective, evidence-delineated health delivery process; the desire to re-create communities within the context of the emerging paradigm; and the need to realign the organizational formats in more functional ways.

> **Shared governance represents the effort of systems to configure themselves in ways that engage stakeholders in a collective construction of a preferable future.**

Health care cannot be viewed in the same context it once was. The sickness-driven, event-based delivery of services has failed to meet society's health needs. Indeed, the current infrastructure has merely extended the mechanism and means of supporting and treating an extended illness-based delivery system. In the long term, illness-based, intervention-oriented healthcare organizations will not be able to survive. In fact, they will simply become unaffordable. As we build a more effective framework for health care, all the structures, support systems, and relationships that once defined the delivery of health care will come crashing down. The question then becomes, what new structures, support systems, and relationships will emerge to meet health needs in the new sociotechnical paradigm?

Although we are quite clearly in the first phases of a long and arduous journey of transformation for health care, shared governance has already proved capable of creating structures and relationships that reflect the expectations of the emerging age. It clearly has the potential to reengage those individuals in health systems who are undergoing dramatic and even painful changes. Consequently, it also has the potential to play a major role in the new healthcare paradigm, because in the final analysis it is the energy and commitment of the stakeholders at every level that will sustain the health systems during the protracted and continuously unfolding evolution toward excellence.

REFERENCES

Batson, V. (2004). Shared governance in an integrated health care network. *AORN Journal, 80*(3), 493–512.

Butterfoss, F. (2007). *Coalitions and partnerships in community health*. Chicago: John Wiley.

Carroll, L., & Ameson, P. (2003). Communication in a shared governance hospital: Managing emergent paradoxes. *Communication Studies, 54*(1), 35.

Cassey, M. (2007). Keeping up with existing and emerging technologies. *Nursing Economics, 25*(2), 121–125.

Farmer, R., & Lawrenson, R. (2004). *Epidemiology and public health medicine*. Chicago: Wiley-Blackwell.

Hildreth, P. M., & Kimble, C. (2004). *Knowledge networks: Innovation through communities of practice*. Hershey, PA: Idea Group.

Malloch, K., & Porter-O'Grady, T. (2005). *The quantum leader: Applications for the new world of work*. Sudbury, MA: Jones and Bartlett.

Malloch, K., & Porter-O'Grady, T. (2006). *Introduction to evidence-based practice in nursing and healthcare*. Sudbury, MA: Jones and Bartlett.

Mazur, D. J. (2003). *The new medical conversation: Media, patients, doctors, and the ethics of scientific communication*. Lanham, MD: Rowman & Littlefield.

McAlearney, A. (2002). *Population health management*. Chicago: Health Administration Press.

Moanojovich, M. (2005). Nurse–physician communication: An organizational accountability. *Journal of Nursing Scholarship, 23*(2), 72–78.

Motes, P. S., & Hess, P. M. (2007). *Collaborating with community-based organizations through consultation and technical assistance*. New York: Columbia University Press.

Porter-O'Grady, T. (2004). Embracing conflict: Building a healthy community. *Healthcare Management Review, 29*(3), 181–187.

Porter-O'Grady, T., & Afable, R. (2003, May/June). The technology of partnership. *Health Progress,* 41–52.

Thielst, C. (2007). Regional health information networks and the emerging organizational structures. *Journal of Healthcare Management, 52*(3), 146–150.

Tourish, D., & Hargie, O. (2004). *Key issues in organizational communication.* New York: Routledge.

Zuber, R. (2005). Compliance with the Medicare conditions of participation: Keeping OASIS data private. *Home Healthcare Nursing, 23*(11), 707–709.

SUGGESTED READING

Condon, P. (2007). *Design charrettes for sustainable communities.* Washington, DC: Island Press.

Young, W. (2001). *Creating sustainable community programs.* Westport, CT: Praeger.

Index

A

accountability, 36, 54, 60–61, 156–159
  breadth of, 222–223
  delegation of, 182–183
  as foundation of systems, 137–138
  responsibility and transition, 30–33
acute care, 132
  designing services along service
    continuum, 62
adaptive systems principles, 42
administrators, 117–118
agenda, controlling, 200
agreement regarding common problem-
  solving steps, 127
air quality, 326
applications of operations and systems
  model, 9–10
approachability, importance of, 172
areas of accountability, distinctions
  between, 175
assistant administrators, 117–118
assistant directors, 117–118
assistant managers, 117–118
assistant supervisors, 117–118
associate administrators, 117–118
assumed outcomes vs. outcome
  measurement, 7
assumption of provider competency, vs.
  competency/improvement report
  cards, 7

authority, in transformation of
  organization, 95
availability of resources, importance of,
  134

B

balance between service accountability,
  system accountability, 61
banking, 306
behavioral health, 132
belief about people, nature of work in
  organization, 47
benefits statement, 189–190
boundaries, determination of, 95–96
brainstorming, 189–190, 291
  agreement regarding, 127
  rules for, 127
broad-based horizontal relationships
  between systems, need for, 332
budget, 134, 189–190, 194–196
  availability issues, 92–93
  capital project presentations, 195
  primary of financial accountability,
    195–196
  target setting, 196
bulletins, 260
burn unit, 132
bylaws of medical staff, 239–245

C

calendars, 291
cancer services, 132
capital budget process, 194–196
   capital project presentations, 195
   primary of financial accountability, 195–196
   target setting, 196
capital plan, consistency of project with, 189–190
care delivery integration, 105–136
   communication linkages, 124
   continuum of care, 109–110
   continuum of care services, 132
   defining linkages, 114–115
   delineating pathways, 119–120
   information pathways, 123–124
   interactions within system, 128–129
   linage defining system, 111–114
      horizontal linkage, 112–113
      provider linkage, 113–114
   linkages, 127–128
   management layers, 117–118
   need for information, 122–123
   new payment requisites, 110–111
   new strategies, implications for, 107–109
   organization around patient, 129–131
   organizing around patient populations, 114
   patient pathway, 106–107
   relational service design, 110–111
   shared vision, propagation of, 115–116
   structural linkages, 117–118
   system functionality, maintaining, 131–135
   systems linkages, 120
   value standards, 118–119
career goals, 22–23
CEO. See chief executive officer
chair-elect mentor, acting as, 200
chair of board of trustees, 217
chair of operations council, 217
chair of service council, 217
challenges to effectiveness, 228–229

change process, in transformation of organization, 101–102
change quotient, 22–23
changes in healthcare marketplace, 6–7
changes in incentives, 240–242
changing concepts of management, 171–173
changing context of healthcare service, 9–10
chaos theory, 102
characteristics of outmoded organizational model, 53
characteristics of shared governance, 175
chart location, 258
charting process, 258
checks and balances, 231–232
chief executive officer, 117
   role of, 217–218
   support from, 203–204
chief information officer, 285
   board support for new information infrastructure, 296–297
   changing role of, 294–297
chief of medical staff, 217
chief operating officer, 117
children, establishing system of services for, 326
CHINs. See community health information networks
clarification of operations council accountability, 190–193
clarification of role, function, and role in accountability, 32–33
clarity of issues, 188–190
clinical advisory group, role of, 294
clinical connections in delivery system, 111–112
clinical interdisciplinary advisory group, establishment of, 294
clinical standards vs. customer satisfaction, 20
clinical support, 316–317
clinical teams, 49–50
coach behaviors, 172
command and control systems, as vestiges of outdated system, 25–26

commitment, 91–92
communications, 260–264. *See also*
    virtual office
    critical communication in shared
        governance system, 260–262
    linkages, 124
community
    health system, informational linkage
        and, 318
    organizing around, 329–331
community connection, making, 321–324
community dream, 326–327
community health information networks,
    318–320
community hospital system approach,
    provider partnerships and, 237–271
    changes in incentives, 240–242
    communications, 260–264
        critical communication in shared
            governance system, 260–262
        conflict resolution, 262
    formal medical staff, 237–238
    future for physician partners in
        shared governance, 269–270
    future vision, changes in preparation
        for managed care and, 250
    governance for new vision, 262–268
        prioritization of organizational
            strategies, 264
        shared governance and value-
            driven care, 266–268
    implementing experience, 250–252
    incentives, alignment of, 241
    inclusion of physicians in hospital
        decision making, 259–260
    informal medical staff structures as
        barriers, 239–240
    integration of physicians into system,
        252–259
        medical staff and decision making,
            256–257
        medical staff, governance, and
            operations, 255
        medical staff integration into
            pathways, 256

physicians and critical path,
    258–259
physicians at point of service, 258
physicians roles in corporate
    shared governance councils,
    254–255
inviting medical staff, 252
operating objectives for physicians,
    259–260
physician disconnection from
    systems perspective, 242–245
physicians, strategies to win over, 255
physician's view of barriers to shared
    governance, 239–245
questions for physician's shared
    governance, 268
vision for whole-systems shared
    governance, 245–252
    structuring, 248–250
community involvement in health care,
    309–334
    health issues, 309–310
    information infrastructure, 313–321
        clinical support, 316–317
        community health information
            networks, 318–320
        creating useful information
            systems, 312–315
        information for evaluation, 317
        political structure linkage, 320–321
        reduced provider competition, 317
        supporting point of service, 316
    linkage among; to all clinical partners
        in system, 313
    making community connection,
        321–324
    membership communities,
        professions as, 310–311
    partnership activities, 325
        children, establishing system of
            services for, 326
        community-driven service,
            331–332
        concept of health, broadening of,
            327–329

focusing staff in community-centered work, 325–326
organizing around community, 329–331
shared governance, 327
community practice vs. critical pathway standards, 7
competition, 8
moving to systems level, 11
complaints, linkage revealed by, 116
complex adaptive systems, 115–117
building infrastructure for, 11
rules, 5
shared governance, shared decision making in, 5
complexity theory, 102
complicated vs. simplified organizational structures, 20
components of information management in shared governance organization, 273
computer technology, increased role in education of children, 16
computers, 306
concept of health, broadening of, 327–329
conceptualization of information, 279–280
conflict between physicians, administrators, 247
conflict resolution, 262
conflict with old organizational design, 77
conglomerates, new types of, 24
consensus-based decision making, 197–199
consensus-building techniques, 197
consulting partners, role of, 218–221
consumer-driven care, 18–19
contemporary payment models, 240
contemporary systems theory, 11
contextual accountability, 175, 176
contextual decisions, 60–61
continuous contract renegotiation, 111
control, challenging aspects of, 203
COO. See chief operating officer
corporate culture, 22–23
cost analysis, 189–190
cost of health care, increase in, 8, 14–15
councils, 53–54, 57–58

chair duties and powers, 200
as decision-making body, 51
member responsibilities, 146
membership selection, 145
in shared governance model, authority to make decisions, 53
as unit of organized decision making, 53–55
cross-section of community, connecting with health system, 326
cultural mindset, as barrier to collaboration, partnership, 239
culture, corporate, 22–23
curing vs. healing, 6
customer focus, transition to, 20
cycle of learning connecting practice, performance, goals of, 126

D

deadlines for motivating, guiding work, 93
decentralizing structure of organization, 28
deconstruction of hospitals, 10
defined service limits, 111
defining linkages, 114–115
defining work of patient care council, 147–148
delegation of accountability, 182–183
delineating pathways, 119–120
demand for change, 11
demand, managing, 16–17
democracy, shared governance, distinguished, 45
departmental, silo-based approaches to work, inefficiency of, 21–22
design team. See shared governance steering group
development, in transformation of organization, 94–95
diagnosis-related group, 240
dialogue, role in accountability, 32–33
digital information infrastructure, 70–71
requirements of, 124–125
directors, 117–118
discharge, 242
distinction of accountability, 175

distribution of structure, power, relationships, need for, 4
diversity, effect on system's strength, effectiveness, 5
documentation, by profession vs. multidisciplinary patient record, 20
DRG. *See* diagnosis-related group

E

early hospital discharge, 242
education of board, on information system matters, 296–297
educational system, inadequacy of, 15–16
effectiveness in shared governance, 231
electronic forms, work flow improvements supported by, 291
electronic idea exchange, brainstorming, 291
electronic mail system, 291
electronic opinion surveys, 291
emergency meetings, 200
emphasis on treatment, vs. emphasis on prevention, 6
empowerment
    components in development of, 171
    defined, 172
    in point of service organization, 26–27
    of providers, supporting, 278
equity, 36, 54
    through inclusive processes, 30
evidence-based practice, various meanings of, 269–270
evidence-based quality outcomes, 111
evidence-driven clinical protocol, critical pathway, 258–259
evolving nature of work, 10–15
    economic and financial shifts, 13–15
        growing healthcare costs, 14–15
    technology, 12–13
        instant access, 12–13
expanding nursing practice council, 161–162
expectations, maintaining, 172
external approval structures in shared governance, 53

external environment, current, future, 22–23
external, internal environmental factors creating conditions requiring shifts, 11

F

family health, 132
fee-for-service, 240, 250
feelings of others, showing sensitivity to, 172
financial accountability, 195–196
fiscal resources, 177, 190–191
fix-it mindset, inappropriateness for addressing constant change, 11
flowcharting, 102
fluoride in water supply, 326
focused work group, in transformation of organization, 78–80
focusing staff in community-centered work, 325–326
formal medical staff, 237–238
foundation of operations council, 178–188
    making operations council work, 187
    operations council membership, 184–187
    operations council process, 188
    purpose of operations council, 180–183
    role of operations council, 183–184
    support for management role, 180
fragmentation of care, 11
free-standing facility, vs. integrated facility/systems, 6
functional partnerships strategy, tactics, 312–313
future for physician partners in shared governance, 269–270
future vision, changes in preparation for managed care, 250

G

Gantt charts, 102
gerontology, designing services along service continuum, 62
globalization, 24, 39, 173
    local impact of, 11
governance, 207–235
    breadth of accountability, 222–223

challenges to effectiveness, 228–229
checks and balances, 231–232
culture, importance of, 232–233
enhancing effectiveness in shared
    governance, 231
governing boards in transition,
    209–210
interface with medical staff, 230
as leadership, 210
linking system, 207–208
linking with function, 210–213
new notions of leadership, 208–209
for new vision, 262–268
    prioritization of organizational
        strategies, 264
    shared governance and value-
        driven care, 266–268
question of systems, 223–224
role of chief executive officer,
    217–218
role of consulting partners, 218–221
senior-level managers, transfer of
    work formerly done by into
    councils, pathways, 229–230
stakeholder engagement, 214–217
    governance council membership,
        217
strategic cascade, 224–228
translating board accountability,
    213–214
governance council, 59, 67–71, 216,
    224–228
    accountability, 221–222
    decision-making body, issues,
        216–217
    information support, 70–71
    membership, 69–70, 217
    physician relationship, 230
governance culture, importance of,
    232–233
governing boards, in transition, 209–210
gridding out, 102
group assignments, 200
group scheduling, 291
guidelines for designing information
    system, 319–320

H
health care cost, increase in, 8, 14–15
healthcare-related activities, share of
    gross domestic products, 15
healthcare marketplace changes, 6–7
healthcare structure changes, 16–22
    consumer-driven care, 18–19
    managing demand, 16–17
    overcoming medical separatism, 17–18
    quality/patient safety movement, 19–21
    user-driven healthcare models, 17
    value-driven care delivery, 21–22
hierarchical infrastructures, 4
high profit margins vs. value-driven
    returns, 6
HMOs, pressure for reform, 8
home services, 132
horizontal integration, 77
horizontal linkage, 112–113
horizontal relationships, requirement of
    adult-to-adult interchanges, 175
horizontal sharing of power, 239
hospital occupancy, 6
human community, developments of new
    relationships, intersecting structures
    in, 2
human resources, 177, 191

I
I&O data. See intake and output data
IHN. See integrated health network
immunization campaigns, 14
implementation of transformation of
    organization, 85–87
implication of shared governance
    principles, structures, 273–280
incentives, alignment of, 241
inclusion of physicians in hospital
    decision making, 259–260
individual differences in transformation
    of organization, 94
individual facilities, corporate
    accountability across, 179
informal medical staff structures as
    barriers, 239–240
information

access in transformation of
organization, 95
development as evolution, 305–306
for evaluation, 317
flow among shared governance
entities, 281–284
self-directed workgroups, 282–284
as lifeblood of shared government
organization, 122
need for, 122–123
as resource, 275–276
information management philosophy,
287–289
information management steering
committee
chair of, 294
establishment by operations council,
293
information management strategies,
289–290
accountability in, 293–294
information management system,
273–307, 312–315
chief information officer
board support for new information
infrastructure, 296–297
changing role of, 294–297
design, approach to, 298–299
devising information management
strategies, accountability in,
293–294
implication of shared governance
principles and structures, 273–280
information as resource, 275–276
information development as
evolution, 305–306
information flow among shared
governance entities, 281–284
self-directed workgroups, 282–284
information management philosophy,
287–289
information project team, 284
integrated health network core
system design, 297–305
linkages and relationships, 280
new information infrastructure, 273

real-time information access, 286–287
development of superusers, 287
roles, 293–294
shifting control, in shared governance
model, 276–277
culture, 278
information, 279–280
relationships, systemness, creation
by, 280
structure, 277–278
training, 278
strategies, 289–290
structures for information
management, 273–280
tactical implementation (sample
projects), 290–293
clinical information system,
292–293
virtual office, 291–292
trouble with vendor partners, 285–286
information network, 261
information pathways, 123–124
information project team, 284
information sharing, 70–71
information support, governance council,
70–71
initial developmental process, shared
governance steering group, 84–85
inpatient care, vs. continuum-based
health care, 7
institution centered, community
centered, 6
insurance, 306
intake and output data, 258
integrated care delivery, 105–136
building continuum of care, 109–110
building linkages, 127–128
communication linkages, 124
continuum of care services, 132
defining linkages, 114–115
delineating pathways, 119–120
information pathways, 123–124
interactions within system, 128–129
linage defining system, 111–114
horizontal linkage, 112–113
provider linkage, 113–114

management layers, 117–118
   need for information, 122–123
   new payment requisites, 110–111
   new strategies, implications for,
      107–109
   organization around patient, 129–131
   organizing around patient
      populations, 114
   patient pathway, 106–107
   relational service design, 110–111
   shared vision, propagation of,
      115–116
   structural linkages, 117–118
   system functionality, maintaining,
      131–135
   systems linkages, 120
   value standards, 118–119
integrated health network, 246
   core system design, 297–305
integrated interdisciplinary shared
   decision-making format, 105–136
integrating process in transformation of
   organization, 75–77
integrating relationships, defined, 29
integration of physicians into system,
   252–259
      corporate shared governance
         councils, physicians roles in,
         254–255
      governance, 255
      medical staff, 256–257
      physicians at point of service, 258
      physicians, critical path for, 258–259
interactions within system, 128–129
interdependence, 34–35
   building, 35
interdisciplinary shared governance, 4–8,
   39–74, 90
   adaptive systems principles, 42
   building on foundations, 39–41
   constructs, 71
   councils, 57–58
      as unit of organized decision
         making, 53–55
      decisions, 56–57

distinguishing system accountability
   and service accountability, 59–61
governance council, 67–71
   information support, 70–71
locus of control decision making, 57
operations council, 65–67
outmoded organizational
   characteristics, 53
patient care council, 62–65
point of care, 44–45
premises of shared governance, 45–47
professional staff, shared governance
   as appropriate model for
   structuring, 41
service pathway leadership, 58
shared governance, 55–56
   principles of, 54
system councils, 59
teams, 47–53
   population-based continuum,
      51–53
   service team, 50–51
   types of, 49–51
interface with medical staff, 230
interfacing with medical staff, 162–164
investment in system, 33–34
inviting medical staff, 252

K
knowledge
   explosion of, 173
   as medium of exchange, 4
   as newest form of capital, 2
   organizational dependent on, 173
   technology, interdependence of, 173
knowledge creation/management, 1–39
   accountability, 30–33
   changing healthcare structures and
      models, 16–22
   consumer-driven care, 18–19
   context for healthcare service,
      changes in, 9–10
   customer focus, transition to, 20
   equity, relationship to quality, 27–30
   healthcare marketplace, changes in,
      6–7

interdependence, 34–35
interdisciplinary shared governance, 4–8
intersecting structures in human community, developments of, 2
investment in system, 33–34
learning organization, creation of, 26–27
locus of control, transfer to point of service, 25–26
managing demand, 16–17
nature of work, evolution of, 10–15
    economic and financial shifts, 13–15
    growing healthcare costs, 14–15
    technology, 12–13
overcoming medical separatism, 17–18
political issues, 22–23
quality/patient safety movement, 19–21
relationship building, partnership in, 23–25
responsibility, transition to accountability, 30–33
shared governance, demand for, 25–26
social reengineering, 15–16
structural issues, 22–23
traditional structure, problems with, 11
user-driven healthcare models, 17
value-driven care delivery, 21–22
value of workers' knowledge and competence, 2–4
knowledge workers, 173–175
    healthcare system constructed predominantly of, 7

L
lack of voting, in consensus decision making, 198
language of shared governance, 56
leadership, 208–209
    facilitating council's decision making, 64
    governance as, 210
    in health care, 7
    managership, distinguished, 8

learning, alteration by technology, 15
learning lab, impact of, 297
learning organization, creating, 26–27
levels of management, 176–178
linage defining system, 111–114
    horizontal linkage, 112–113
    provider linkage, 113–114
linear administrative hierarchies, diminishment in value, 10–11
linkages, 207–208
    to all clinical partners in system, 313
    building, 127–128
    characteristics of, 116
    defining, 114–115
    with external community, 176–177
    between governance and function, 210–213
    to other councils, 202–203
    relationships, 280
local, regional political structure, linkage to, 320–321
locus of control, 56–57
    decision making, 57
    to point of service, transfer of, 25–26
    shift in, 3

M
management accountability, 175–176, 177
management, changing concepts of, 171–173
management council, 169–206. *See also* operations council
management layers, 117–118
management of knowledge, 1–39
    accountability, 30–33
    changing context for healthcare service, 9–10
    customer focus, transition to, 20
    equity, relationship to quality, 27–30
    evolving nature of work, 10–15
        economic and financial shifts, 13–15
        growing healthcare costs, 14–15
        technology, 12–13
    healthcare marketplace, changes in, 6–7

healthcare structures and models,
changes in, 16–22
consumer-driven care, 18–19
managing demand, 16–17
overcoming medical separatism,
17–18
quality/patient safety movement,
19–21
user-driven healthcare models, 17
value-driven care delivery, 21–22
human community and new
relationships, intersecting
structures in, 2
interdependence, 34–35
building, 35
interdisciplinary shared governance,
4–8
investment in system, 33–34
learning organization, creating, 26–27
managing demand, 17
ownership in system, 33–34
partnership and relationship building,
23–25
point of service, transfer of locus of
control to, 25–26
principles for new age, 22–34
responsibility, accountability,
transition, 30–33
shared governance, demand for,
25–26
social reengineering, 15–16
structural/political issues, 22–23
traditional structure, problems with, 11
value of, and workers' competence, 2–4
managers, 117–118
history of directing, controlling, 174
managership, leadership, distinguished, 8
master path diagram, 129–130
material resources, 177, 191
medical model of health care, changes in,
16–22
medical school, residency, boundaries to
behavior in, 240
medical separatism, overcoming, 17–18
medical staff
decision making, 256–257

governance and operations, 255
integration into pathways, 256
meetings, 261
organization and traditional structure,
effect on hospital system, 263
membership communities, professions
as, 310–311
membership criteria, shared governance
steering group, 82–84
mental health, designing services along
service continuum, 62
mentor of chair-elect, acting as, 200
mentor of coach behaviors, 172
microsystem, interdisciplinary point of
service, 137–168
accountability, 156–159
council member responsibilities, 146
council membership selection,
principles of, 145
nursing shared governance, to whole-
systems shared governance,
160–164
expanding nursing practice
council, 161–162
interfacing with medical staff,
162–164
patient care council, 140–148,
156–159
defining work of patient care
council, 147–148
patient care council membership,
144–147
purpose of patient care council,
143–144
patient care, foundations of health
service, 138–140
patient care integration, 164–167
physician involvement in shared
governance, principles of, 162
physicians on patient care council,
role of, 164
service pathway council, 148–159
accountability, 152–159
patient care council accountability,
156–159
work of, 155–156

shared governance, principles of, 138
team accountability, 148–159
minutes from unit team meetings, 261
mistakes, helping people learn from, 172
models of healthcare, changes in, 16–22
    consumer-driven care, 18–19
    managing demand, 16–17
    overcoming medical separatism,
        17–18
    quality/patient safety movement,
        19–21
    user-driven healthcare models, 17
    value-driven care delivery, 21–22
multiple knowledges, technologies,
    interdependence of, 173
multiple vs. limited customer contacts, 20

N
national, state, and local reform, 7
nature of work, evolving, 10–15
    economic and financial shifts, 13–15
        growing healthcare costs, 14–15
    technology, 12–13
        instant access, 12–13
need for information, 122–123
negotiation, function, role in
    accountability, 32–33
network upgrade, 291
new ideas, listening to, 172
new information infrastructure, 273
new reality for organizations, 8–9
new strategies, implications for, 107–109
newer configurations, making
    organizations, people ready for, 10
newsletters, 260
Newtonian vs. quantum thinking, 11
nonbudgeted projects, 189–190
nonproductive downtime, 11
nursing management council, 179
    operations council vs., 179
nursing shared governance, 87–89,
    160–164
    expanding nursing practice council,
        161–162
    interfacing with medical staff,
        162–164

O
old, new decision processes contrasted,
    189
operating budget process, 193–194
operating objectives for physicians,
    259–260
operations council, 65–67, 169–206
    accountability statement, 190–193
    capital budget process, 194–196
        capital project presentations, 195
        primary of financial accountability,
            195–196
        target setting, 196
    changing concepts of management,
        171–173
    clarifying operations council
        accountability, 190–193
    clarity of issues, 188–190
    commitment, 196–197
    consensus-based decision making,
        197–199
    consensus building techniques, 197
    control, challenging aspects of, 203
    council chair duties and powers, 200
    distinction of accountability, 175
    empowerment, components in
        development of, 171
    foundation of operations council,
        178–188
        making operations council work,
            187
        operations council membership,
            184–187
        operations council process, 188
        purpose of operations council,
            180–183
        role of operations council, 183–184
        support for management role, 180
    and governance council, 59
    knowledge worker, 173–175
    linkage to other councils, 202–203
    management accountability, 175–176,
        177
    membership, 185
    mentor of coach behaviors, 172

nursing management council vs.
operations council, 179
old vs. new decision processes, 189
operating budget process, 193–194
operations council accountability
statement, 190–193
operations council commitment,
196–197
operations council membership, 185
presentation guidelines, 189–190
service integrator and coordinator
roles, comparison of, 181
shared organizational vision, 199–201
support accountability, 201–202
support from chief executive officer,
203–204
systems accountability, 201–202
technology-driven systems, 173–175
translation strategies into tactics for
organization, 66
two levels of management, 176–178
option design, selection, 189–190
organization around patient, 129–131
organizational readiness to respond, 11
organizational transformation, 75–103
authority, 95
boundaries, determination of, 95–96
change process, SGSG and, 101–102
decision making, 95
development, 94–95
focused work group, 78–80
implementation, 85–87
inadequacy of structure, 77–78
individual differences, 94
information access, 95
integrating process, 75–77
interdisciplinary shared governance, 90
limitations, 92
budgetary availability, 92–93
deadlines for motivating, guiding
work, 93
workload, 93
nursing shared governance, 87–89
planning process, 96–98
expectations, 96–97
functional components, 97

roles, positions, delineation of,
97–98
rules of engagement, 90–92
shared governance steering group,
80–85
initial developmental process, 84–85
membership criteria, 82–84
training, 94–95
outmoded organizational characteristics,
53
ownership, 31, 36, 54
investment in system, 33–34

P
paper records, limitations of, 274
parallel decision-making processes, as
obstacle to empowerment, 150
partnerships, 36, 54
growth in, 25
in relationship building, 23–25
patient as recipient vs. as participant, 7
patient care
as central activity of health system, 62
foundations of health service, 138–140
integration, 164–167
patient care council, 57, 62–65, 140–148,
156–159, 174
areas of accountability, 157, 159
defining work of patient care council,
147–148
membership, 144–147
operations council, and governance
council, 59
patient care council membership,
144–147
purpose of patient care council,
143–144
patient pathways, 106–107
patient populations, organizing around, 114
patient safety movement, 19–21
payment requisites, 110–111
performance-driven payment schemes,
emergence of, 11
pharmacists, 313
philosophy of information management,
289

physician agreement, 189–190
physician-centered vs. patient/family-
    centered, 6
physician integration, 237–271
    changes in incentives, 240–242
    communications, 260–264
        critical communication in shared
            governance system, 260–262
    conflict resolution, 262
    disconnection from systems
        perspective, 242–245
    formal medical staff, 237–238
    future for physician partners in
        shared governance, 269–270
    future vision, changes in preparation
        for managed care, 250
    governance for new vision, 262–268
        prioritization of organizational
            strategies, 264
        shared governance and value-
            driven care, 266–268
    implementing experience, 250–252
    incentives, alignment of, 241
    inclusion of physicians in hospital
        decision making, 259–260
    informal medical staff structures as
        barriers, 239–240
    integration of physicians into system,
        252–259
        critical path, 258–259
        medical staff, 255–257
        at point of service, 258
        roles in corporate shared
            governance councils, 254–255
    inviting medical staff, 252
    operating objectives for physicians,
        259–260
    physician's view of barriers to shared
        governance, 239–245
    questions for physician's shared
        governance, 268
    strategies, 255
    vision for whole-systems shared
        governance, 245–252
        structuring, 248–250
physicians, 6

conflicts, 240
critical path, 258–259
disconnection from systems
    perspective, 242–245
input/agreement, 189–190
involvement in shared governance,
    principles of, 162
loss of clinical control, 230
move to other area hospitals, 239
on patient care council, role of, 164
vs. physicians plus physician
    extenders, 6
at point of service, 258
political power, related to personality
    strength, 239
role, 230
roles in corporate shared governance
    councils, 254–255
strategies to win over, 255
summary authority, locus of control,
    230
traditional, 108, 230
view of barriers to shared
    governance, 239–245
planning process, 96–98
    expectations, 96–97
    functional components, 97
    roles and positions, delineation of,
        97–98
point of care, 44–45
point of service
    locus of control to, transfer of, 25–26
    provider teams, 57
    system building, 9
point of service interdisciplinary
    microsystem, 137–168
    accountability, 156–159
    council member responsibilities, 146
    council membership selection,
        principles of, 145
    fundamentals of patient care council,
        140–148
        defining work of patient care
            council, 147–148
        patient care council membership,
            144–147

purpose of patient care council,
143–144
patient care, 138–140
patient care council, 156–159
patient care integration, 164–167
physician involvement in shared
governance, principles of, 162
physicians on patient care council,
role of, 164
service pathway council, 148–159
accountability, 152–159
patient care council accountability,
156–159
work of, 155–156
shared governance, principles of, 138
team accountability, 148–159
transition from nursing shared
governance to whole-systems
shared governance, 160–164
expanding nursing practice
council, 161–162
interfacing with medical staff,
162–164
pointing finger vs. fixing
structure/process/impact, 20
political issues, 22–23
political structure, linkage to, 320–321
political system, relational equation in,
1–39
population-based continuum, 51–53
portable electronic mail system, 291
power shifts, 1–39
premises of shared governance, 45–47
previously approved project, subproject
of, 189–190
primary care, low/high status and, 6
principles for new age, 22–34
creating learning organization, 26–27
demand for shared governance, 25–26
equity, relationship to quality, 27–30
ownership and investment in system,
33–34
partnership in relationship building,
23–25
transfer of locus of control to point of
service, 25–26

transition from responsibility to
accountability, 30–33
problems with emerging information,
knowledge society, 3–4
problems with traditional structure, 11
professional staff, shared governance as
appropriate model for structuring, 41
professional teams vs. multidisciplinary
customer-focused teams, 20
provider linkage, 113–114
provider partnerships, community
hospital system approach, 237–271
changes in incentives, 240–242
communications, 260–264
conflict resolution, 262
formal medical staff, 237–238
future for physician partners in
shared governance, 269–270
future vision, changes in preparation
for managed care, 250
governance for new vision, 262–268
prioritization of organizational
strategies, 264
shared governance and value-
driven care, 266–268
implementing experience, 250–252
incentives, alignment of, 241
inclusion of physicians in hospital
decision making, 259–260
informal medical staff structures as
barriers, 239–240
integration of physicians into system,
252–259
medical staff and decision making,
256–257
medical staff, governance, and
operations, 255
medical staff integration into
pathways, 256
physicians and critical path,
258–259
physicians at point of service, 258
physicians roles in corporate
shared governance councils,
254–255
inviting medical staff, 252

operating objectives for physicians,
259–260
physician disconnection from
systems perspective, 242–245
physicians, strategies to win over, 255
physician's view of barriers to shared
governance, 239–245
questions for physician's shared
governance, 268
vision for whole-systems shared
governance, 245–252
structuring, 248–250
providers
as partners in decision making, 43–44
as revenue generators vs. providers as
value centers, 6
public expectations, 8
purpose of operations function in system,
66
purpose of patient care council, 143–144

Q
quackery, 17
quality, 19
quality/equity, relationship, 27–30
quality organization, commitment level in,
34–35
quality/patient safety movement, 19–21
quantum thinking, replacement of
vertical, linear thinking, 22
questions for physician's shared
governance, 268

R
reactive medical care, vs. health needs
assessment, 6
real-time information access, 286–287
development of superusers, 287
redesign of systems within integrated
interdisciplinary shared decision-
making format, 105–136
reduced provider competition, 317
reengineering, social, 15–16
referrals, 6
regional political structure, linkage to,
320–321
rehabilitation, 132

relational service design, 110–111
relationship building, partnership in,
23–25
representation, 57–58
residency, boundaries to behavior in, 240
responsibility, accountability, transition,
30–33
right to membership in quality system, 35
risk, 22–23
in commitment to change, 33
encouraging, 172
role of partnership, growth in, 25
roles in information management system,
293–294
roles necessary in sustaining
organization, 28–29

S
safety movement in health care, 19–21
senior-level managers, transfer of work
formerly done by councils, pathways,
229–230
senior statesmen, selection by physicians,
247
senior vice presidents, 117–118
separatism, medical, overcoming, 17–18
service accountability, 61
system accountability, distinguishing,
59–61
service continuum, building, 105–136
service integrator, service coordinator
roles, comparison of, 181
service pathway council, 148–159
accountability, 152–159
patient care council accountability,
156–159
work of, 155–156
service pathway, leadership, 58
service team, 50–51
sewage system, 14
SGSG. *See* shared governance steering
group
shared decision making, 55–56, 105–136
shared governance, 40–41, 327
accountability-based model, 55–56
demand for, 25–26

democracy, distinguished, 45
distinction between role of service
    pathway, 58
principles of, 54, 138
shared governance steering group, 80–85,
    184
    initial developmental process, 84–85
    membership criteria, 82–84
shared organizational vision, 199–201
shared vision, propagation of, 115–116
shifting control, in shared governance
    model, 276–277
    culture, 278
    information, 279–280
    relationships and systemness,
        creation by, 280
    structure, 277–278
    training, 278
signature authority for council,
    executing, 200
silo approach to organizational structure,
    113
    inefficiency of, 21–22
size of decision-making groups, 54
social reengineering, 15–16
social system, relational equation in, 1–39
social workers, 313
solo vs. group practice, 6
spending for health care, 13–14
    lack of control in, 13–14
stakeholder councils, 53–54
stakeholders
    complex adaptive systems to
        integrate, 36
    engagement of, 214–217
        governance council membership,
            217
    identification/inclusion in project
        process, 189–190
    inclusion of chief financial officer,
        185
    sharing role in evaluating
        performance of others, 30–31
    understanding of mission, objectives
        of organization, 215

stewardship of resources in leadership,
    65
stimulating enthusiasm, 172
strategic cascade, 224–228
strategic requirements, meeting, 189–190
structural issues, 22–23
structural linkages, 117–118
structural/political issues, 22–23
structures for information management,
    273–280
structures of health care, changes in,
    16–22
    consumer-driven care, 18–19
    managing demand, 16–17
    overcoming medical separatism,
        17–18
    quality/patient safety movement,
        19–21
    user-driven healthcare models, 17
    value-driven care delivery, 21–22
supervisors, 117–118
support resources, 177, 191
supporting point of service, 316
sustainable outcomes. See quality
system accountability, service
    accountability
    balance between, 61
    distinguishing, 59–61
system competition, 11
system councils, 59
system functionality, maintaining,
    131–135
system resources, 177
systems accountability, 201–202
systems councils, 55
systems linkages, 120
systems redesign within integrated
    interdisciplinary shared decision-
    making format, 105–136
systems resources, 192–193

T
tactical implementation, sample projects,
    290–293
    clinical information system, 292–293

virtual office, 291–292
task-oriented vs. improvement/outcome-oriented, 11, 20
tasks completion mechanism, 223
team accountability, 148–159
team attitudes, 22–23
team coordinators, 117–118
team responsibilities, 48–49
teams, 47–53. *See also* clinical teams
    as basic unit of work in whole-systems organization, 48
    configuration around specific kinds of services, 51
    focused on specific functions or activities, 49–50
    focused on system and relationship issues, 49–50
    population-based continuum, 51–53
    service team, 50–51
technology
    explosion of, 173
    organizational dependent on, 173
technology-driven systems, 173–175
teenage mothers, 326
template elements
    agreement regarding, 127
    examples of, 128
tension between service accountability, system accountability, managing, 61
traditional delivery infrastructure, 10–11
traditional focus, customer focus, 20
traditional structure, problems with, 11
traditional vs. alternative medicine, 6
training, 94–95
transformation of organization, 75–103
    authority, 95
    boundaries, determination of, 95–96
    change process, SGSG and, 101–102
    decision making, 95
    development, 94–95
    focused work group, 78–80
    implementation, 85–87
    inadequacy of structure, 77–78
    individual differences, 94
    information access, 95

integrating process, 75–77
interdisciplinary shared governance, 90
    limitations, 92
        budgetary availability, 92–93
        deadlines for motivating, guiding work, 93
        workload, 93
    nursing shared governance, 87–89
    planning process, 96–98
        expectations, 96–97
        functional components, 97
        roles, positions, delineation of, 97–98
    rules of engagement, 90–92
    shared governance steering group, 80–85
        initial developmental process, 84–85
        membership criteria, 82–84
    training, 94–95
transition from responsibility to accountability, 30–33
transition to customer focus, 20
translating board accountability, 213–214
trauma level 1, 132
turf battles, 11, 22–23

U
underinsured population, increase in, 8
uniform problem solving templates, 291
unit of organized decision making, councils as, 53–55
unit team meetings, minutes from, 261
user-driven healthcare models, 17

V
value-driven care delivery, 21–22
value of knowledge, workers' competence, 2–4
value standards, 118–119
    examples, 118
    formula, 248
variety, effect on system's strength, effectiveness, 5

variety of pathways, 62
vendor partners, 285–286
    trouble with, 285–286
vertical, hierarchical power structures,
    physician familiarity with, 239
vertical integration, 77
vertical organizations, vs. complex
    adaptive systems, 7
virtual office, 291–292
    communication, importance of,
        291–292
    information management strategies,
        292
vision for whole-systems shared
    governance, 115–116, 245–252
    structuring, 248–250
voting, lack of, in consensus decision
    making, 198

W
waste, ignoring vs. designing out, 7
whole-system templating, 125
whole-system thinking, 61
women's health, 132
    designing services along service
        continuum, 62
work, evolving nature of, 10–15
work flow improvements supported by
    portability, electronic forms, 291
work group, in transformation of
    organization, 78–80
work system, relational equation in, 1–39
workers historically unfamiliar with use
    of power, 3
workplace changes within new paradigm,
    170–171